Minimally Invasive Gynecological Surgery

Olav Istre

Editor

Minimally Invasive Gynecological Surgery

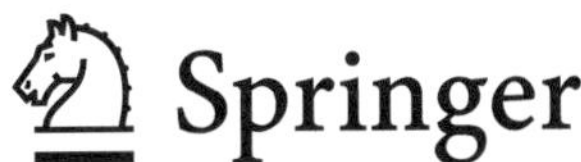 Springer

Editor
Olav Istre, MD, PhD
Fredriksberg
Denmark

ISBN 978-3-662-51002-5   ISBN 978-3-662-44059-9   (eBook)
DOI 10.1007/978-3-662-44059-9
Springer Heidelberg New York Dordrecht London

Springer is part of Springer Science+Business Media (www.springer.com)

Preface

Gynecological surgery has evolved rapidly in the past few years. New surgical and nonsurgical options are emerging for a variety of gynecological conditions, with major emphasis on minimally invasive and noninvasive options. The ORs with their equipment have changed to HD, 3D, and robotic surgery; all of these have major benefits for our patients. Since Harry Reich first described total laparoscopic hysterectomy (LH) in 1988, endoscopic hysterectomies have become a routine procedure in many gynecologic departments, even though open abdominal hysterectomy is still the dominant surgical technique worldwide. In Denmark, for instance, total abdominal hysterectomy (TAH) is the main treatment for enlarged uterus in 53 % of cases (The Danish hysterectomy database 2011). Laparoscopic hysterectomy is performed in 12 % and vaginal route is utilized in 35 % of cases of smaller uterus. Complication rate was 18 % and readmission rate 5.4 %, and repeat surgery was performed in 4 % of cases. Lately there have been issues with the morcelation technique, which is mandatory in big fibroids. These concerns will probably set us back in time; however, the developments will continue as increasingly women will not accept big scars for removal of uterus and fibroids.

This is not acceptable; therefore we will have to spread our knowledge. The main goal of minimally invasive surgery is to avoid a large abdominal incision. This has several benefits to the patient, which include:

- Faster and easier recovery time
- Less pain
- Less blood loss
- Decreased scar tissue formation
- Less complications

In this book we will show some of the new modalities in this field and also the new developments in specific conditions.

It is an honor for me to present to the readers knowledge from some of the most distinguished gynecologist in the world.

Fredriksberg, Denmark — Olav Istre

Contents

Imaging Before Endoscopic Surgery

1

Margit Dueholm

Contents

Abbreviations

2D	Two-dimensional
3D	Three-dimensional
3D-PDA	Three-dimensional power Doppler angiography
3D-TVS	Three-dimensional transvaginal ultrasound
ADC	Apparent diffusion coefficient
CEUS	Contrast-enhanced ultrasound
CT-scanning	Computer tomographic imaging
DCE MRI	Dynamic contrast-enhanced magnetic resonance imaging
DW-MRI	Diffusion-weighted magnetic resonance imaging
FI	Flow index
GIS	Gel infusion sonography
HSG	Hysterosalpingography
HY	Hysteroscopy
HyCoSy	Hysterosalpingo-contrast sonography
IETA	International Endometrial Tumor Analysis group
IOTA group	The International Ovarian Tumor Analysis group
JZ	Junctional zone

M. Dueholm
Department of Obstetric and Gynecology,
Aarhus University Hospital, Brendstupgaardsvej 100,
Aarhus N 8200, Denmark
e-mail: dueholm@dadlnet.dk

O. Istre (ed.), *Minimally Invasive Gynecological Surgery*,
DOI 10.1007/978-3-662-44059-9_1, © Springer-Verlag Berlin Heidelberg 2015

JZ_{diff}	Difference between maximal and minimal junctional zone thickness
JZ_{max}	Maximal junctional zone thickness
K^{trans}	Volume transfer constant
MRgFUS	Magnetic resonance-guided focused ultrasound
MRI	Magnetic resonance imaging
PET-CT	Positron emission tomography – computed tomography
RFA	Radiofrequency ablation of uterine myomas
RMI	Risk of malignancy index
SIS	Saline infusion hydrosonography
TVS	Transvaginal ultrasound
UAE	Uterine artery embolization
VFI	Vascularization-flow index
VI	Vascularization index

1.1 Introduction

During the last centuries diagnostic imaging has been followed by therapeutic imaging. Nowadays, therapeutic imaging is most often endoscopic surgery. Several newer procedures such as uterine artery embolization (UAE), magnetic resonance-guided focused ultrasound (MRgFUS), and radiofrequency ablation of uterine myomas (RFA) are examples of therapeutic imaging, which are not based on endoscopy.

Preoperative imaging should be seen as an integrated part of endoscopy that is absolutely needed to help the surgeon plan the type of surgery, and makes endoscopy safe and cost-effective.

Transvaginal ultrasound (TVS) is an easy accessible technique, and it is the first technique of choice in gynecologic diagnosis before endoscopic surgery. Simple gray-scale TVS is a sufficient imaging technique for most simple endoscopic procedures. A supplement to TVS of power Doppler, saline infusion hydrosonography (SIS) or gel infusion sonography (GIS) and three-dimensional transvaginal ultrasound (3D-TVS) may add valuable information.

TVS has limitations, where magnetic resonance imaging (MRI) should be added with different supplements. MRI is clearly superior to CT scanning for pelvic pathology, and CT scanning is not included in this section.

TVS is a very observer-dependent technique, and introduction of terms and standards increases the diagnostic performance of imaging (Kaijser et al. 2012). Terms and definitions for describing uterine and ovarian pathology have been developed (Leone et al. 2010; Munro et al. 2011; Timmerman et al. 2010). These terms should be adopted in the strategy of preoperative diagnosis and for operative planning.

In this chapter, we will give a schematic overview of these terms and details of the present performance of TVS and MRI before endoscopy and newer imaging procedures.

1.2 Everyday, Perioperative Imaging in Endoscopy

There are large advantages of incorporating image mapping immediately before and during endoscopic surgery. It is important to have an easy access to ultrasound equipment with sufficient resolution in the surgical units. Image documentation on still images may not give the surgeon the same information as is provided with a scan immediately before the surgery. Type 3 myomas may not be seen by either hysteroscopy (HY) or laparoscopy, and may be removed at ultrasonographic guidance at either HY (Lykke et al. 2012) or laparoscopy. Hysteroscopic resection of adenomyosis, asherman, septate uteri, and other uterine anomalies is performed more safely with ultrasound guidance, and perioperative TVS may guide the surgeon in the right direction in a frozen pelvis.

1.3 Standardization on Performance of TVS, GIS and SIS, Doppler – Terms and Definitions

1.3.1 Standardization of TVS

TVS is an operator-dependent technique, and should follow the sequences below:
(a) Optimization of the image. Four important buttons should be used at each examination (magnification, gain, focus, frequency)

(b) A systematic examination technique, as outlined below
(c) Pattern recognition of different pathologic conditions in the female pelvic, which should be described according to standardized terms and documented.

When additional information is needed:

(d) Addition of power Doppler (description according to standard terms and documentation)
(e) Addition of contrast (SIS or GIS) (description according to standard terms and documentation)
(f) Addition of 3D-TVS
(g) Addition of trained ultra-sonographer
(h) Addition of MRI
(i) Image conferences

The uterus is scanned in the sagittal plane from cornu to cornu and in the transverse plane from the cervix to the fundus. During examination assure the buttons are corrected to optimize visualization (magnification, gain, focus, frequency). Having established an overview of the whole uterus, the image is magnified to contain only the uterine corpus. The sagittal plane of the uterus is identified, and systematic scanning of the endometrium is performed using the terminology for the endometrium (Leone et al. 2010) in Table 1.1. The myometrium should be evaluated and described according to Table 1.2. The terms for myometrial lesions are built on terminology in prior studies (Dueholm et al. 2001c; Yaman et al. 1999; Champaneria et al. 2010; Meredith et al. 2009; Bazot et al. 2001), and the classification system for myomas is built on the FIGO system (Munro et al. 2011). The FIGO classification system for myomas is displayed in Fig. 1.1. In abnormal findings in the uterus, power Doppler may be added and described (Tables 1.1 and 1.2).

After evaluation of the uterus, the remaining pelvic area should be evaluated. The ovaries and the uterine horns should be located in the transverse plan. The tubes can be followed from the uterine horns to the iliac vessels and these procedures will normally reveille the ovaries. Each ovary should be scanned in the transverse and sagittal plane from the bottom to top and scanning should be performed in two perpendicular planes. Areas above, beneath and besides the ovaries should be scanned at each side.

The ovaries should be described according to standard terms from the International Ovarian Tumor Analysis (IOTA) group (Timmerman et al. 2000, 2010) (Table 1.3). Again power Doppler may be added in the evaluation of abnormal findings. The urinary bladder and the pouch of Douglas should be evaluated. Sliding of different organs (gentle movement with the probe) should be noted. The urinary bladder, the rectum, and sacrouterine ligaments are also scanned and recorded.

In endometriosis, visualization of the relationship with the vaginal wall and the rectum may be important to diagnose rectal involvement (Hudelist et al. 2011). To evaluate deep rectovaginal endometriosis, the probe should be placed on the posterior cul de sac of the vagina, and when the probe is slowly withdrawn through the vagina the utero sacral ligament, posterior fornix and the rectovaginal septum can be visualized. By gentle movement of the probe the rectal mucosal and the recto sigmoid wall can be identified and evaluated for deep infiltrating endometriosis. Visualization may be increased by large amounts of gel in the vagina.

1.3.2 Saline Infusion Sonography (SIS) and Gel Infusion Sonography (GIS)

Negative contrast agent such as saline or gel can increase the visualization and outline of abnormalities in the uterine cavity at TVS. Polyps, myomas, synekia, cesarean section scars, and uterine anomalies are often more clearly visualized by contrast in the uterine cavity. When saline is used as contrast agent, it is called saline infusion sonography (SIS), while the use of gel as contrast agent is called gel infusion sonography (GIS).

1.3.2.1 Submucous Myomas for Hysteroscopic Surgery

Submucous myomas for hysteroscopic surgery may at GIS/SIS be evaluated as outlined in Table 1.2 and displayed in Fig. 1.2, and may be scored by the STEPW system to predict complexity of surgery (Lasmar et al. 2011) (Table 1.2). The STEPW system consists of the following

Table 1.1 Systematic scanning of the uterine endometrium, with application of common terms and measurements for description of abnormalities

TVS	Terms and measurements
In the sagittal the endometrial thickness is measured	"Double endometrial thickness"
Intracavitary fluid: the thickness of both single layers are measured and the sum is recorded as the maximum measurement in the sagittal plane	Endometrial thickness
Amount of intracavitary fluid: largest measurement in the sagittal plane	Largest measurement of fluid
Echogenicity of fluid	Anechogenic, low-level echogenicity ground glass
	Mixed echogenicity
Endometrial morphology	
Endometrial echogenicity compared to the myometrium	Hyper-, iso- or hypoechogenic
Homogeneous with symmetrical anterior and posterior sides (includes the three-layer pattern, and the homogeneous hyper-, hypo- and isoechogenic endometrium)	Uniform
Heterogeneous, asymmetrical or cystic endometrium	Not uniform
The endometrial midline is described — Straight hyperechogenic interface	Linear
A waved hyperechogenic interface	Non-linear
Irregular interface	Irregular
Absence of a visible interface.	Not defined
The endometrial–myometrial junction	Regular, irregular, interrupted or not defined
An echo formed by the interface between an intracavitary lesion and the endometrium	Bright edge
Intracavitary pathology	
Endometrial thickness including the lesion is measured (not including intracavitary myoma)	
Intracavitary lesions should be measured in three perpendicular diameters (d1, d2, d3)	d1, d2, d3
The volume (V) of the lesion may be calculated from the three orthogonal diameters ($d1 \times d2 \times d3 \times 0.523$)	V
Myoma measurement (Table 1.2)	
Synechiae are defined as strands of tissue crossing the endometrium	Synechia
Color Doppler assessment of the endometrium	
The color content of endometrium can be scored: (1) no color flow; (2) with minimal color; (3) moderate color; (4) abundant color is presented	Color score 1 to 4
Vascular pattern:	
Scattered (dispersed color signals within the endometrium but without visible origin at the myometrial–endometrial junction) or not scattered vessels	Scattered, not scattered
Dominant vessel: one vessel passing the endomyometrial junction	Dominant, not dominant
Caliber of vessels	Large or small
Vessels may be single (double) or multiple, with focal or multifocal origin or there might be circular flow	Single (double), multiple focal, multifocal, circular flow
Branching of vessels	Orderly or disorderly/chaotic
GIS or SIS	
The endometrial outline	
Appears regular	Smooth
Multiple thickened "undulating" areas, "moguls" with a regular profile	Endometrial folds
Deep indentations or	Polypoid
Surface is cauliflower like or sharply toothed ("spiky")	Irregular

Table 1.1 (continued)

Intracavitary lesions:	
Extended: Lesion involves ≥ 25 % of the endometrial surface	Extended
Localized: Lesion involves < 25 % of the endometrial surface	Localized
Pedunculated: *a/b* ratio is <1; Sessile: : *a/b* ratio is ≥ 1	Pedunculated, sessile
a/b ratio between the diameter of the base level of the endometrium (*a*)	
Maximal transverse diameter of the lesion (*b*)	
The echogenicity of a lesion is defined as "uniform" (homogenic) or	Uniform
"Nonuniform" (heterogenic), which includes cystic lesions	Not uniform
The outline of the lesion is defined as "regular"	Regular
or "irregular" (e.g. spiky or cauliflower like)	Irregular

five parameters, where a score of 0–2 is given according to Table 1.2:

(a) *Size*: Myomas (largest diameter)
(b) *Topography*: Defined by the third of the uterine cavity where the myoma is situated (lower, middle and upper third).
(c) *Extension of the base of the myoma*: Base of myoma covers (one-third of the wall, one- to two-thirds of the wall, and more than two-thirds of the wall).
(d) *Penetration of the myoma into the myometrium*: Type 0,1,2 myoma
(e) *Wall*: when the fibroid is on the lateral wall, one extra point is added.

The total sum score predicts complexity of hysteroscopic surgery.

1.3.3 Three-Dimensional Transvaginal Ultrasound (3D-TVS)

3D-TVS is just a collection of 2D images added together in a volume, which allow reconstruction and evaluation of the scan in different planes. Resolution at 3D will never be better, than at the original 2D images. In the presence of poor image quality at 2D, a collection of images of poor quality at 3D will seldom be helpful. Most important feature at 3D–TVS is the ability to "reconstruct" the uterus to provide a coronal view.

Procedure: For 3D-TVS of the uterus, volumes are obtained at a mid-sagittal view of the uterus. The image settings at 2D should be optimized, and magnified to an optimal image with a minimum amount of free space around the region of interest (uterus). The volume box for sampling of the 3D images should be applied again with a limited amount of free space around the uterus. Both the patient and the probe should not be moved during collection of the volumes.

To obtain a reconstruction of the coronal plane, the volume of the uterus should be perfectly aligned along the mid long axis in the sagittal plane and along the axis of the uterine horns in the transverse planes. This can be achieved by the Z-technique (Abuhamad et al. 2006), which include three steps (Fig. 1.3).

The time spent on producing a perfect coronal view is less than 1 min after limited training (Abuhamad et al. 2006). A perfect coronal view and a simple scroll through the images in the C-plan may in clinical practice supply most additional information given by 3D-TVS.

There is a substantial learning curve and time involved to manage all the different features in post-processing, which limits the common use in clinical practice. However, two or three features can easily be learned and may in most clinical situations cover the need.

At SIS a 3D volume of the uterus can be obtained (3D-SIS), which allow reconstructing the outline of the uterine cavity. However, an optimal reconstruction without acoustic shadows from an intrauterine catheter is achieved with gel in the uterine cavity, and the catheter should be removed before volume sampling (3D-GIS). 3D-GIS may be helpful in some clinical situations especially in indefinite coronal view at 3D-TVS (Mavrelos et al. 2011; Caliskan et al. 2010; Makris et al. 2007; de Kroon et al. 2004).

Table 1.2 Qualitative assessment of myometrium and myometrial lesions (myomas and adenomyosis)

	Definition	Term, measurement
Uterine contour	Normal: pear shape; globular: globally enlarged; bernoccolute: uterus with irregular external profile	Normal, globular, bernocculuto
Uterine volume	Length (d1), anterior posterior diameter (d2) and transverse diameter (d3)	$(d1 \times d2 \times d3 \times 0.523)$
Uterine perimetrial outline	Regular: smooth with a regular shape; irregular: not smooth contour	Regular, irregular, not defined
Myometrial wall	Measurement of anterior and posterior wall thickness in sagittal plane	Symmetrical, asymmetrical maximal thickness of wall
Myometrial echogenicity	Homogenous	Uniform
	Heterogenous, or cystic	Non-uniform
	Regular cystic or not regular cystic	Cystic
Junctional zone	Hypoechogenic inner subendometrial halo	Regular, irregular, interrupted, not defined
Myometrial lesions		**Presence, number, shape**
Contour	Clear hypo or hyperechoic external contour (rim)	Rim defined, not defined
Margins	Defined margins	Regular, irregular
Echogenicity	Hypo, iso, hyperechogenic (+/− shadows)	Uniform
	Heterogenic mixed echo, cystic areas, lacunae, stripes, shadows	Not uniform
Site		Anterior, posterior wall
Location		Middle site or lateral (right, left, corneal or intra ligamentar)
		Fundus, corpus, isthmus, cervix
	The minimal distance between the perimetrium and the outer portion of myoma (dm). The minimal distance between the endometrium and the inner portion of the myometrium (de)	dm de
	Submucous myomas extension of the base: proportion of wall covered	$\leq 1/3$; $1/3$–$2/3$;$>2/3$
Type	Submucous (sm)	Type: 0,1,2
	(Type 0), myoma completely within the cavity; (Type 1) with $\geq 50\,\%$ of the endocavitary portion protruding into the cavity; and (Type 2), with the endocavitary part of myoma $<50\,\%$	
	Other (O)	Type: 3,4,5,6,7,8
	Contacts endometrium; 100 % intramural	Type 3
	Intramural	Type 4
	Subserosal $\geq 50\,\%$ intramural	Type 5
	Subserosal $<50\,\%$ intramural	Type 6
	Subserosal pedunculated	Type 7
	Other (Specify, e.g. cervical, parasitic)	Type 8
	Hybrid impact on both endometrium and serosa	Type: 0–5
Size	The three largest perpendicular diameters (a1, a2, a3) mm	a1, a2, a3
	$1/6 \times \pi \times a1 \times a2 \times a3$	Volume
	$P = 6\,A^2\,(B/2 - A/3)/B^3$ B largest diameter perpendicular to the uterine cavity and A part of this diameter in the uterine cavity	P = Proportion of myoma volume in uterine cavity
Doppler morphology	Regular vessels or irregular vessels	Regular or irregular
	Branching: regular, irregular, no branching	Regular branching

Table 1.2 (continued)

		Definition					Term, measurement
		Scattered dispersed color signal					Scattered
		Many vessels					Multiple pattern
		Caliper, number					Large, small, few, many
		Homogenic vessels, size					Homogenic
		Peripheral					Circular or not circular flow
		Color score: (1) no color flow; (2) with minimal color; (3) moderate color; (4) abundant color is presented					Color score 1–4
STEPW		Submucous classification for complexity of hysteroscopic surgery					
	Score	Size	Topography	Extension of base	Myoma type	Lateral wall	
	0	<2	Low	<1/3	0 (100 %)	+1	
	1	2–5	Middle	1/3–2/3	1 (>50 %)		
	2	>5	Upper	>1/3	2 (<50 %)		
	$\sum$	+	+	+	+	+	$\sum$ Total score (SUM)
SUM	0–4	Low complexity hysteroscopy					
	5–6	High complexity hysteroscopy, two steps, medical preoperative treatment					
	7–9	Consider alternatives					

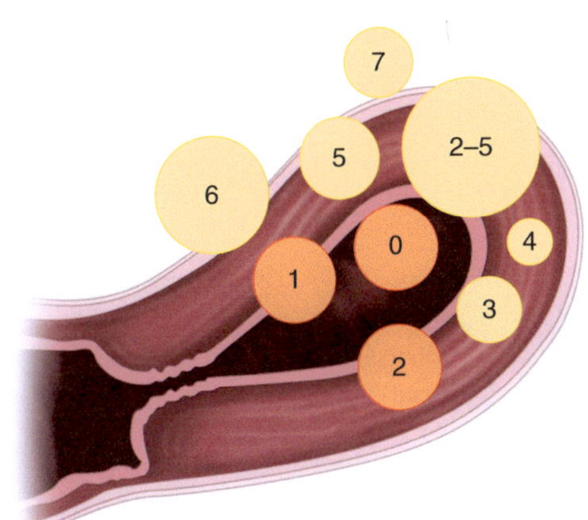

Fig. 1.1 In the FIGO system intracavitary myomas are classified by the traditional European Society for Gynaecological Endoscopy (ESGE) (type 0–2), and in addition intramural myomas are classified (type 3 to 7). Myomas with impact on both the endometrium and serosa are classified as type 2–5

1.3.4 Three-Dimensional Power Doppler Angiography (3D-PDA)

A three-dimensional power Doppler angiography (3D-PDA) can be performed to study the distribution, pattern, and vascular branching of the vascular vessels. Power Doppler is simply applied to the volume box and a 3D volume is obtained. The technique also allow for a more objective reproducible (Raine-Fenning et al. 2003) assessment of uterine vascularization, although the measurement is dependent on machine settings (Raine-Fenning et al. 2008).

1.3.5 Dynamic Contrast-Enhanced MRI (DCE MRI) and Diffusion-Weighted MRI (DW MRI)

Tissue perfusion in pelvic masses and uterine masses can be evaluated by DCE MRI (Nakai et al. 2008; Paldino and Barboriak 2009). In tissue with high perfusion there will be high signal intensity in T2-weighted images after injection of contrast, while tissue without perfusion will have low intensity at T2-weighted images. Tissue perfusion can be assessed in two ways: a semi-quantitative method (dependent on individual system and patients) which analyze the changes in signal intensity, and a quantitative method using a pharmacokinetic system and patient-independent model.

Diffusion-weighted (DW) MRI is based on diffusion motion of water molecules. Signals are

Table 1.3 Terms in definition of ovaries and ovarian mass

	Definitions	Measurements and terms
Size, site	Ovarian measurement: three perpendicular planes largest 3 diameters (mm) (a1, a2, a3)	a1,a2,a3
Ovarian volume		$(a1 \times a2 \times a3 \times 0.523)$.
Outline of ovary		Regular, irregular
Morphology of ovarian tissue		
	Follikels (numbers (n) and size in largest perpendicular diameters (A1, A2, A3) (mm)	N, A1, A2, A3
Antral follicle count	Count follicles between cycle days 2 and 4	Antral follicle count
	Include all antral follicles of 2–10 mm in diameter (most reliable in 3D volume) in both ovaries	
	Ovarian stroma	Homogenic
		Heterogenic
Measurements of ovarian mass (inconsistent in normal ovarian function)	Measurement of the ovarian mass in three perpendicular planes (b1, b2, b3) largest diameter in mm	b1, b2, b3
Morphology of mass	Echogenicity of solid component	Heterogenic or homogenic
	Solid: high echogenicity suggesting presence of tissue	Cystic or solid or
		Cystic-solid
Cystic content		Anechogenic
		Low level
		Ground glass
		Hemorrhagic
		Mixed
	Septum complete/incomplete	Complete
	Thin strands of tissue running across the cyst cavity	Incomplete
	An incomplete septum is not completed in some scanning planes	
	The thickness of thickest septum (S) is measured	Thickness septum (S)
Locules	Numbers of locules (L) is counted	L
Internal wall		Smooth, irregular
	Any solid projection from the cystic wall ≥ 3 mm	Solid papillary projections
	Measurement of largest solid component in three perpendicular planes (height(h), base(ba1), base(ba2))	Height(h), base(ba1), base(ba2)
Cyst type	(No septae and no solid parts)	Unilocular
	No septae, but solid parts	Unilocular solid
	More than one septae, no solid parts	Multilokular
	More than one septae, and solid parts	Multilokular solid
		Not classifiable
Doppler assessment	Color score: (1) no color flow; (2) with minimal color; (3) moderate color; (4) abundant color is presented	Color score 1–4
Ascitis	Presence of ascites is noted, largest pouch of fluid in pouch of Douglas is measured (F) in a saggital plane largest diameter (mm)	F

dependent on microscopic water diffusivity, and decrease in the presence of factors that restrict water diffusion, such as cell membranes and the viscosity of the fluid. Signals are influenced by changes in the balance between extracellular and intracellular water molecules, and changes in cytologic morphology including the nuclear-to-cytoplasm ratio and cellular density. The technique can easily be added to any routine MR protocol.

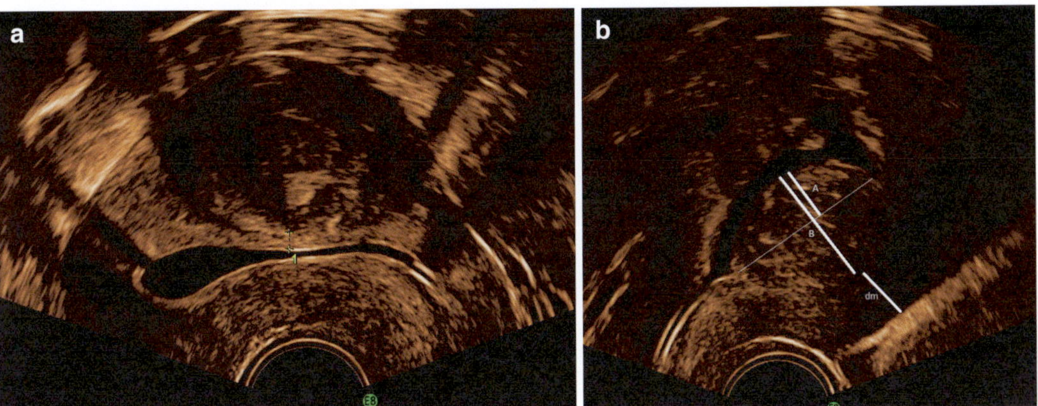

Fig. 1.2 A myoma type 2–5 (**a**) with impact on the serosa and endometrium (SIS), and (**b**) a myoma type 2 with measurement of the proportion of the myoma in the uterine cavity (P). *B* is largest diameter perpendicular to the uterine cavity and *A* is part of this diameter in the uterine cavity $P = 6\,A^2\,(B/2 - A/3)/B^3$

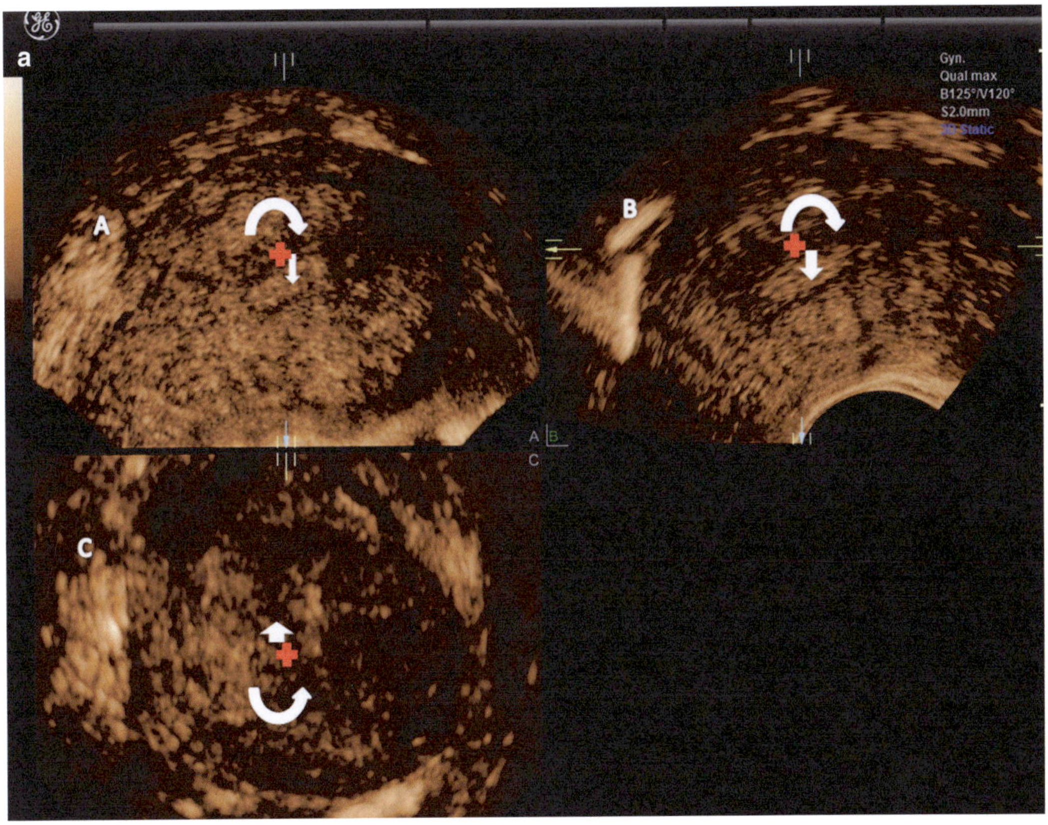

Fig. 1.3 (**a**) Step *A*. The reference/rotational point (+) is placed in the midlevel of the endometrial stripe in the sagittal plane. Z rotation is used to align the long axis of the endometrial stripe along the horizontal axis in the sagittal plane of the uterus. Step *B*. The reference/rotational point (+) is placed in the midlevel of the endometrial stripe in the transverse plane. The Z rotation is used to align the endometrial stripe with the horizontal axis in the transverse plane of the uterus Step *C*. Z rotation is applied on plane C to display the mid coronal plane in the traditional orientation in plane C. (**b**) In the C plane is the coronal view displayed (VCI-settings). (**c**) Postprocessor rendering is performed

                                                        M. Dueholm

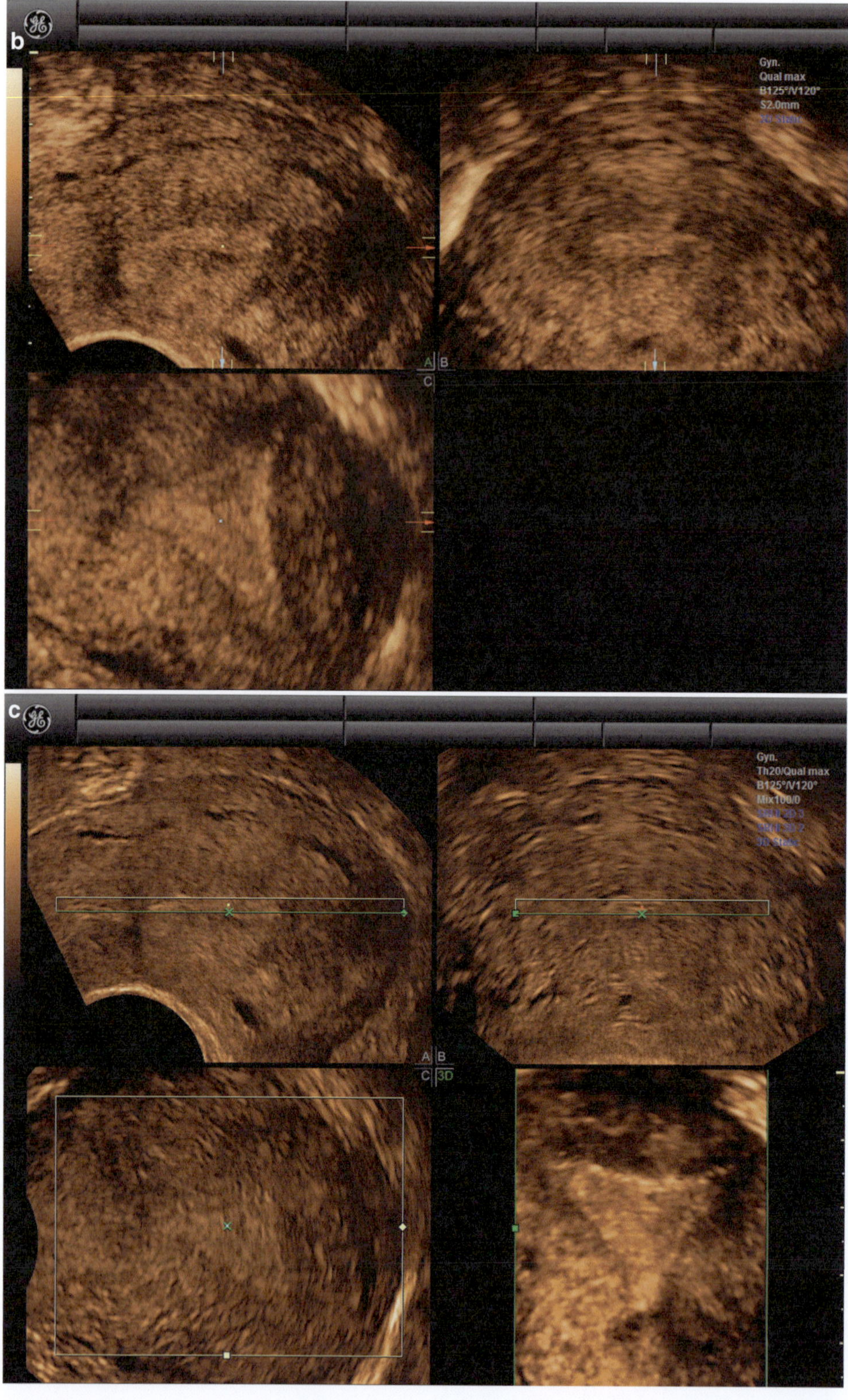

Fig. 1.3 (continued)

1.3.6 Contrast Enhanced Ultrasound (CEUS)

CEUS is an alternative upcoming method with use in other specialties (Piscaglia et al. 2012), to evaluate perfusion after different treatment modalities. CEUS has been used when HIFU has been monitored by TVS, and seems to be a promising low cost method (Zhou et al. 2007). Enhancement in the tissue is observed after contrast injection supported with in-built or off-line software to measure the degree of enhancement. The time of enhancement and the distribution is observed.

1.4 Diagnosis of Uterine Pathology

1.4.1 Abnormal Uterine Bleeding

The newly established FIGO system – the PALM-COIN ((P) polyp, (A) adenomyosis, (L) leiomyoma, (M) malignancy/hyperplasia-(C) Coagulopathy, (O) Ovulatory dysfunction, (I) Iatrogenic, and (N) Not classified) system – has been elaborated (Munro et al. 2011).

A patient with abnormal uterine bleeding should be categorized according to this system. The PALM – part of the system – is mainly based on ultrasound and pathologic evaluation of the endometrium. The COIN – part of the system – is evaluated by the patient history and laboratory analysis.

1.4.2 Endometrial Pathology

1.4.2.1 Premenopausal Bleeding

TVS, GIS, or SIS are very efficient methods to rule out pathology in the uterine cavity as polyps and myomas in premenopausal bleeding. To rule out polyps and myomas, TVS seems to miss one in five endometrial polyps (de Kroon et al. 2003; Dueholm et al. 2001a, b), while SIS is in line with hysteroscopy (HY). TVS is able to identify myomas, but a differentiation between myomas of type 1–3 most often

require GIS/SIS, which is important for selection of myomas for either laparoscopic or hysteroscopic treatment (Dueholm et al. 2002a). Patients with symptomatic focal pathology will have a time-efficient planning of HY by TVS supplied with SIS or GIS. This will provide clear information of the size, number and type of pathology in the uterine cavity, and thereby patients can be selected for outpatient mini-hysteroscopy at an office setting, two-generation endometrial ablation, inpatients resectoscopic surgery, and also to surgeons with the required experience. Small intrauterine pathology with diameter below 2 cm (Bettocchi et al. 2004; Cicinelli 2010) is removed at outpatient mini-hysteroscopy. The complexity of resectoscopic hysteroscopic myoma surgery can be predicted by the findings at SIS/GIS and scored by the STEPW system (Table 1.2). Complex surgery (score five or more) should be performed by experienced surgeons, and a two-step procedure and preoperative medical treatment should be considered. UAE or laparoscopic myomectomy should be taken into account at scores of more than 7–9.

1.4.2.2 Postmenopausal Bleeding

TVS is the first investigation in postmenopausal bleeding. The endometrium should be investigated and described according to Table 1.1. Figure 1.4 shows examples of heterogenic (a) and cystic endometrium (b). In the presence of a sharp well-defined midline echo with endometrial thickness of ≤3 or ≤4 mm only 2 % respective 5 % of endometrial cancers will be missed (Timmermans et al. 2010). At an endometrial thickness >3–4 mm endometrial sampling is performed (Timmermans et al. 2010).

Neither systematic reviews nor international guidelines have been able to reach consensus regarding the sequence in which TVS, SIS/GIS endometrial samples and HY should be implemented in the diagnostic set-up (van Hanegem et al. 2011).

HY is more efficient than endometrial samples (van Hanegem et al. 2011) and there is lower efficiency of endometrial sampling in the presence of focal changes of the endometrium

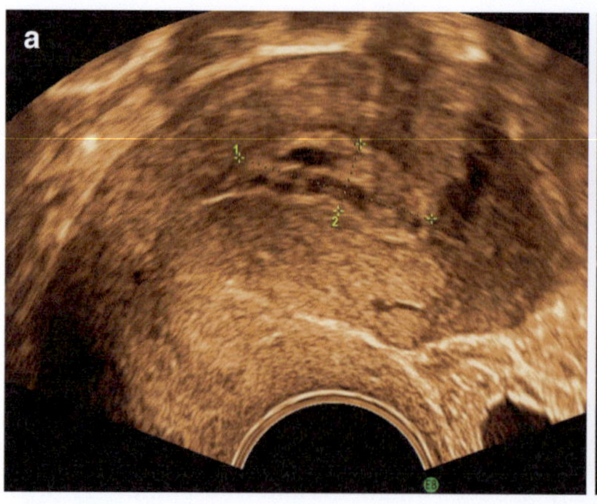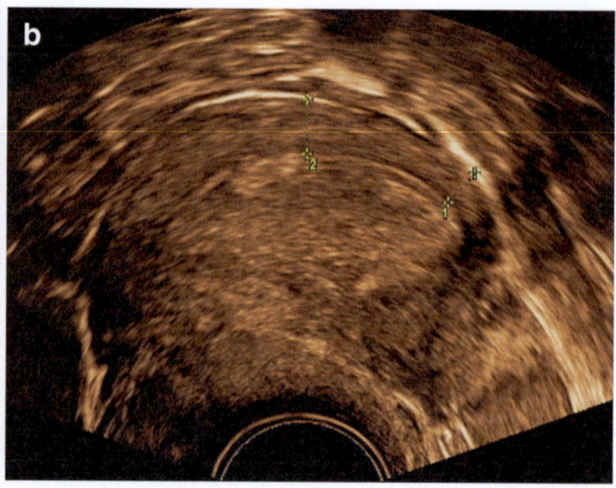

Fig. 1.4 A cystic polyp is seen in (**a**) with cystic regular endometrium, clear margins and bright line. A single small vessel was seen at Doppler. In (**b**) endometrial cancer, with a thickened heterogenic endometrium with regular endomyometrial junction at the posterior wall, (*marked*), but irregular not defined margins at the anterior wall

(Epstein et al. 2001; Angioni et al. 2008). This has motivated a supplement of SIS to TVS at endometrial thickness >5 mm, and to offer HY to patients with focal pathology at SIS (Epstein et al. 2002). The size of focal pathology can be clearly depicted at SIS/GIS and allows selection of office mini-hysteroscopy (Lotfallah et al. 2005; Cicinelli et al. 2003) for most minor pathology.

There has been limited attention on implementation of imaging for staging malignancy in a time-efficient diagnostic set up not only to diagnosis but also to fulfilled minimally invasive laparoscopic treatment of both benign and malignant pathology. Preoperative staging has the advantage of an efficient operative planning of a minimal invasive surgical procedure. An efficient preoperative diagnosis has been either additional TVS or MRI (Kinkel et al. 1999, 2009). HY may give important information of tumor type and cervical involvement (Cicinelli et al. 2008; Avila et al. 2008). The aspect of staging has to be implemented in the diagnostic set up during the next years.

1.4.2.3 Diagnosis of Myometrial Pathology

The diagnostic criteria for differentiation between the most common different myometrial abnormalities are outlined in Table 1.4, and examples are given in Fig. 1.5.

Unclassified ovarian and pelvic masses should primarily be seen by a trained sonographer. MRI may be indicated, and should be performed by a MRI specialist in pelvic MRI (Sect. 1.3.5).

TVS has the same diagnostic efficiency as MRI in experienced hands in differentiation between myomas and adenomyosis (Champaneria et al. 2010). However, MRI may be superior when experienced sonographers are not at hand, in indefinite cases at TVS, and when adenomyosis are present together with myomas (Bazot et al. 2001; Dueholm et al. 2001c).

1.4.2.4 Selection of Patients with Myomas for Endoscopy and Image-Guided Procedures

Selection of patients for different newer myoma treatment modalities is a developing specialty. The most common alternatives are UAE, RFA, and MRgFUS. The efficiency of UAE is well established, with good long-term outcome (Walker and Barton-Smith 2006).

MRgFUS is the only technique which is totally noninvasive. Focused ultrasound is applied to myomas guided by MRI, and myomas are ablated by thermal energy. This technique has efficient long- to midterm outcome (Stewart et al. 2007), and even pregnancy rates are encouraging (Rabinovici et al. 2010). The main disadvantage is the dependence on a costly new technology,

Table 1.4 TVS and MRI characteristics of most common myometrial masses

TVS	
Regular defined margin, edge shadows, echo dense, homogeneous, hypoechogenic, circular flow, regular or scattered vessels	Typical leiomyoma
Regular well-defined margins, edge shadows, heterogenic echogenicity with anechogenic, or mixed echogenicity and circular flow, regular or scattered vessels	Atypical leiomyoma
Irregular heterogenic echogenicity, irregular anechoic areas of necrosis, irregular margins, vessels irregular, regular or scattered	Neoplasme suspect myometrial lesion
Globular uterus, with asymmetric myometrial walls. Margins: Irregular poorly described. Echogenicity: heterogeneity, hypo- or hyperechogenicity. Distinct features: Linear striations, indistinct endomyometrial junction, hyperechogenic dots, anechogenic lacunae or cysts and irregular widening of the junctional zone. Vessels: Perpendicular vessels and limited circular flow	Probably adenomyosis
MRI	
Low signal intensity on T2-weighted images, and possible high intensity rim	Leiomyoma
Cystic degeneration: cystic, high intensity (T2) and myxoid degeneration: lobular, septate process, high intensity (T2), red degeneration: heterogenic mass of ten high intensity at the rim, late enhancement	Atypical leiomyoma
Large regular asymmetric uterus without myomas, ill-defined low signal intensity myometrial areas, heterotopic endometrial tissue (foci of increased high signal intensity in the junctional zone (JZ)). Ratio max >40 (JZmax/myometrial thickness), maximal junctional zone thickness. (JZmax) of 12 mm, (JZdif) difference of >5 mm between maximum and minimum JZ thickness (degree of irregularity)	Adenomyosis
Large broad based bulky polypoid mass, filling the uterine cavity, heterogeneous hypointense signal on T1-weighted images and hyperintense signal (T2), hemorrhage, (areas of elevated T1 signal), necrosis (foci of hyperintense signal (T2) myometrial invasion and heterogenic enhancement)	Carcinosarcoma/ adenosarcomas
Large heterogeneously enhancing mass, with central (T2) hyperintensity (necrosis). Hemorrhage (areas of elevated T1 signal), calcifications may be present. Early contrast enhancement, marginal irregularity (50 %). Alternatively, homogeneously low-signal mass, similar to a leiomyoma	Leiomyosarcomas

and that the technique only is applicable in limited numbers of myoma cases (Taran et al. 2010; Behera et al. 2010).

Needle-guided ablation can be performed with cryotherapy, focused ultrasound, and RFA. At RFA a needle is introduced into the fibroids guided by ultrasound, and radiofrequency energy is applied to the needle causing ablation of the fibroid. There is limited experience with this technique (Iversen et al. 2012; Kim et al. 2011; Garza Leal et al. 2011), but the midterm outcome is promising, and RFA seems to be a low cost simple alternative to MRgFUS.

In the individual patient the total numbers of myomas and their correct location have to be mapped before selection of patients for endoscopic treatment, UAE, RFA, or MRgFUS. It is without larger problems done by TVS when image quality is good. However, in the presence of several myomas (four or more), there might

be more myomas in the acoustic shadows at TVS and MRI should be considered (Dueholm et al. 2002b). Patients with several to numerous small myomas could most efficiently be treated by UAE, while laparoscopic myomectomy is most often preferred for patients with larger subserous myomas (type 6–7), where none of the newer methods are optimal.

Submucous myomas with score below 5 in the STEMW system are treated with hysteroscopic resection, but there are often both submucous and intramural myomas. Submucous myomas are not optimally treated by MRgFUS or RFA (Iversen et al. 2012; Taran et al. 2010), but they are not any hindrance for UAE. However, there might be more infectious morbidity and prolonged discharge (Walker et al. 2004; Spies et al. 2002), and HY may be needed in the follow-up period after treatment.

TVS is a very efficient technique to roughly sort patients for modern image techniques, but

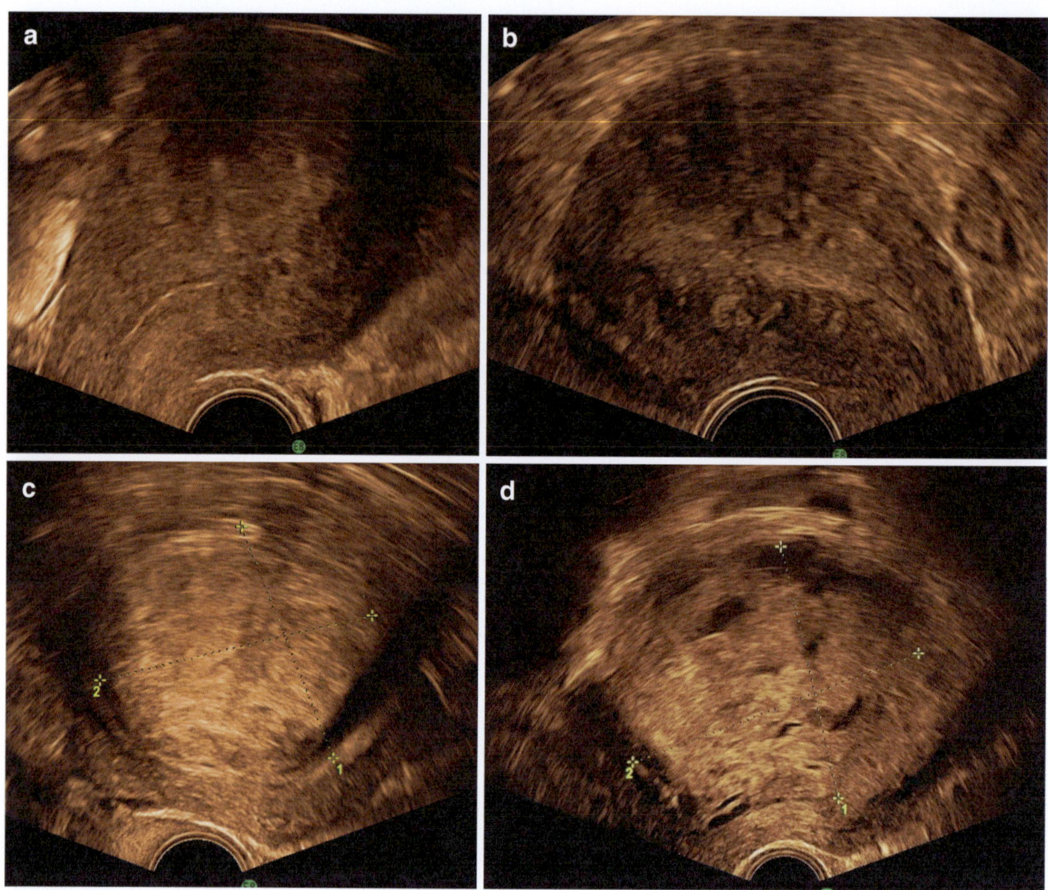

Fig. 1.5 Two typical examples of adenomyosis at TVS are displayed in (**a**) and (**b**). Both have irregular margins and not uniform echogenicity, and linear striation (**a**) with clear islands of ectopic endometrium and cysts, while the presence of adenomyosis in (**b**) is characterized with muscular hypertrofia, and small anechoic lacunae. (**c**) A typical well circumscribed myoma with regular margins, a hyperechoic rim, and uniform echogenicity. (**d**) An atypical myoma hyaline degenerated myoma with regular margins without a rim not uniform echogenicity, with irregular cystic spaces

MRI should be performed before definite treatment with UAE, MRgFUS, or RFA. It may have a higher efficiency for selection of patients than ultrasound (Spielmann et al. 2006), which probably is very observer-dependent. However, most important is valuable information on myoma vascularity given by MRI (see Sect. 1.3.5).

1.4.3 Adnexal Masses

TVS is the standard imaging for adnexal masses (ACOG 2007). These masses should in premenopausal women be described according to Table 1.3 which display the IOTA terms. Premenopausal adnexal masses should be handled according to the traditional risk of malignancy index (RMI) (RCOG.(11)) or IOTA rules (Table 1.5). (The two left column are the IOTA rules, and the left three display RMI in table 1.5.) In premenopausal women, newer studies (Kaijser et al. 2012; Timmerman et al. 2010) seem to show higher efficiency of the IOTA system (Van et al. 2012a, b). Corpus luteums, endometriomas, dermoids, fibroids, and hydrosalpinges are recognized by the specific pattern in the hands of trained sonographers (Sokalska et al. 2009). Figure 1.6 displays examples of adnexal masses.

RMI, which include Ca-125 may still provide the highest diagnostic efficiency in postmenopausal women (RCOG.(11)). Ca-125 has a low specificity in premenopausal women

Table 1.5 Classification of ovarian mass (IOTA rules left, RMI right)

IOTA rules		RMI		
B features	*M features*	Menopausal status (*M*)	Premenopausal	0
Benign	*Suspect tumor*		Postmenopausal (hysterectomy >50 years)	3
				M score
(1) Unilocular cyst;	(1) Irregular solid tumor;	Ultrasound score (*U*)	Unilokular	0
			> Bilokular	1
(2) Presence of solid components (largest solid component is <7 mm in largest diameter)	(2) Ascites; and		Solid areas	1
			Bilateral	1
(3) Acoustic shadows	(3) At least four papillary structures;		Excrescences	1
			Ascites	1
(4) Smooth multilocular tumor less than 100 mm in largest diameter; and	(4) Irregular multilocular – solid tumor (largest diameter >100 mm)		Extra-ovarian disease	1
(5) No detectable blood flow (color Doppler)	(5) Very high color content (color Doppler)	$\sum U$ score		$\sum U$ score
If one or more M features were present in the absence of a B feature, we classified the mass as malignant (rule 1)	If one or more B features were present in the absence of an M feature, we classified the mass as benign (rule 2)	Ca-125	Value	Ca-125
Not classifiable				
If both M features and B features were present, or if none of the features was present, the simple rules were inconclusive (rule 3)		RMI	RMI = M-Score × U-Score × CA-125	

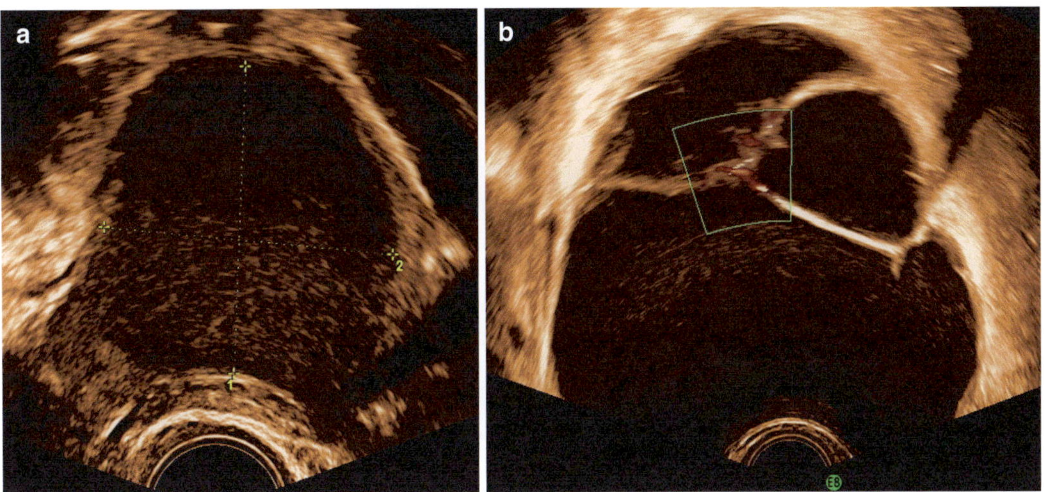

Fig. 1.6 A typical endometrioma (**a**) unilocular with ground glass appearance. (**b**) Benign mucinous cystadenoma, regular, multilocular cyst without solid components, with septae and minimal color score (2)

opposed to postmenopausal women. The simple rules (Table 1.5) will either classify the mass as benign, malignant, or not classifiable. Patients with adnexal masses classified as malignant should be treated by oncologists, while not classified tumors should be evaluated by specially trained sonographers (Ameye et al. 2012). For tumors, that are not classified the value of addition of 3D-TVS is questionable, although 3D-TVS was superior to conventional TVS for the prediction of malignant cases in a single study (Geomini et al. 2007). However, MRI may help in distinction between malignant and benign tumors (Dodge et al. 2012; Spencer and Ghattamaneni

2010; Spencer et al. 2010), which may be optimized further by DW MRI (Chou et al. 2012). For evaluation of tumor stage and recurrence CT, positron emission tomography – computed tomography (PET CT) may identify extra-ovarian disease (Dodge et al. 2012). Laparoscopy may be preferred (Whiteside and Keup 2009), when operative treatment is needed in adnexal masses classified as benign. Unclassified cysts have to be removed without spill, and oncologic expertise should be at hand.

1.4.4 Power Doppler at TVS for Evaluation of Uterus and Adnexal Mass

Power Doppler at TVS displays the overall vascularity and the pattern of the vessels.

The evaluation of color score is an additional parameter to the pattern palette at gray-scale evaluation in distinction between benign and malignant adnexal mass (Timmerman et al. 2010).

The power Doppler findings may vary in benign and malignant uterine mass (Hata et al. 1997; Szabo et al. 2002). In general, tumor vessels have an irregular chaotic pattern with numerous small and larger vessels and irregular branching, but several tumors have only scattered vessels (Szabo et al. 2002).

The circular flow around myomas is different from the perpendicular flow in adenomyosis (Chiang et al. 1999) in distinction between adenomyosis and myomas.

In the assessment of endometrial pathology, vessel pattern may have distinct features. The single vessel pattern indicate polyps and circular flow myomas, while an increased color score, and multiple vessel pattern (Alcazar et al. 2003; Epstein et al. 2002) are present in two-thirds of cases with endometrial malignancy. Examples are displayed in Fig. 1.7.

Calculation of vascularization index, flow index, and vascularization-flow index can be performed in a volume area of the 3D volume in the (VOCAL) post-processing system and may give an objective measurement of the color content, which is an observer-independent technique to evaluate increased tumor flow in the

endometrium (Alcazar and Galvan 2009; Alcazar et al. 2006). However, quantification of vascularity at TVS is problematic, as this is dependent on standard settings of the software in different ultrasound machines (Alcazar 2008).

1.4.5 Dynamic Contrast-Enhanced MRI (DCE MRI) and Diffusion-Weighted MRI (DW MRI)

The features of DCE MRI are used in diagnosis and staging of malignant tumors (Kinkel et al. 2009; Bipat et al. 2003) and in indistinct pelvic mass (Kinkel et al. 2005). Unclassified ovarian and pelvic masses should primarily be seen by a trained sonographer, and when MRI is indicated, it should be performed by a MRI specialist in pelvic MRI. In distinction between degenerating leiomyomas and sarcomas early enhancement at MRI may suggest sarcomas (Goto et al. 2002; Shah et al. 2012; Wu et al. 2011). Moreover a combination of T2-weighted images and diffusion-weighted images is often helpful (Namimoto et al. 2009), as restricted diffusion is often seen in sarcomas. However, restricted diffusion may also be present in cellular leiomyomas, and No imaging technique has a high efficiency for a diagnosis of sarcomas. DW MRI may improve staging in endometrial and cervical cancer. It can also be helpful in characterizing complex adnexal masses and in depicting recurrent tumor after treatment of various gynecologic malignancies (Thoeny et al. 2012; Li et al. 2013; Chou et al. 2012).

1.4.5.1 DCE MRI in Therapeutic Imaging

DCE MRI is used to evaluate perfusion in myomas before and after UAE, RFA, and MRgFUS. Myomas with high extend of hyalinization and low vessel density had poor enhancement at DCE MRI (Shimada et al. 2004). The main object of all these newer methods is to achieve degenerative changes in myomas. Myomas without enhancement have often already had a spontaneous degeneration. Thus, myomas without significant perfusion may not benefit from UAE or MRgFUS (Nikolaidis et al. 2005; Al Hilli

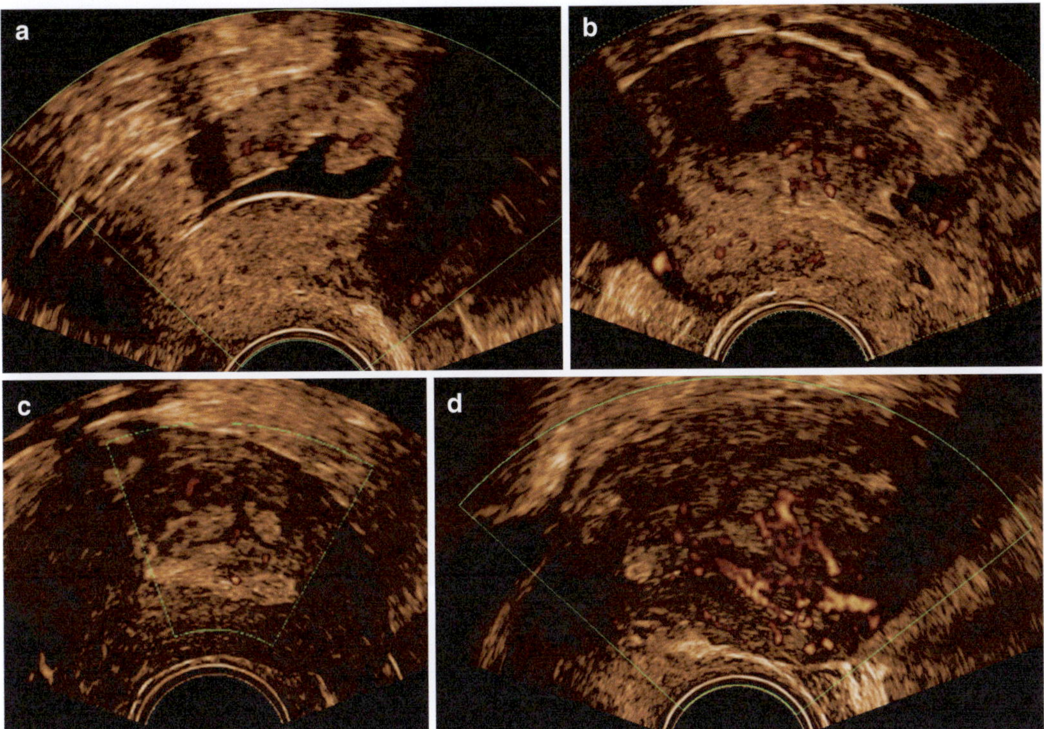

Fig. 1.7 Polyp (**a**), localized lesion with regular outline and one single small dominant vessel. (**b**) Adenomyosis, scattered, inhomogenic vessels in adenomyosis with large cystic areas in the myometrium and indistinct endomyometrial junction. (**c**) Endometrial cancer with heterogenic endometrium, irregular interrupted endomyometrial junction and scattered, not dominant large vessels. (**d**) An endometrial cancer with typical not scattered, not dominant multifocal vessels with abundant color score (4), and irregular branching

and Stewart 2010; Cura et al. 2006). Moreover, residual perfusion after treatment seems to be the most determined point for long-term effect of UAE or MRgFUS (Machtinger et al. 2012; Scheurig-Muenkler et al. 2012; Katsumori et al. 2008). At MRgFUS perfusion is normally evaluated immediately after treatment, and permanent efficient outcome is dependent on percentage of residual perfused myoma (Fig. 1.8). Contrast at MRI should never be used in patients with impaired renal function, where it may have serious complication (Marenzi et al. 2012) – and in these patients DW MRI can be used.

1.5 Evaluation of Congenital Uterine Abnormalities

In 3D TVS, the advantage of the coronal view makes it simple to diagnose the presence of either an arcuate, septate or bicorn uterus (Faivre et al. 2012). GIS may be added in indefinite findings. In the presence of more complex fusions anomalies especially in children, transabdominal ultrasound is the image modality, and MRI may add important information, as the resolution of MRI is higher than transabdominal ultrasound in the female pelvic.

1.6 Fertility Investigation

In the evaluation of subfertility TVS is the first step performed for evaluation of pathology in the uterus and ovary and for exclusion of a hydrosalpinx. Hydrosalpinx affects implantation in the endometrium (Strandell et al. 2001) and should be removed before fertility treatment (Camus et al. 1999). TVS is performed in the early follicular faze and may exclude most common uterine causes for subfertility (NICE.(04)). HY or SIS has higher diagnostic efficiency, and SIS may

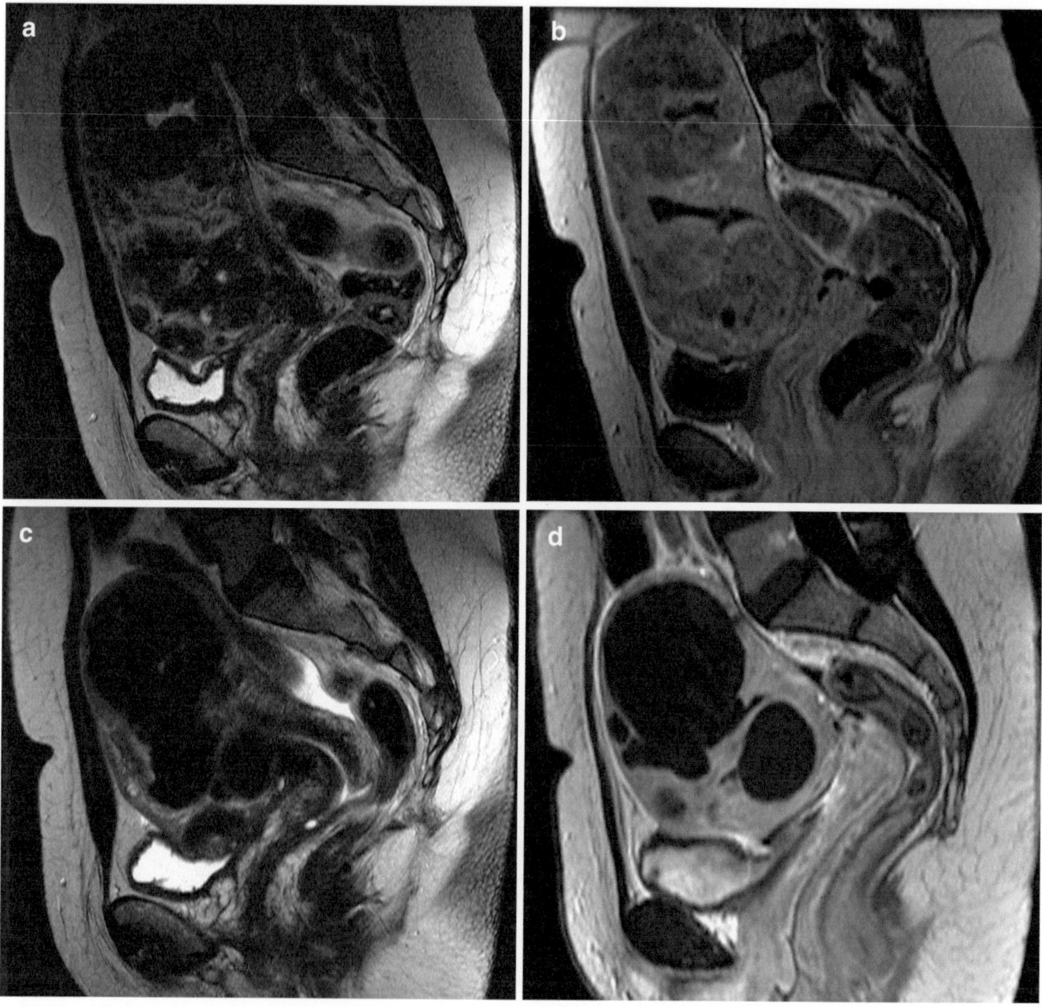

Fig. 1.8 T2-weighted MRI of myoma, (**a**) before UAE without contrast; (**b**) after contrast, where there is enhancement in myoma (*light colors*); (**c**) T2-weighted image 6 months after embolization with marked reduced volume of myoma; (**d**) 6 months after UAE after contrast, and there is no enhancement in myoma (*black*) – indicating complete embolization

be incorporated in the evaluation of tuba patency (see Sect. 1.6.1).

1.6.1 Tuba Factor

Traditionally tuba patency assessed by hysterosalpingography (HSG) has been replaced by hysterosalpingo-contrast sonography (HyCoSy). After a conventional scanning, a small uterine balloon catheter is placed in the uterine cavity, and the balloon inflated with saline is positioned just above the internal orificium. Saline is infused, and SIS is performed (Sect. 1.3.2). The intrauterine portion of the tube (proximal part) is localized. A contrast media containing air bubbles is introduced, and the passage of air bubbles through the proximal tube is observed at both sites. Free spill from the tube to the abdomen may be observed, but is not always optional. Passage of bubbles through the proximal tube, no hydrosalpinx observed and free fluid in the abdomen, after the examination has a high diagnostic efficiency for diagnosis of tuba patency (Chan et al. 2005; Holz et al. 1997).

The diagnostic efficiency of HyCoSy is dependent on training, and close to 50 scans is reported for sufficient efficiency (Dijkman et al. 2000). There might be slight but not substantial advantages of 3D-PDA (Sladkevicius et al. 2000; Kiyokawa et al. 2000). 3D-PDA may allow to capture a full volume of the tube and observe the spill, which seems to be the most optimal way to document the findings.

An alternative is transvaginal hydro laparoscopy, which will be dealt with in another chapter of the book.

1.7   Observer Variation

Endoscopy is a very observer-dependent technique, and the ability to recognizes and differentiate between normal and pathologic anatomy is part of the technical skill. This has raised attention on the difference in evaluation of anatomic structures even by trained surgeons (Buddingh et al. 2012). There is demonstrated considerable observer variation in the evaluation of adherences and endometriosis (Corson et al. 1995), and even for common benign diagnosis at HY (Kasius et al. 2011).

At TVS observer variation between different observers is substantial for diagnosis of adnexal mass (Sladkevicius and Valentin 2013), different abnormalities in the uterine cavity even in trained observers (Van den Bosch et al. 2012), and may be substantial when it comes to findings as adenomyosis (Dueholm et al. 2002c).

The observer variation at gynecologic MRI might also be substantial between MRI specialist with special training in pelvic pathology and other MRI specialists (Bazot et al. 2003).

Observer variation may be reduced by implementation of standard terms for definition, standards for image training, documentation and image conferences on findings. This is an important aspect to improve the diagnosis and treatment. There are large advances of TVS performed by surgeons in outpatient office settings, and with additional imaging added as outlined above. However, the widespread use may have an impact on image quality, and implementation

of standardized terms should be elaborated in all imaging including endoscopy. Findings should be documented and conferences of imaging before and during endoscopy are quite obvious actions, which may increase the quality of surgery.

References

Abuhamad AZ, Singleton S, Zhao Y et al (2006) The Z technique: an easy approach to the display of the mid-coronal plane of the uterus in volume sonography. J Ultrasound Med 25:607–612

ACOG (2007) ACOG practice bulletin. Management of adnexal masses. Obstet Gynecol 110:201–214

Alcazar JL (2008) Three-dimensional power Doppler derived vascular indices: what are we measuring and how are we doing it? Ultrasound Obstet Gynecol 32:485–487

Alcazar JL, Galvan R (2009) Three-dimensional power Doppler ultrasound scanning for the prediction of endometrial cancer in women with postmenopausal bleeding and thickened endometrium. Am J Obstet Gynecol 200:44–46

Alcazar JL, Castillo G, Minguez JA et al (2003) Endometrial blood flow mapping using transvaginal power Doppler sonography in women with postmenopausal bleeding and thickened endometrium. Ultrasound Obstet Gynecol 21:583–588

Alcazar JL, Ajossa S, Floris S et al (2006) Reproducibility of endometrial vascular patterns in endometrial disease as assessed by transvaginal power Doppler sonography in women with postmenopausal bleeding. J Ultrasound Med 25:159–163

Al Hilli MM, Stewart EA (2010) Magnetic resonance-guided focused ultrasound surgery. Semin Reprod Med 28:242–249

Ameye L, Timmerman D, Valentin L et al (2012) Clinically oriented three-step strategy to the assessment of adnexal pathology. Ultrasound Obstet Gynecol 140:582–591

Angioni S, Loddo A, Milano F et al (2008) Detection of benign intracavitary lesions in postmenopausal women with abnormal uterine bleeding: a prospective comparative study on outpatient hysteroscopy and blind biopsy. J Minim Invasive Gynecol 15:87–91

Avila ML, Ruiz R, Cortaberria JR et al (2008) Assessment of cervical involvement in endometrial carcinoma by hysteroscopy and directed biopsy. Int J Gynecol Cancer 18:128–131

Bazot M, Cortez A, Darai E et al (2001) Ultrasonography compared with magnetic resonance imaging for the diagnosis of adenomyosis: correlation with histopathology. Hum Reprod 16:2427–2433

Bazot M, Darai E, de Clement GS et al (2003) Fast breath-hold T2-weighted MR imaging reduces interobserver variability in the diagnosis of adenomyosis. AJR Am J Roentgenol 180:1291–1296

Behera MA, Leong M, Johnson L et al (2010) Eligibility and accessibility of magnetic resonance-guided focused ultrasound (MRgFUS) for the treatment of uterine leiomyomas. Fertil Steril 94:1864–1868

Bettocchi S, Ceci O, Nappi L et al (2004) Operative office hysteroscopy without anesthesia: analysis of 4863 cases performed with mechanical instruments. J Am Assoc Gynecol Laparosc 11:59–61

Bipat S, Glas AS, van der Velden J et al (2003) Computed tomography and magnetic resonance imaging in staging of uterine cervical carcinoma: a systematic review. Gynecol Oncol 91:59–66

Buddingh KT, Morks AN, ten Cate Hoedemaker HO et al (2012) Documenting correct assessment of biliary anatomy during laparoscopic cholecystectomy. Surg Endosc 26:79–85

Caliskan E, Ozkan S, Cakiroglu Y et al (2010) Diagnostic accuracy of real-time 3D sonography in the diagnosis of congenital Mullerian anomalies in high-risk patients with respect to the phase of the menstrual cycle. J Clin Ultrasound 38:123–127

Camus E, Poncelet C, Goffinet F et al (1999) Pregnancy rates after in-vitro fertilization in cases of tubal infertility with and without hydrosalpinx: a meta-analysis of published comparative studies. Hum Reprod 14:1243–1249

Champaneria R, Abedin P, Daniels J et al (2010) Ultrasound scan and magnetic resonance imaging for the diagnosis of adenomyosis: systematic review comparing test accuracy. Acta Obstet Gynecol Scand 89:1374–1384

Chan CC, Ng EH, Tang OS et al (2005) Comparison of three-dimensional hysterosalpingo-contrast-sonography and diagnostic laparoscopy with chromopertubation in the assessment of tubal patency for the investigation of subfertility. Acta Obstet Gynecol Scand 84:909–913

Chiang CH, Chang MY, Hsu JJ et al (1999) Tumor vascular pattern and blood flow impedance in the differential diagnosis of leiomyoma and adenomyosis by color Doppler sonography. J Assist Reprod Genet 16:268–275

Chou CP, Chiou SH, Levenson RB et al (2012) Differentiation between pelvic abscesses and pelvic tumors with diffusion-weighted MR imaging: a preliminary study. Clin Imaging 36:532–538

Cicinelli E (2010) Hysteroscopy without anesthesia: review of recent literature. J Minim Invasive Gynecol 17:703–708

Cicinelli E, Parisi C, Galantino P et al (2003) Reliability, feasibility, and safety of minihysteroscopy with a vaginoscopic approach: experience with 6,000 cases. Fertil Steril 80:199–202

Cicinelli E, Marinaccio M, Barba B et al (2008) Reliability of diagnostic fluid hysteroscopy in the assessment of cervical invasion by endometrial carcinoma: a comparative study with transvaginal sonography and MRI. Gynecol Oncol 111:55–61

Corson SL, Batzer FR, Gocial B et al (1995) Intra-observer and inter-observer variability in scoring laparoscopic diagnosis of pelvic adhesions. Hum Reprod 10:161–164

Cura M, Cura A, Bugnone A (2006) Role of magnetic resonance imaging in patient selection for uterine artery embolization. Acta Radiol 47:1105–1114

de Kroon CD, de Bock GH, Dieben SW et al (2003) Saline contrast hysterosonography in abnormal uterine bleeding: a systematic review and meta-analysis. BJOG 110:938–947

de Kroon CD, Louwe LA, Trimbos JB et al (2004) The clinical value of 3-dimensional saline infusion sonography in addition to 2-dimensional saline infusion sonography in women with abnormal uterine bleeding: work in progress. J Ultrasound Med 23:1433–1440

Dijkman AB, Mol BW, van der Veen F et al (2000) Can hysterosalpingocontrast-sonography replace hysterosalpingography in the assessment of tubal subfertility? Eur J Radiol 35:44–48

Dodge JE, Covens AL, Lacchetti C et al (2012) Management of a suspicious adnexal mass: a clinical practice guideline. Curr Oncol 19:e244–e257

Dueholm M, Forman A, Jensen ML et al (2001a) Transvaginal sonography combined with saline contrast sonohysterography in evaluating the uterine cavity in premenopausal patients with abnormal uterine bleeding. Ultrasound Obstet Gynecol 18:54–61

Dueholm M, Lundorf E, Hansen ES et al (2001b) Evaluation of the uterine cavity with magnetic resonance imaging, transvaginal sonography, hysterosonographic examination, and diagnostic hysteroscopy. Fertil Steril 76:350–357

Dueholm M, Lundorf E, Hansen ES et al (2001c) Magnetic resonance imaging and transvaginal ultrasonography for the diagnosis of adenomyosis. Fertil Steril 76:588–594

Dueholm M, Lundorf E, Olesen F (2002a) Imaging techniques for evaluation of the uterine cavity and endometrium in premenopausal patients before minimally invasive surgery. Obstet Gynecol Surv 57:388–403

Dueholm M, Lundorf E, Hansen ES et al (2002b) Accuracy of magnetic resonance imaging and transvaginal ultrasonography in the diagnosis, mapping, and measurement of uterine myomas. Am J Obstet Gynecol 186:409–415

Dueholm M, Lundorf E, Sorensen JS et al (2002c) Reproducibility of evaluation of the uterus by transvaginal sonography, hysterosonographic examination, hysteroscopy and magnetic resonance imaging. Hum Reprod 17:195–200

Epstein E, Ramirez A, Skoog L et al (2001) Dilatation and curettage fails to detect most focal lesions in the uterine cavity in women with postmenopausal bleeding. Acta Obstet Gynecol Scand 80:1131–1136

Epstein E, Skoog L, Isberg PE et al (2002) An algorithm including results of gray-scale and power Doppler ultrasound examination to predict endometrial malignancy in women with postmenopausal bleeding. Ultrasound Obstet Gynecol 20:370–376

Faivre E, Fernandez H, Deffieux X et al (2012) Accuracy of three-dimensional ultrasonography in differential diagnosis of septate and bicornuate uterus compared with office hysteroscopy and pelvic magnetic resonance imaging. J Minim Invasive Gynecol 19:101–106

Garza Leal JG, Hernandez Leon I, Castillo SL et al (2011) Laparoscopic ultrasound-guided radiofrequency volumetric thermal ablation of symptomatic uterine leiomyomas: feasibility study using the halt 2000 ablation system. J Minim Invasive Gynecol 18:364–371

Geomini PM, Coppus SF, Kluivers KB et al (2007) Is three-dimensional ultrasonography of additional value in the assessment of adnexal masses? Gynecol Oncol 106:153–159

Goto A, Takeuchi S, Sugimura K et al (2002) Usefulness of Gd-DTPA contrast-enhanced dynamic MRI and serum determination of LDH and its isozymes in the differential diagnosis of leiomyosarcoma from degenerated leiomyoma of the uterus. Int J Gynecol Cancer 12:354–361

Hata K, Hata T, Maruyama R et al (1997) Uterine sarcoma: can it be differentiated from uterine leiomyoma with Doppler ultrasonography? A preliminary report. Ultrasound Obstet Gynecol 9:101–104

Holz K, Becker R, Schurmann R (1997) Ultrasound in the investigation of tubal patency. A meta-analysis of three comparative studies of Echovist-200 including 1007 women. Zentralbl Gynakol 119:366–373

Hudelist G, English J, Thomas AE et al (2011) Diagnostic accuracy of transvaginal ultrasound for non-invasive diagnosis of bowel endometriosis: systematic review and meta-analysis. Ultrasound Obstet Gynecol 37:257–263

Iversen H, Lenz S, Dueholm M (2012) Ultrasound-guided radiofrequency ablation of symptomatic uterine fibroids: short-term evaluation of effect of treatment on quality of life and symptom severity. Ultrasound Obstet Gynecol 40:445–451

Kaijser J, Bourne T, Valentin L et al (2013) Improving strategies for diagnosing ovarian cancer: a summary of the International Ovarian Tumor Analysis (IOTA) studies. Ultrasound Obstet Gynecol 41:9–20

Kasius JC, Broekmans FJ, Veersema S et al (2011) Observer agreement in the evaluation of the uterine cavity by hysteroscopy prior to in vitro fertilization. Hum Reprod 26:801–807

Katsumori T, Kasahara T, Kin Y et al (2008) Infarction of uterine fibroids after embolization: relationship between postprocedural enhanced MRI findings and long-term clinical outcomes. Cardiovasc Intervent Radiol 31:66–72

Kim CH, Kim SR, Lee HA et al (2011) Transvaginal ultrasound-guided radiofrequency myolysis for uterine myomas. Hum Reprod 26:559–563

Kinkel K, Kaji Y, Yu KK et al (1999) Radiologic staging in patients with endometrial cancer: a meta-analysis. Radiology 212:711–718

Kinkel K, Lu Y, Mehdizade A et al (2005) Indeterminate ovarian mass at US: incremental value of second imaging test for characterization—meta-analysis and Bayesian analysis. Radiology 236:85–94

Kinkel K, Forstner R, Danza FM et al (2009) Staging of endometrial cancer with MRI: guidelines of the European Society of Urogenital Imaging. Eur Radiol 19:1565–1574

Kiyokawa K, Masuda H, Fuyuki T et al (2000) Three-dimensional hysterosalpingo-contrast sonography (3D-HyCoSy) as an outpatient procedure to assess infertile women: a pilot study. Ultrasound Obstet Gynecol 16:648–654

Lasmar RB, Xinmei Z, Indman PD et al (2011) Feasibility of a new system of classification of submucous myomas: a multicenter study. Fertil Steril 95:2073–2077

Leone FP, Timmerman D, Bourne T et al (2010) Terms, definitions and measurements to describe the sonographic features of the endometrium and intrauterine lesions: a consensus opinion from the International Endometrial Tumor Analysis (IETA) group. Ultrasound Obstet Gynecol 35:103–112

Li W, Zhang Y, Cui Y et al (2013) Pelvic inflammatory disease: evaluation of diagnostic accuracy with conventional MR with added diffusion-weighted imaging. Abdom Imaging 38:193–200

Lotfallah H, Farag K, Hassan I et al (2005) One-stop hysteroscopy clinic for postmenopausal bleeding. J Reprod Med 50:101–107

Lykke R, Clevin L, Dueholm M (2012) A new technique for hysteroscopic resection of intramural myomas. J Gynecol Surg 28:147–149

Machtinger R, Inbar Y, Cohen-Eylon S et al (2012) MR-guided focus ultrasound (MRgFUS) for symptomatic uterine fibroids: predictors of treatment success. Hum Reprod 27:3425–3431

Makris N, Kalmantis K, Skartados N et al (2007) Three-dimensional hysterosonography versus hysteroscopy for the detection of intracavitary uterine abnormalities. Int J Gynaecol Obstet 97:6–9

Marenzi G, Cabiati A, Milazzo V et al (2012) Contrast-induced nephropathy. Intern Emerg Med 7(Suppl 3):181–183

Mavrelos D, Naftalin J, Hoo W et al (2011) Preoperative assessment of submucous fibroids by three-dimensional saline contrast sonohysterography. Ultrasound Obstet Gynecol 38:350–354

Meredith SM, Sanchez-Ramos L, Kaunitz AM (2009) Diagnostic accuracy of transvaginal sonography for the diagnosis of adenomyosis: systematic review and metaanalysis. Am J Obstet Gynecol 201:107.e1-6

Munro MG, Critchley HO, Fraser IS (2011) The FIGO classification of causes of abnormal uterine bleeding in the reproductive years. Fertil Steril 95:2204–2208

Nakai A, Koyama T, Fujimoto K et al (2008) Functional MR imaging of the uterus. Magn Reson Imaging Clin N Am 16:673–684, ix

Namimoto T, Yamashita Y, Awai K et al (2009) Combined use of T2-weighted and diffusion-weighted 3-T MR imaging for differentiating uterine sarcomas from benign leiomyomas. Eur Radiol 19:2756–2764

NICE. Fertility: assessment and treatment for people with fertility problems. National Institute for Clinical

Excellence (1-2-2004) [cited 1-11-2012]. Available from: http://www.rcog.org.uk

Nikolaidis P, Siddiqi AJ, Carr JC et al (2005) Incidence of nonviable leiomyomas on contrast material-enhanced pelvic MR imaging in patients referred for uterine artery embolization. J Vasc Interv Radiol 16:1465–1471

Paldino MJ, Barboriak DP (2009) Fundamentals of quantitative dynamic contrast-enhanced MR imaging. Magn Reson Imaging Clin N Am 17:277–289

Piscaglia F, Nolsoe C, Dietrich CF et al (2012) The EFSUMB guidelines and recommendations on the Clinical Practice of Contrast Enhanced Ultrasound (CEUS): update 2011 on non-hepatic applications. Ultraschall Med 33:33–59

Rabinovici J, David M, Fukunishi H et al (2010) Pregnancy outcome after magnetic resonance-guided focused ultrasound surgery (MRgFUS) for conservative treatment of uterine fibroids. Fertil Steril 93:199–209

Raine-Fenning NJ, Campbell BK, Clewes JS et al (2003) The reliability of virtual organ computer-aided analysis (VOCAL) for the semiquantification of ovarian, endometrial and subendometrial perfusion. Ultrasound Obstet Gynecol 22:633–639

Raine-Fenning NJ, Nordin NM, Ramnarine KV et al (2008) Evaluation of the effect of machine settings on quantitative three-dimensional power Doppler angiography: an in-vitro flow phantom experiment. Ultrasound Obstet Gynecol 32:551–559

RCOG. management of suspected ovarian masses in premenopausal women.GTG62. Royal College of Obstetricians and Gynaecologists (1-11-2011) [cited 25-10-2012]. Available from http://www.rcog.org.uk

Scheurig-Muenkler C, Koesters C, Grieser C et al (2012) Treatment failure after uterine artery embolization: prospective cohort study with multifactorial analysis of possible predictors of long-term outcome. Eur J Radiol 81:e727–e731

Shah SH, Jagannathan JP, Krajewski K et al (2012) Uterine sarcomas: then and now. AJR Am J Roentgenol 199:213–223

Shimada K, Ohashi I, Kasahara I et al (2004) Triple-phase dynamic MRI of intratumoral vessel density and hyalinization grade in uterine leiomyomas. AJR Am J Roentgenol 182:1043–1050

Sladkevicius P, Valentin L (2013) Intra- and inter-observer agreement when describing adnexal masses using the International Ovarian Tumour Analysis (IOTA) terms and definitions: a study on three-dimensional (3D) ultrasound volumes. Ultrasound Obstet Gynecol 41:318–327

Sladkevicius P, Ojha K, Campbell S et al (2000) Three-dimensional power Doppler imaging in the assessment of Fallopian tube patency. Ultrasound Obstet Gynecol 16:644–647

Sokalska A, Timmerman D, Testa AC et al (2009) Diagnostic accuracy of transvaginal ultrasound examination for assigning a specific diagnosis to adnexal masses. Ultrasound Obstet Gynecol 34:462–470

Spencer JA, Ghattamaneni S (2010) MR imaging of the sonographically indeterminate adnexal mass. Radiology 256:677–694

Spencer JA, Forstner R, Cunha TM et al (2010) ESUR guidelines for MR imaging of the sonographically indeterminate adnexal mass: an algorithmic approach. Eur Radiol 20:25–35

Spielmann AL, Keogh C, Forster BB et al (2006) Comparison of MRI and sonography in the preliminary evaluation for fibroid embolization. AJR Am J Roentgenol 187:1499–1504

Spies JB, Spector A, Roth AR et al (2002) Complications after uterine artery embolization for leiomyomas. Obstet Gynecol 100:873–880

Stewart EA, Gostout B, Rabinovici J et al (2007) Sustained relief of leiomyoma symptoms by using focused ultrasound surgery. Obstet Gynecol 110:279–287

Strandell A, Lindhard A, Waldenstrom U et al (2001) Hydrosalpinx and IVF outcome: cumulative results after salpingectomy in a randomized controlled trial. Hum Reprod 16:2403–2410

Szabo I, Szantho A, Csabay L et al (2002) Color Doppler ultrasonography in the differentiation of uterine sarcomas from uterine leiomyomas. Eur J Gynaecol Oncol 23:29–34

Taran FA, Hesley GK, Gorny KR et al (2010) What factors currently limit magnetic resonance-guided focused ultrasound of leiomyomas? A survey conducted at the first international symposium devoted to clinical magnetic resonance-guided focused ultrasound. Fertil Steril 94:331–334

Thoeny HC, Forstner R, De KF (2012) Genitourinary applications of diffusion-weighted MR imaging in the pelvis. Radiology 263:326–342

Timmerman D, Valentin L, Bourne TH et al (2000) Terms, definitions and measurements to describe the sonographic features of adnexal tumors: a consensus opinion from the International Ovarian Tumor Analysis (IOTA) Group. Ultrasound Obstet Gynecol 16:500–505

Timmerman D, Ameye L, Fischerova D et al (2010) Simple ultrasound rules to distinguish between benign and malignant adnexal masses before surgery: prospective validation by IOTA group. BMJ 341:c6839

Timmermans A, Opmeer BC, Khan KS et al (2010) Endometrial thickness measurement for detecting endometrial cancer in women with postmenopausal bleeding: a systematic review and meta-analysis. Obstet Gynecol 116:160–167

Van CB, Timmerman D, Valentin L et al (2012a) Triaging women with ovarian masses for surgery: observational diagnostic study to compare RCOG guidelines with an International Ovarian Tumour Analysis (IOTA) group protocol. BJOG 119:662–671

Van HC, Van CB, Bourne T et al (2012b) External validation of diagnostic models to estimate the risk of malignancy in adnexal masses. Clin Cancer Res 18:815–825

Van den Bosch T, Valentin L, Van SD et al (2012) Detection of intracavitary uterine pathology using offline analysis of three-dimensional ultrasound volumes: interobserver agreement and diagnostic accuracy. Ultrasound Obstet Gynecol 40:459–463

van Hanegem N, Breijer MC, Khan KS et al (2011) Diagnostic evaluation of the endometrium in post-menopausal bleeding: an evidence-based approach. Maturitas 68:155–164

Walker WJ, Barton-Smith P (2006) Long-term follow up of uterine artery embolisation–an effective alternative in the treatment of fibroids. BJOG 113:464–468

Walker WJ, Carpenter TT, Kent AS (2004) Persistent vaginal discharge after uterine artery embolization for fibroid tumors: cause of the condition, magnetic resonance imaging appearance, and surgical treatment. Am J Obstet Gynecol 190:1230–1233

Whiteside JL, Keup HL (2009) Laparoscopic management of the ovarian mass: a practical approach. Clin Obstet Gynecol 52:327–334

Wu TI, Yen TC, Lai CH (2011) Clinical presentation and diagnosis of uterine sarcoma, including imaging. Best Pract Res Clin Obstet Gynaecol 25:681–689

Yaman C, Sommergruber M, Ebner T et al (1999) Reproducibility of transvaginal three-dimensional endometrial volume measurements during ovarian stimulation. Hum Reprod 14:2604–2608

Zhou XD, Ren XL, Zhang J et al (2007) Therapeutic response assessment of high intensity focused ultrasound therapy for uterine fibroid: utility of contrast-enhanced ultrasonography. Eur J Radiol 62:289–294

Hysteroscopic Instrumentation

Olav Istre and Andreas Thurkow

Contents

2.1 Introduction

The first successful hysteroscopy was reported by Pantaleoni in 1869. In the last two decades, technical developments led to major improvements in diagnostic hysteroscopy and hysteroscopic surgery. Diagnostic hysteroscopy is currently the "gold standard" investigation of diseases involving the uterine cavity (Fraser 1993; Nagele et al. 1996) and hysteroscopic surgery is currently the standard treatment of intrauterine pathology, such as endometrial polyps (Polena et al. 2005; Preutthipan and Herabutya 2005; Savelli et al. 2003), submucous fibroids (Rosati et al. 2008; Timmermans and Veersema 2005), uterine septa (Colacurci et al. 2002; Perino et al. 1987) and intrauterine adhesions (Al-Inany 2001). Appropriate instrumentation, together with distension media like CO_2, saline and nonsaline solutions are of vital importance in hysteroscopic procedures.

O. Istre, MD, PhD, DMSc (✉)
Minimal Invasive Gynecology,
University of Southern Denmark, Odense, Denmark

Aleris-Hamlet Hospital, Scandinavia
e-mail: oistre@gmail.com

A. Thurkow, MD
Division of Gynaecological Endoscopy and Minimal
Invasive Gynaecological Surgery, Department
of Ob/Gyn, St Lucas Andreas Hospital Amsterdam,
Amsterdam, The Netherlands
e-mail: thurkow@mac.com

O. Istre (ed.), *Minimally Invasive Gynecological Surgery*,
DOI 10.1007/978-3-662-44059-9_2, © Springer-Verlag Berlin Heidelberg 2015

2.2 Diagnostic Hysteroscopy

Diagnostic hysteroscopy can be carried out as an outpatient procedure, taking only a few minutes, with success rates up to 98 % (Wieser et al. 1998). Outpatient hysteroscopy saves the patients' inconvenience, cost, undue stress and concern. Further advantages of outpatient hysteroscopy include its safety, expeditious performance, and high diagnostic accuracy (Glasser 2009).

An additional advantage above other diagnostic options for the uterine cavity (ultrasound, sonohysterography, MRI) is the possibility of performing therapeutic interventions in the same session in appropriate cases and situations.

2.2.1 Distension Medium in Hysteroscopy

The most commonly used distension media in hysteroscopy is saline. Saline is equal (Litta et al. 2003; Shankar et al. 2004) or better (Pellicano et al. 2003) in terms of patient discomfort and satisfaction and provides a superior view to CO_2, as bubbles and bleeding impede the view more often when CO_2 is used (Litta et al. 2003; Shankar et al. 2004; Pellicano et al. 2003). If the choice is made to convert to a see-and-treat procedure, saline has the advantage of compatibility with bipolar equipment allowing for immediate treatment. It is not advisable to use nonelectrolytic distension fluids (e.g. glycine 1.5 %, sorbitol-mannitol) associated with monopolar equipment, as these are limited to shorter use due to a higher risk of hyponatremia and brain edema (Istre et al. 1994).

2.2.2 Instruments for Hysteroscopy

1. Rigid 3.5–5.5 mm endoscope (Agdi and Tulandi 2009)
   Distension medium: *saline*
2. Office Continuous Flow Hysteroscope (Karl Storz GmbH, Tuttlingen, Germany; Olympus Surgery Technologies Europe GmbH, Hamburg, Germany; Richard Wolf GmbH, Knittlingen, Germany, etc.). Based on 1.9–3.0 mm rod lens systems with an outer diameter of 4.0–5.5 mm.

   Equipped with or without an operative 5-Fr canal (multiple 5-Fr mechanical instruments and 5-Fr bipolar electrodes are available) (Bettocchi et al. 2003).
3. Versascope (Gynecare division of Johnson & Johnson). 3.5 mm endoscope with a disposable sheath containing a collapsed working channel (5–7 Fr), which is distended during introduction of an instrument.

2.2.2.1 Rigid Versus Flexible Hysteroscopes

There are two different hysteroscope systems on the market: rigid and flexible hysteroscopes. The diameter of flexible hysteroscopes is smaller than that of rigid hysteroscopes and their rounded tip allows it to bend according to need, but rigid endoscopes have superior optical quality as the fiber optic pattern is clearly seen with the flexible hysteroscopes. Although more pain is associated with the "bigger" diameter rigid hysteroscopes, this is well compensated by the superior optical quality allowing for faster examination (on average 50s less (>70 %)) (Unfried et al. 2001) at higher success rates (100 % versus 87.5 %) (Unfried et al. 2001), and at a lower price than flexible endoscopes.

2.2.3 Tricks for Hysteroscopic Insertion

1. *Rotate the scope 90°*
   The internal cervical os is oval shaped with a diameter of approximately 4–5 mm. The "new" small-diameter hysteroscopes imitate this oval profile keeping the total diameter between 4 and 5 mm. Rotate the scope 90° on the endo-camera to align the longitudinal axis of the scope with the transverse axis of the internal cervical os. Doing so facilitates a painless entry (Bettocchi et al. 2003).
2. *Keep the cervical canal in the lower half of the screen*
   If you look through a hysteroscope the view is deflected by 12–30° (depending on the scope). In this way the structures in the middle of the

screen are actually positioned 12–30° lower. To ensure a painless entry keep the cervical canal in the lower half of the screen during insertion. In this way the scope will be located in the middle of the canal, avoiding stimulation of the muscle fibers (Bettocchi et al. 2003).

3. *Use 30° lenses*

For a correct examination of the uterine cavity and to reduce patient discomfort it is advisable to use 30° lenses. If the tip of the scope is placed 1–1.5 cm from the fundus, a view of the whole cavity and tubal ostiae can be gained by rotating the instrument on its axis, without any other lateral movement of the scope being required, which might cause pain to the patient (Bettocchi et al. 2003).

2.3 Hysteroscopic Surgery

Hysteroscopic surgery is now widely used to treat a variety of intrauterine diseases. In the scope of this article we discuss the instrumentation used for the following pathology: intrauterine synechiae, polyps and myoma, and the uterine septum followed by the hysteroscopic techniques used for ablation of the endometrium.

2.3.1 View Angle of the Telescope

The angle of the telescope on the resectoscope is usually 12° to always keep the loop within the viewing field (Mencaglia et al. 2009). By using a wider field of vision some companies offer resectoscopes with 0° or 30°, but care has to be taken to use these dedicated scopes that cannot be changed with just any other in order to avoid the above-mentioned viewing problems.

2.3.2 Distension Media in Hysteroscopic Surgery

The choice of the distension medium in hysteroscopic surgery depends on the type of equipment used. In the first days of hysteroscopic surgery only nonelectric/mechanical or monopolar equipment was available and mainly hypotonic,

electrolyte-free solutions were used to distend the uterine cavity. These solutions, when absorbed in large volumes, potentially cause hyponatremia and hypervolemia leading to neurotoxic coma or even death. In 1999 the first bipolar resectoscope was introduced (Loffer 2000). Bipolar systems show an improved safety profile through the use of physiological saline (contains electrolytes, 0.9 % NaCl), which prevents the drop in serum sodium associated with nonelectrolytic solutions used with monopolar equipment (Berg et al. 2009). The electrical current passes through multiple tissues before its return to the generator in the monopolar technique, in the bipolar technique the electrical current is restricted between the two loops of the electrode, thereby decreasing electrical/thermal injury to adjacent tissues. The "plasma effect" makes the bipolar more effective than the monopolar system. With bipolar equipment the generator produces a high initial voltage spike that establishes a voltage gradient in a gap between the bipolar electrodes. When the activated bipolar electrode is not in contact with the tissue, the electrolyte solution in the uterus dissipates it. When the loop is sufficiently close to tissue, the high bipolar voltage spike arc between the electrodes converts the conductive sodium chloride solution into a nonequilibrium vapor layer or "plasma effect." Once formed, this plasma effect can be maintained at lower voltages (Mencaglia et al. 2009). This suggests bipolar equipment to be superior to monopolar equipment, however current data show no differences in terms of safety and effectiveness (Garuti and Luerti 2009).

2.4 Intrauterine Synechiae

2.4.1 Instruments for Hysteroscopic Adhesiolysis

1. 5-F mechanical instrument (office hysteroscope) equipped with hysteroscopic scissors (Karl Storz GmbH, Tuttlingen, Germany; Olympus Surgery Technologies Europe GmbH, Hamburg, Germany; Richard Wolf GmbH, Knittlingen, Germany; Gynecare Johnson & Johnson Versascope) (Pabuccu et al. 2008).

Distension medium: *saline*

2. A 7–9 mm working element along with sheath and 4 mm 30° telescope (Karl Storz GmbH, Tuttlingen, Germany; Olympus Surgery Technologies Europe GmbH, Hamburg, Germany; Richard Wolf GmbH, Knittlingen, Germany; Gynecare Johnson & Johnson) equipped with a hysteroscopic monopolar or bipolar (Collin's) knife (Roy et al. 2010). A monopolar or bipolar loop could also be used, but is less versatile due to the fact that more working space is needed.

   Distension medium: *glycine (1.5%) or saline resp.*

3. Versapoint Twizzle bipolar electrode (Gynecare Johnson & Johnson).

   Distension medium: *saline.*

2.4.2 Diagnosis

Hysteroscopy.

2.4.3 Discussion

The use of hysteroscopic scissors avoids the possibility of energy-related damage to the endometrium. However, several studies have reported successful outcomes of adhesiolysis by using electrosurgery, which suggests that with proper application significant damage is unlikely (Cararach et al. 1994; Chervenak and Neuwirth 1981; Decherney and Polan 1983). Electrosurgery has the advantage over scissors by achieving better hemostasis, thus providing an improved optical clarity of the operative field (Yu et al. 2008).

2.5 Uterine Septum

2.5.1 Instruments for Metroplasty

1. 26 F resectoscope fitted with monopolar or bipolar 90° knife electrode and with a 0–12° telescope (Karl Storz GmbH, Tuttlingen, Germany; Olympus Surgery Technologies Europe GmbH, Hamburg, Germany; Richard Wolf GmbH, Knittlingen, Germany; Ethicon Gynecare Inc., Johnson & Johnson) (Colacurci et al. 2007).

   Distension medium: *sorbitol, mannitol, saline*

2. Continuous flow small-diameter hysteroscope (maximum diameter 5 mm) (Karl Storz GmbH, Tuttlingen, Germany; Olympus Surgery Technologies Europe GmbH, Hamburg, Germany; Richard Wolf GmbH, Knittlingen, Germany; Ethicon Gynecare Inc., Johnson & Johnson) fitted with a 0–30° telescope of 1.9–2.9 mm caliber equipped with a 1.6 mm single-fiber, twizzle-tip electrode passed through the 5 F working channel of the hysteroscope and connected with an electro-surgical generator (Versapoint Bipolar System) (Colacurci et al. 2007).

   Distension medium: *saline*

2.5.2 Background

To date, many data are available regarding the treatment of septate uterus performed by means of a traditional 26 F resectoscope fitted with a unipolar knife requiring nonelectrolytic solutions to distend the uterine cavity. Despite the excellent results, this technique was associated with serious complications such as mechanical trauma to the cervix, thermal injuries and fluid intravasation. In recent years technological improvements have led to the introduction of small-diameter hysteroscopes not exceeding 5 mm in diameter fitted with bipolar electrodes that work in saline solution, which allow simple and safe treatment of many intrauterine diseases, thus reducing the risk of severe complications.

The efficacy on reproductive outcome after metroplasty has never been proven in random-ized controlled trials. A similar multicenter trial is now being performed in several centers in the Netherlands[50].

2.5.3 Diagnosis

Three-dimensional ultrasound.

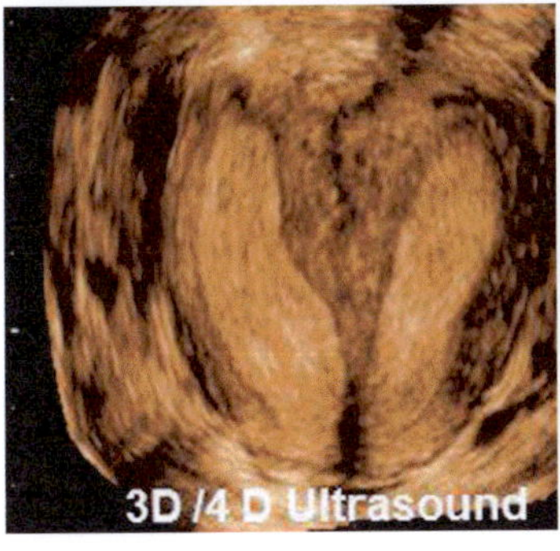
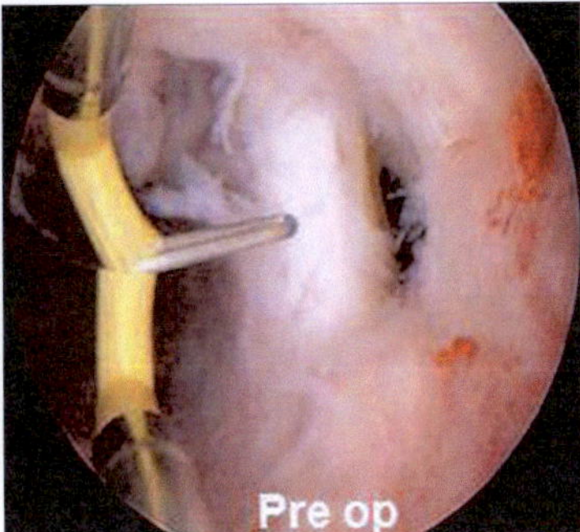
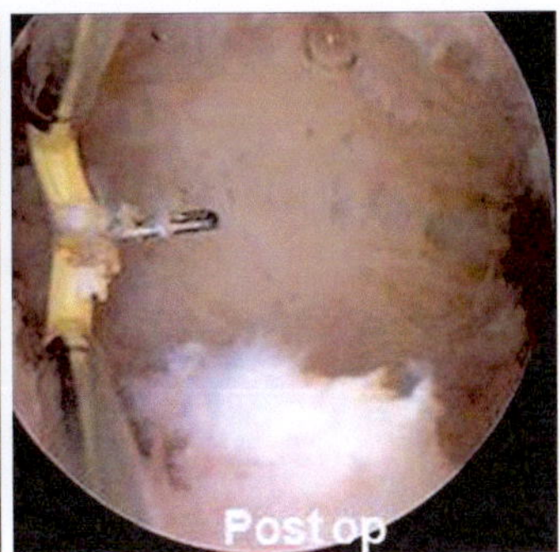

Uterine septum

2.5.4 Conclusion

No difference is seen with regard to reproductive outcome between both electrosurgical techniques mentioned before, so the choice of technique depends on the cost of instrumentation, operating time, and rate of complication. The resectoscopes offer that advantage of no requirement for disposable or specific equipments because the unipolar electrosurgery unit is usually available in most operating rooms and also nonexpensive and readily feasible. On the other hand, because of the shorter operating time, the easier feasibility, the lower incidence of complications, and the general improved safety, in experienced hands the small-diameter hysteroscope technique is a valuable and valid alternative to resectoscopy and should be preferred for the septate uterus class Vb (Colacurci et al. 2007).

2.5.5 Instruments for Polypectomy and Myomectomy

1. Outpatient setting: a 1.9–3 mm rigid optic with 0, 12° or 30° fore oblique lens and an outer sheath executed with a 5-french operating channel and continuous flow, with a maximum diameter of 4.5–5.5 mm. Equipped with either a graper forceps or scissors (mechanically), with bipolar electrodes (electrosurgical) (Van et al. 2009), an intrauterine morcellator (Smith & Nephew Trueclear® or Hologic Myosure® system) or with a polypsnare (Cook) (Timmermans and Veersema 2005).

2. Day case setting: a continuous flow operative hysteroscope (Karl Storz GmbH, Tuttlingen, Germany; Olympus Surgery Technologies Europe GmbH, Hamburg, Germany; Richard Wolf GmbH, Knittlingen, Germany; Ethicon Gynecare Inc., Johnson & Johnson or Smith and Nephew, Andover, MA, USA) with a 7- or 9-mm operative sheath and a 0° or 12° optic. Equipped with either a mechanical device (intrauterine morcellator: Smith & Nephew or Hologic Myosure®, scissors or forceps) or electrosurgical device (monopolar or bipolar electrodes) (Van et al. 2009).

3. Resectoscopes:
   (a) TCRis resectoscope (Olympus Surgery Technologies Europe GmbH, Hamburg), ch. 26 model WA 22061 with 12 optic 22001A with various loop sizes and types. Dedicated electrogenerator.
   (b) Gynecare 9 mm resectoscope with Versapoint loop (Ethicon Gynecare Inc., Johnson & Johnson), various loop sizes. Dedicated electrogenerator.
   (c) Storz bipolar resectoscope (Karl Storz GmbH, Tuttlingen, Germany).
   (d) Wolf Princess bipolar and monopolar 7 mm resectoscope or Wolf Resection Master with automatic chip aspiration (Richard Wolf GmbH, Knittlingen, Germany).
   all using NaCl 0.9 % (Braun) as irrigant (Berg et al. 2009).
   Resection of polyp with the loop resectoscope
   Resection of fibroid with the loop resectoscope

2.5.6 Background

There are many different resectoscopes available for treatment of endometrial polyps and fibroids. The current standard of treatment is resectoscopic surgery under general or epidural anesthesia. Marketing of small-diameter operative hysteroscopes, uterine distention by liquid delivered at controlled pressure, visualization supported by videocamera, and the vaginoscopic approach rendered hysteroscopic polypectomy toward a one-stop diagnostic and therapeutic step, safely and effectively accomplished in an office setting (Bettocchi et al. 2002; Garuti et al. 2004; Sesti et al. 2000).

2.5.7 Diagnosis

Transvaginal ultrasound, saline infusion sonography, diagnostic hysteroscopy.

Transvagial ultrasound

2.5.8 Discussion

Mechanical or electrosurgical outpatient polypectomy is equally safe and effective and does not differ in terms of operating time or induced pelvic discomfort (Garuti et al. 2008). Bipolar electrodes appear to have a safer profile compared with monopolar electrodes because of the unchanged serum sodium (Berg et al. 2009). Small versus big loops. A smaller loop will cut more superficially and remove a smaller amount of tissue. Subsequently, it may be necessary to resect twice at the same level to remove the basal layer, and this may increase operating time (Berg et al. 2009).

The differences between the various systems for the resection of fibroids need further evaluation (efficacy, speed, safety), although the learning curve seems to be shorter for mechanical myomectomy (van Dongen et al. 2008) and therefore this technique might be more appropriate for less experienced physicians.

2.5.9 Instruments for Hysteroscopic Endometrial Ablation

1. 9 mm (Perez-Medina et al. 2002)/26Fr (Gupta et al. 2006) resectoscope (Karl Storz GmbH & Co., Tuttlingen, Germany) equipped with a 4 mm cutting loop.

   Distension medium: Glycine 1.5 % for monopolar or saline for bipolar surgery
2. Rollerball electrodes, available in 2.5 and 5 mm (Chang et al. 2009).

   Distension medium: Glycine 1.5 %
3. Weck-Baggish hysteroscope (Weck; ER Squibb and Sons, New York, NY)

   Equipped with a Neodynium:Yttrium-Aluminium Garnet (Nd-YAG)

   (Surgical Laser Technology, Malvern, PA) (Garry et al. 1995; Shankar et al. 2003).

   Distension medium: saline

2.5.10 Background

There are two techniques of endometrial resection/ablation: hysteroscopic guided or first-generation endometrial ablation and nonhysteroscopic second-generation endometrial ablation. The first-generation endometrial ablation techniques are considered the gold standard for endometrial ablation, these techniques include transcervical endometrial resection by resectoscope, rollerball electrocoagulation and laser ablation (Papadopoulos and Magos 2007). Second-generation endometrial techniques include thermal balloon ablation, microwave endometrial ablation, hydrotherm ablation, electrode ablation, and cryoablation (Overton et al. 1997). In experienced hands, a significant difference in efficacy between first and second-generation ablation techniques for the treatment of heavy menstrual bleeding has not been found. Second-generation techniques however are less operator-dependent, easier and appear to have a lower complication rate (van Dongen et al. 2008).

2.5.11 Description of the First-Generation Techniques

2.5.11.1 Loop Endometrial Resection

Bipolar continuous flow resectoscopes provide an effective resection of the endometrium and underlying superficial myometrium. This technique can still be used when the endometrium is not pharmacologically or mechanically prepared (Papadopoulos and Magos 2007).

2.5.11.2 Laser Ablation

The Nd-YAG laser is a fiber laser with a tissue penetration of 5–6 mm. This renders him very suitable for intrauterine surgery. The power settings for the laser generator are usually between 40 and 80 W giving a power density of 4,000–6,000 W/cm^2 (Baggish and Sze 1996).

Two techniques are used for laser ablation. The first technique is described by Goldrath and is known as the dragging technique. Tissue vaporization is created by keeping the laser fiber in contact with the endometrium (Goldrath et al. 1981). The second technique is known as the blanching technique and involves no contact of the laser fiber with the endometrium. There is no consensus as to which technique is superior, but most important is to keep the distal tip of the laser fiber always in view and to move it rapidly enough to avoid excessive coagulation and resultant thermal necrosis of the full thickness of the uterine wall or extrauterine structures (Papadopoulos and Magos 2007).

2.5.11.3 Rollerball Endometrial Ablation

The rollerball electrocoagulates the endometrium to a depth of just under 4 mm (Duffy et al. 1992). The mainly used cutting current is 120 W at a setting of blend 1. To ensure deep enough tissue destruction, the rollerball should be moved slowly over the endometrium. The optimum speed is reached when a white halo of desiccated tissue appears in front of the rollerball. If you move too fast, the endometrium will not turn white. Conversely, too slow increases the risk for uterine perforation. Keep the rollerball clean, as debris adherent to it will act as an insulator resulting in suboptimal outcome (Papadopoulos and Magos 2007).

2.5.11.4 Vaporization Systems

A similar effect as described under rollerball endometrial ablation is reached by vaporization techniques, which produce tissue destruction through vaporization rather than by desiccation:

- 0° Vaporization Electrode (Versapoint generator, Johnson & Johnson Gynecare)
- "Mushroom" bipolar vaporizing electrode (TCRis generator Olympus).

Both systems have the advantage of increased safety through bipolar electrosurgery with saline as distension medium (see Uterine septum).

2.5.11.5 Combined Cutting Loop Resection and Rollerball Ablation

Various authors use a combination of a cutting loop and a rollerball for endometrial ablation. The rollerball is used at the fundus and cornual or angular areas and the loop at the walls of the uterus (Cooper et al. 1999; Litta et al. 2006; Perino et al. 2004; Rosati et al. 2008).

2.5.12 Diagnosis

Transvaginal ultrasound, office hysteroscopy, and endometrial biopsy (Gupta et al. 2006; Litta et al. 2006; Perino et al. 2004; Rosati et al. 2008).

2.5.13 Discussion

Studies showed no significant difference in menstrual improvement and patient satisfaction for the three different first-generation techniques (Papadopoulos and Magos 2007). Loop resection provides tissue for histology and is suitable even when endometrium is thick, but requires the most skill and therefore bares the greatest risk of uterine perforation. The rollerball is easier to learn and faster than the laser, but it provides no tissue for histology and fails to treat submucous fibroids. The laser can vaporize small fibroids and polyps, but is the most expensive and slowest of all three techniques (Papadopoulos and Magos 2007). Therefore, the choice of technique should depend on the operator's preference.

Although glycine 1.5 % has been used traditionally for resectoscopic procedures, alternative-irrigating solutions should now be actively sought. Moreover, the data available motivate cautious monitoring of the inflow pressure applied and the fluid absorption during transcervical resectoscopic surgery.

New hysteroscopes and resectoscopes with continuous flow designs have greatly facilitated diagnostic and therapeutic hysteroscopy. Saline is the ideal distending medium for hysteroscopic procedures in which mechanical or bipolar instruments are used; Regardless of the medium chosen, careful fluid monitoring is essential.

References

Agdi M, Tulandi T (2009) Outpatient hysteroscopy with combined local intracervical and intrauterine anesthesia. Gynecol Obstet Invest 69:30–32

Al-Inany H (2001) Intrauterine adhesions. An update. Acta Obstet Gynecol Scand 80:986–993

Baggish MS, Sze EH (1996) Endometrial ablation: a series of 568 patients treated over an 11-year period. Am J Obstet Gynecol 174:908–913

Berg A, Sandvik L, Langebrekke A, Istre O (2009) A randomized trial comparing monopolar electrodes using glycine 1.5 % with two different types of bipolar electrodes (TCRis, Versapoint) using saline, in hysteroscopic surgery. Fertil Steril 91:1273–1278

Bettocchi S, Ceci O, Di VR, Pansini MV, Pellegrino A, Marello F, Nappi L (2002) Advanced operative office hysteroscopy without anaesthesia: analysis of 501 cases treated with a 5 Fr. bipolar electrode. Hum Reprod 17:2435–2438

Bettocchi S, Nappi L, Ceci O, Selvaggi L (2003) What does 'diagnostic hysteroscopy' mean today? The role of the new techniques. Curr Opin Obstet Gynecol 15:303–308

Cararach M, Penella J, Ubeda A, Labastida R (1994) Hysteroscopic incision of the septate uterus: scissors versus resectoscope. Hum Reprod 9:87–89

Chang PT, Vilos GA, Abu-Rafea B, Hollett-Caines J, Abyaneh ZN, Edris F (2009) Comparison of clinical outcomes with low-voltage (cut) versus high-voltage (coag) waveforms during hysteroscopic endometrial ablation with the rollerball: a pilot study. J Minim Invasive Gynecol 16:350–353

Chervenak FA, Neuwirth RS (1981) Hysteroscopic resection of the uterine septum. Am J Obstet Gynecol 141:351–353

Colacurci N, De FP, Fornaro F, Fortunato N, Perino A (2002) The significance of hysteroscopic treatment of congenital uterine malformations. Reprod Biomed Online 4(Suppl 3):52–54

Colacurci N, De FP, Mollo A, Litta P, Perino A, Cobellis L, De PG (2007) Small-diameter hysteroscopy with Versapoint versus resectoscopy with a unipolar knife for the treatment of septate uterus: a prospective randomized study. J Minim Invasive Gynecol 14:622–627

Cooper KG, Bain C, Parkin DE (1999) Comparison of microwave endometrial ablation and transcervical resection of the endometrium for treatment of heavy menstrual loss: a randomised trial. Lancet 354: 1859–1863

Decherney A, Polan ML (1983) Hysteroscopic management of intrauterine lesions and intractable uterine bleeding. Obstet Gynecol 61:392–397

Duffy S, Reid PC, Sharp F (1992) In-vivo studies of uterine electrosurgery. Br J Obstet Gynaecol 99:579–582

Fraser IS (1993) Personal techniques and results for outpatient diagnostic hysteroscopy. Gynecol Endosc 2:29–33

Garry R, Shelley-Jones D, Mooney P, Phillips G (1995) Six hundred endometrial laser ablations. Obstet Gynecol 85:24–29

Garuti G, Luerti M (2009) Hysteroscopic bipolar surgery: a valuable progress or a technique under investigation? Curr Opin Obstet Gynecol 21:329–334

Garuti G, Cellani F, Colonnelli M, Grossi F, Luerti M (2004) Outpatient hysteroscopic polypectomy in 237 patients: feasibility of a one-stop "see-and-treat" procedure. J Am Assoc Gynecol Laparosc 11:500–504

Garuti G, Centinaio G, Luerti M (2008) Outpatient hysteroscopic polypectomy in postmenopausal women: a comparison between mechanical and electrosurgical resection. J Minim Invasive Gynecol 15:595–600

Glasser MH (2009) Practical tips for office hysteroscopy and second-generation "global" endometrial ablation. J Minim Invasive Gynecol 16:384–399

Goldrath MH, Fuller TA, Segal S (1981) Laser photovaporization of endometrium for the treatment of menorrhagia. Am J Obstet Gynecol 140:14–19

Gupta B, Mittal S, Misra R, Deka D, Dadhwal V (2006) Levonorgestrel-releasing intrauterine system vs. transcervical endometrial resection for dysfunctional uterine bleeding. Int J Gynaecol Obstet 95:261–266

Istre O, Bjoennes J, Naess R, Hornbaek K, Forman A (1994) Postoperative cerebral oedema after transcervical endometrial resection and uterine irrigation with 1.5 % glycine. Lancet 344:1187–1189

Kowalik CR, Mol BW, Veersema S, Goddijn M (2010). Critical appraisal regarding the effect on reproductive outcome of hysteroscopic metroplasty in patients with recurrent miscarriage. Arch Gynecol Obstet 282(4):465

Kowalik CR, Goddijn M, Emanuel MH, Bongers MY, Spinder T, de Kruif JH, Mol BW, Heineman MJ (2011). Metroplasty versus expectant management for women with recurrent miscarriage and a septate uterus. Cochrane Database Syst Rev 6:CD008576. Review

Litta P, Bonora M, Pozzan C, Merlin F, Sacco G, Fracas M, Capobianco G, Dessole S (2003) Carbon dioxide versus normal saline in outpatient hysteroscopy. Hum Reprod 18:2446–2449

Litta P, Merlin F, Pozzan C, Nardelli GB, Capobianco G, Dessole S, Ambrosini A (2006) Transcervical endometrial resection in women with menorrhagia: long-term follow-up. Eur J Obstet Gynecol Reprod Biol 125:99–102

Loffer FD (2000) Preliminary experience with the VersaPoint bipolar resectoscope using a vaporizing electrode in a saline distending medium. J Am Assoc Gynecol Laparosc 7:498–502

Mencaglia L, Lugo E, Consigli S, Barbosa C (2009) Bipolar resectoscope: the future perspective of hysteroscopic surgery. Gynecol Surg 6:15–20. http://link.springer.com/search?query=mencaglia&search-within=Journal&facet-journal-id=10397.

Nagele F, O'Connor H, Davies A, Badawy A, Mohamed H, Magos A (1996) 2500 Outpatient diagnostic hysteroscopies. Obstet Gynecol 88:87–92

Overton C, Hargreaves J, Maresh M (1997) A national survey of the complications of endometrial destruction for menstrual disorders: the MISTLETOE study. Minimally Invasive Surgical Techniques–Laser, EndoThermal or Endoresection. Br J Obstet Gynaecol 104:1351–1359

Pabuccu R, Onalan G, Kaya C, Selam B, Ceyhan T, Ornek T, Kuzudisli E (2008) Efficiency and pregnancy outcome of serial intrauterine device-guided hysteroscopic adhesiolysis of intrauterine synechiae. Fertil Steril 90:1973–1977

Papadopoulos NP, Magos A (2007) First-generation endometrial ablation: roller-ball vs loop vs laser. Best Pract Res Clin Obstet Gynaecol 21:915–929

Pellicano M, Guida M, Zullo F, Lavitola G, Cirillo D, Nappi C (2003) Carbon dioxide versus normal saline as a uterine distension medium for diagnostic vaginoscopic hysteroscopy in infertile patients: a prospective, randomized, multicenter study. Fertil Steril 79:418–421

Perez-Medina T, Haya J, Frutos LS, Arenas JB (2002) Factors influencing long-term outcome of loop endometrial resection. J Am Assoc Gynecol Laparosc 9:272–276

Perino A, Mencaglia L, Hamou J, Cittadini E (1987) Hysteroscopy for metroplasty of uterine septa: report of 24 cases. Fertil Steril 48:321–323

Perino A, Castelli A, Cucinella G, Biondo A, Pane A, Venezia R (2004) A randomized comparison of endometrial laser intrauterine thermotherapy and hysteroscopic endometrial resection. Fertil Steril 82:731–734

Polena V, Mergui JL, Zerat L, Darai E, Barranger E, Uzan S (2005) Long-term results of hysteroscopic resection of endometrial polyps in 367 patients. Role of associated endometrial resection. Gynecol Obstet Fertil 33:382–388

Preutthipan S, Herabutya Y (2005) Hysteroscopic polypectomy in 240 premenopausal and postmenopausal women. Fertil Steril 83:705–709

Rosati M, Vigone A, Capobianco F, Surico D, Amoruso E, Surico N (2008) Long-term outcome of hysteroscopic endometrial ablation without endometrial preparation. Eur J Obstet Gynecol Reprod Biol 138:222–225

Roy KK, Baruah J, Sharma JB, Kumar S, Kachawa G, Singh N (2010) Arch Gynecol Obstet 281(2):355–61. doi:10.1007/s00404-009-1117-x. Epub 2009 May 20.

Savelli L, De IP, Santini D, Rosati F, Ghi T, Pignotti E, Bovicelli L (2003) Histopathologic features and risk factors for benignity, hyperplasia, and cancer in endometrial polyps. Am J Obstet Gynecol 188:927–931

Sesti F, Marziali M, Santomarco N (2000) Hysteroscopic surgery for endometrial polyps using a bipolar microelectrode. Int J Gynaecol Obstet 71:283–284

Shankar M, Naftalin NJ, Taub N, Habiba M (2003) The long-term effectiveness of endometrial laser ablation: a survival analysis. Eur J Obstet Gynecol Reprod Biol 108:75–79

Shankar M, Davidson A, Taub N, Habiba M (2004) Randomised comparison of distension media for outpatient hysteroscopy. BJOG 111:57–62

Timmermans A, Veersema S (2005) Ambulatory transcervical resection of polyps with the Duckbill polyp snare: a modality for treatment of endometrial polyps. J Minim Invasive Gynecol 12(1):37–39

Unfried G, Wieser F, Albrecht A, Kaider A, Nagele F (2001) Flexible versus rigid endoscopes for outpatient hysteroscopy: a prospective randomized clinical trial. Hum Reprod 16:168–171

van Dongen H, Emanuel MH, Wolterbeek R, Trimbos JB, Jansen FW (2008) Hysteroscopic morcellator for removal of intrauterine polyps and myomas: a randomized controlled pilot study among residents in training. J Minim Invasive Gynecol 15(4):466–471, Epub 18 Apr 2008. PMID: 18588849 [PubMed – indexed for MEDLINE]

Van DH, Janssen CA, Smeets MJ, Emanuel MH, Jansen FW (2009) The clinical relevance of hysteroscopic polypectomy in premenopausal women with abnormal uterine bleeding. BJOG 116:1387–1390

Wieser F, Kurz C, Wenzl R, Albrecht A, Huber JC, Nagele F (1998) Atraumatic cervical passage at outpatient hysteroscopy. Fertil Steril 69:549–551

Yu D, Wong YM, Cheong Y, Xia E, Li TC (2008) Asherman syndrome–one century later. Fertil Steril 89:759–779

Olav Istre and Thomas Tiede Vellinga

Contents

O. Istre, MD, PhD, DMSc (✉)
Head of Gynecology Aleris-Hamlet Hospital,
Scandinavia Professor in Minimal Invasive
Gynecology University of Southern Denmark,
Fredriksberg, Denmark
e-mail: oistre@gmail.com

T.T. Vellinga, MD
Surgical Department, Leiden University,
Leiden, The Netherlands
e-mail: thomas.vellinga@hotmail.com

3.1 Introduction

Uterine anomalies result from a defect in the development or fusion of the paired Mullerian ducts during embryogenesis and are the most common types of malformations of the female reproductive system. The septate uterus is the most common structural uterine anomaly and results from failure of the partition between the two fused Mullerian ducts to resorb (Taylor and Gomel 2008). Congenital malformations may be associated with recurrent pregnancy loss, preterm labor, abnormal fetal presentation, and infertility (Heinonen et al. 1982). The overall frequency of uterine malformations was 4.0 % (Raga et al. 1997). Infertile patients (6.3 %) had a significantly ($P<.05$) higher incidence of Mullerian anomalies, in comparison with fertile patients (3.8 %). Septate (33.6 %) and arcuate (32.8 %) uteri were the most common malformations observed (Raga et al. 1997). The septate uterus is associated with the highest incidence of reproductive failure among the Mullerian anomalies (Fedele et al. 1993). Thirty-eight percent to 79 % of pregnancies in women with septate uteri ended in miscarriage (Raga et al. 1997; Homer et al. 2000). Such outcomes are thought to be a result of poor blood supply, rendering the septum inhospitable to the implanting embryo (Fedele et al. 1996). Diagnosis is established with hysterosalpingography, magnetic resonance imaging, and ultrasound. The diagnostic accuracy of hysterosalpingography in patients with septate

O. Istre (ed.), *Minimally Invasive Gynecological Surgery*,
DOI 10.1007/978-3-662-44059-9_3, © Springer-Verlag Berlin Heidelberg 2015

uteri has been reported to be between 20 and 60 % (Braun et al. 2005; Pellerito et al. 1992). Transvaginal ultrasonography is more accurate, with a sensitivity of 100 % and a specificity of 80 % in the diagnosis of the septate uterus (Pellerito et al. 1992). Three-dimensional sonography (3DULS) is associated with an even higher diagnostic accuracy of 92 % (Wu et al. 1997) and hysterosonography, with a 100 % diagnostic accuracy in the largest series published to date

(Alborzi et al. 2002). The benefit of 3DULS is the view of the uterus in the coronal plane, which allows the operator to distinguish between arcuate, septate, and bicornuate uteri, thereby eliminating the need for simultaneous laparoscopy (Figs. 3.1 and 3.2). In this review we describe the diversity of clinical presentations, management strategies, and report the obstetric outcomes observed in our series of 114 women with uterine septa.

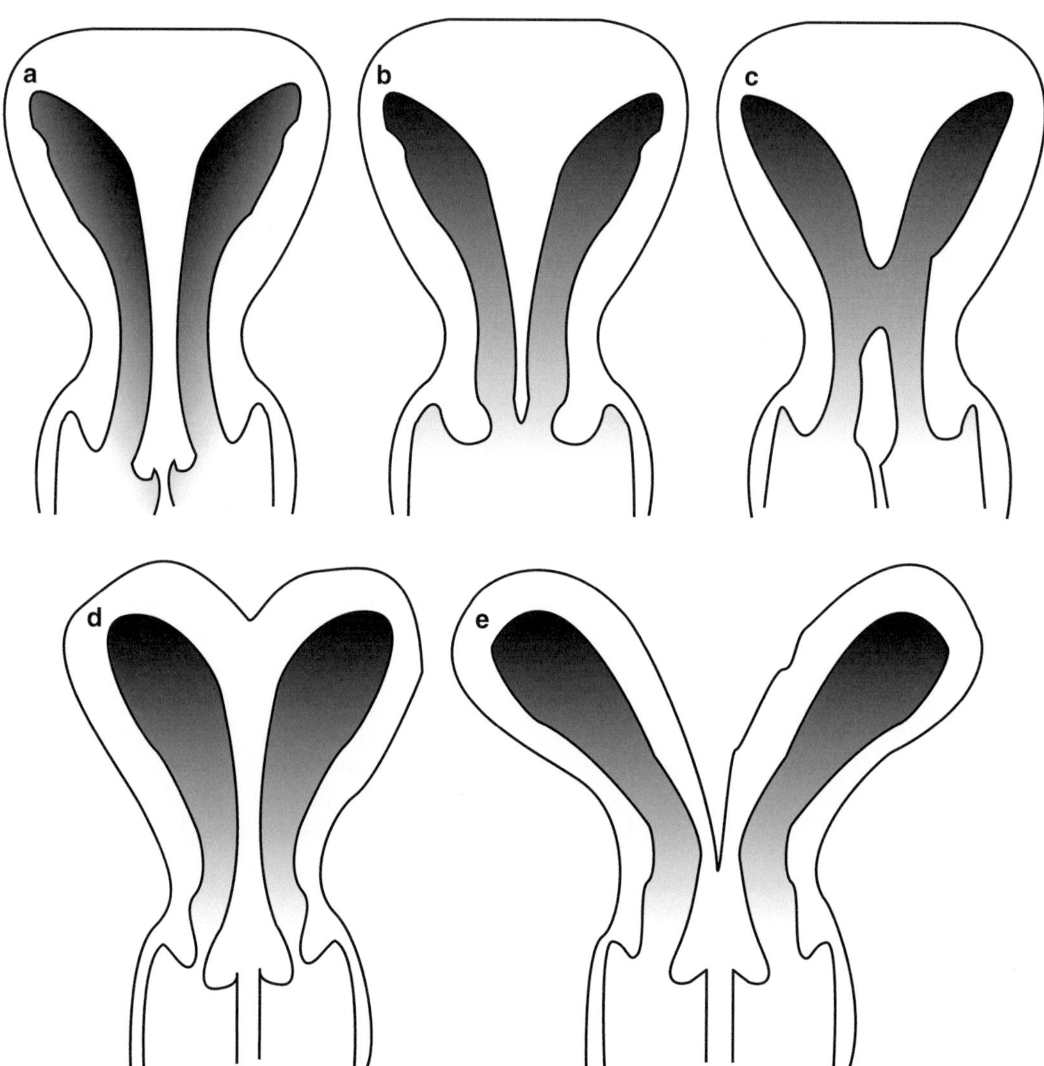

Fig. 3.1 Different types of uterine malformations. (**a**) Uterus septus cervix duplex vagina septa. (**b**) Uterus septus cervix septa. (**c**) Uterus communicans septus cervix septa vagina septa. (**d**) Uterus bicornis duplex vagina septa. (**e**) Uterus didelphys cervix duplex vagina septa

3.2 Materials and Methods

A total of 114 women were investigated and their fertility outcome was followed for an average of 2 years. Patients with some degree of Mullerian malformation, as detected at their local gynecologist on transvaginal ultrasound or at our department during admission for any condition connected to the anomaly, were included in our study. The patients were assessed using B-mode, 3D ultrasound examinations using a Voloson 730 Expert (General Electric Healthcare, Zipf,

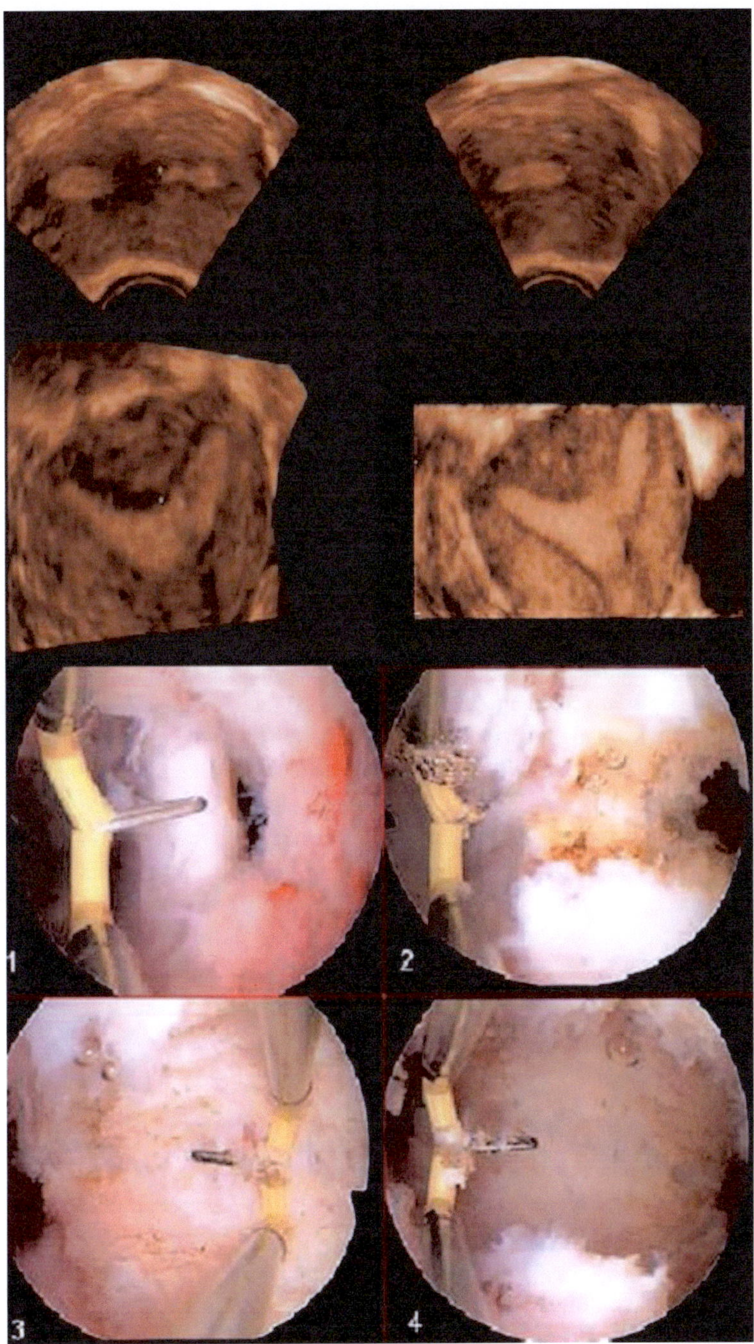

Fig. 3.2 Three-dimensional ultrasound and metroplasty of the uterine septum

Austria) with a vaginal multifrequency probe (5–9 Hertz). An initial B-Mode examination provided morphologic evaluation of the pelvic organs, including uterine size and endometrium thickness, followed by a saline infusion sonography in most of the patients with findings suggestive of a uterine septum. The operations were performed under general anesthesia using the following surgical technique for all patients. During hysteroscopy, the automatic pressure cuff (Olympus, Center Valley, PA) maintained an infusion pressure of 100 mmHg, and suction of 10–15 mmHg was applied to the outflow tube to achieve a sufficient flow. The TCRis resectoscope (Olympus), Ch. 26 model WA 22061 with 12 optic 22001A (Hamburg, Germany), using NaCl 0.9 % (Braun, Melsungen, Germany) as irrigant, with a needle of 5 mm was then used to perform the metroplasty. The needle was used with a bipolar cutting current of 280 W to incise the lower segments of the septum from side to side until the tubal ostia were visualized. The high power is needed for the ignition of the plasma only. A couple of milliseconds after the ignition, the generator automatically regulates the power down to normal values around 100 W. The septum excision was stopped approximately 10 mm from the line between the two ostia. In six patients, a total uterine septum was identified. In these cases, the incision was made horizontally toward the other obliterated cavity, starting just after the internal ostium. In cases with a double cervix the same procedure was performed leaving the cervices intact (Fig. 3.1). The received information was entered in statistical software (SPSS, version 14, SPSS 22 Inc., Chicago, IL). Patient characteristics of the study groups were analyzed with one way analysis of variance in case of normally distributed continuous variables, and Pearson's chi-square test in case of dichotomous data. Confidence intervals for difference in means were calculated. Pearson's chi-square was also used to analyze differences of preference among the study groups. A paired-samples t test was used to compare expected visual analog scale scores for both investigations. All tests were two-sided and P values $< .05$.

3.3 Results

One hundred fourteen women underwent hysteroscopic examination in case of larger than 1/4 of the uterine size septum a resection was performed, with a mean age of 31 (19–42 years). Eight small septum was found to be small and not in need of resection. Uterine septa were found as part of the workup for the following events: infertility workup (33.3 %), first trimester miscarriage (22.8 %), three or more miscarriages (22.8 %), Cesarean section (11.4 %), premature delivery (7.9 %), normal delivery (1.8 %) (Table 3.1). We evaluated the septum size in the 114 women. Ten (8.8 %) had a septum consisting one-quarter of their uterus, 18 (15.8 %) a septum one-half of their uterus, and 86 (75.4 %) a septum larger than one-half of their uterus. Six women had a total septum and were included in the septum larger than one-half of their uterus group. The different diagnostic events leading to diagnosis of the uterine septum per septum size is presented in Table 3.2. The uterine septum was successfully resected in all 106 women. No intra- or postoperative complications were noted. One hundred and three out of 114 women desired a future pregnancy. Seventy-two (69.9 %) of these women achieved a successful pregnancy after metroplasty, with 63 (87.5 %) subsequent term deliveries, and 9 (12.5 %) premature deliveries. Twenty-two (30.6 %) of the 72 women who had live births delivered by Cesarean section. Twenty-four (23.3 %) women who desired future fertility did not become pregnant, and 7 (6.8 %) had a spontaneous miscarriage. Eleven women were not interested in future fertility; however, they opted for surgery at time of diagnosis. In examining the outcomes in women divided up by group of septum diagnosis, we found the following rates of live birth following metroplasty: infertility workup (56.3 %), miscarriage (77.6 %), normal/premature delivery (80 %), and Cesarean section (66.7 %) (Table 3.1). We found different pregnancy outcomes after metroplasty of the various septum sizes as is presented in Table 3.2. To compare the pregnancy outcome after metroplasty of a different septum size the material was divided in two groups: one group with a septum size of

Table 3.1 Pregnancy outcome after metroplasty

Diagnosis following	Infertility workup	Miscarriage[a]	Normal/premature delivery	C-section	Total group
Pregnancy outcome:	38 (33.3 %)	52 (45.6 %)	11 (9.7 %)	13 (11.4 %)	114
Live birth	18 (56.3 %) (3 premature)	38 (77.6 %) (4 premature)	8 (80 %) (1 premature)	8 (66.7 %) (1 premature)	72 (69.9 %)
Miscarriage	3	4	–	–	7 (6.8 %)
No pregnancy	11	7	2	4	24 (23.3 %)
Desired fertility	32	49	10	12	103 (100 %)
Undesired fertility	6[b]	3	1	1	11

[a]Twenty-six women were diagnosed following a first miscarriage and 26 following three or more miscarriage
[b]No desired fertility at that time, but opted for surgery

Table 3.2 Event leading to diagnosis and pregnancy outcome after metroplasty for different septumw sizes, $n = 114$

	Septum size ¼	Septum size ½	Septum size >½
Diagnostic event:	10 (8.8 % of n)	18 (15.8 % of n)	86 (75.4 % of n)
Infertility workup	4 (40 %)	7 (39 %)	27 (31 %)
First trimester miscarriage	4 (40 %)	4 (22 %)	18 (21 %)
Premature delivery	–	2 (11 %)	7 (8 %)
Normal delivery	–	1 (6 %)	1 (1 %)
Three or more miscarriage	1 (10 %)	3 (17 %)	22 (26 %)
C-section	1 (10 %)	1 (6 %)	11 (13 %)
Pregnancy outcome after metroplasty:			
No pregnancy	7 (70 %[a])	6 (40 %[a])	11 (14.1 %[a])
Live birth	3 (30 %[a])	5 (33.3 %[a])	64 (82 %[a])
Miscarriage	–	4 (26.7 %[a])	3 (3.8 %[a])
Desired fertility	10 (100 %)	15 (100 %) (3 had no desire)	78 (100 %) (8 had no desire)

[a]The percentages are derived from the 100 % value of desired fertility

one-quarter or one-half and one other group with a septum size larger than one-half of their uterus. The pregnancy outcome of a septum size one-quarter or one-half is significantly different from the pregnancy outcome after metroplasty of septum larger than one-half of the uterus (chi-square: $P < .001$). There were only four women in our study with the combination of a septum consisting one-quarter of their uterus and the diagnosis following a first trimester miscarriage. After metroplasty none of these women became pregnant, although all four had desired fertility. ANOVA linear regression showed no significant difference of age in the different events leading to diagnosis ($P¼.708$) and no significant difference in age and pregnancy outcome ($P¼.160$).

3.4 Discussion

In our study we performed hysteroscopic metroplasty solely based on ULS findings. No patients underwent laparoscopy. No intra or postoperative complications occurred. Based on our experience in this study we believe metroplasty of the uterine septum can be safely performed as an office procedure. This corresponds to the study of Ghi et al. (2009), demonstrating ULS and 3DULS to be extremely accurate (positive predictive value 96.3 % and negative predictive value 100 %) for the diagnosis and classification of congenital uterine anomalies. They suggest women diagnosed with malformations amenable to treatment with a resectoscope may avoid a diagnostic pelviscopy by using operative hysteroscopy with the addition of 3DULS. In the present study we used this strategy of diagnosis and management as 3DULS was followed by operative hysteroscopy. Our findings indicated an excellent prognosis for successful pregnancy after metroplasty of the uterine septum. Seventy-two women (69.9 %) delivered a healthy baby. This was consistent with previous studies. Homer et al. (2000) found in their review a live birth rate of 64 % in a total of 658 patients. In our study the live birth rate was different per diagnostic event. We found a lower live birth rate after metroplasty when the septum was diagnosed during infertility workup (56.3 %), thus indicating multiple factors were contributing to the patient's infertility. In approximately 40 % of these patients other factors (e.g., male factor, tubal factors) were found during infertility workup. The lower live birth rate with unexplained infertility and a uterine septum is seen in other studies as well: Homer et al. (2000) found a crude pregnancy rate of 48 %, Pabuccu and Gomel (2004) found a live birth rate of 29.5 %, and Mollo et al. (2009) a live birth rate of 34.1 %. The overall live birth rate of 64 % observed by Homer et al. and our live birth rates with the other diagnostic events. This suggests again that when the uterine septum is diagnosed during infertility workup, there are coexisting factors such as genetic, infective, endocrine, immune, or thrombophilic factors that play a role in their infertility (Rai and Regan 2006). Therefore, in the past, removal of the uterine septum in these cases was subject to debate. The lower live birth rate after metroplasty makes it questionable to perform correction of the uterine septum, as these patients may benefit from concentrating on other infertility treatments. However, in certain cases, prophylactic resection of the uterine septum continues to be recommended: women with long-standing (>6 months) unexplained infertility in whom an extensive workup has ruled out other factors, women above 35 years of age, women undergoing laparoscopy and hysteroscopy for other reasons (septal incision at the same time is opportune and appears logical), and

women pursuing assisted reproductive technologies (Homer et al. 2000). Mollo et al. (2009) have recently addressed this question. They concluded metroplasty in women with unexplained infertility and a uterine septum improved their live birth rate compared with women with unexplained infertility and no septate uterus. The live birth rate was 34.1 % after metroplasty in the septate uterus group compared with 18.9 % when there was no uterine septum present (chi-square: $P<.05$). We found women with prior miscarriages leading to diagnosis of a uterine septum had the highest live birth rate after metroplasty. Previous studies also reported a significant improvement after metroplasty in this group. Homer et al. (2000) found the overall miscarriage rate dropped from 88 to 5.9 % after hysteroscopic metroplasty. In our study, four women had a septum size of one-quarter of their uterus diagnosed after a first trimester miscarriage; despite desired fertility, none of these four women achieved a live birth following metroplasty. Further studies with larger numbers are required to evaluate the need of metroplasty in this group of women. The highest rate of live births after metroplasty in our study was in the group of women with the largest septum (larger than one-half of the uterus). In this group, 82 % had a live birth compared with 33.2 and 30 % when the septum is one-half or one-quarter of their uterus, respectively (chi-square: $P<.05$). If a septum extends over more than one-half of the uterine cavity we strongly recommend metroplasty. There is no reason to wait for these women to prove bad obstetric outcome before surgical management. Outpatient hysteroscopic metroplasty of the uterine septum is a minor procedure with rare complications. In conclusion, our data demonstrate three-dimensional ultrasound followed by hysteroscopic metroplasty of uterine septa to be a safe and effective office procedure. Women with a septum more than one-half of their uterus have a very high chance of developing a successful pregnancy after metroplasty. Women with miscarriages leading to diagnosis of a uterine septum have the highest live birth rate after metroplasty.

References

Alborzi S, Dehbashi S, Parsanezhad ME (2002) Differential diagnosis of septate and bicornuate uterus by sonohysterography eliminates the need for laparoscopy. Fertil Steril 78:176–178

Braun P, Grau FV, Pons RM, Enguix DP (2005) Is hysterosalpingography able to diagnose all uterine malformations correctly? A retrospective study. Eur J Radiol 53:274–279

Fedele L, Arcaini L, Parazzini F, Vercellini P, Di NG (1993) Reproductive prognosis after hysteroscopic metroplasty in 102 women: life-table analysis. Fertil Steril 59:768–772

Fedele L, Bianchi S, Agnoli B, Tozzi L, Vignali M (1996) Urinary tract anomalies associated with unicornuate uterus. J Urol 155:847–848

Ghi T, Casadio P, Kuleva M, Perrone AM, Savelli L, Giunchi S et al (2009) Accuracy of three-dimensional ultrasound in diagnosis and classification of congenital uterine anomalies. Fertil Steril 92: 808–813

Heinonen PK, Saarikoski S, Pystynen P (1982) Reproductive performance of women with uterine anomalies. An evaluation of 182 cases. Acta Obstet Gynecol Scand 61:157–162

Homer HA, Li TC, Cooke ID (2000) The septate uterus: a review of management and reproductive outcome. Fertil Steril 73:1–14

Mollo A, De FP, Colacurci N, Cobellis L, Perino A, Venezia R et al (2009) Hysteroscopic resection of the septum improves the pregnancy rate of women with unexplained infertility: a prospective controlled trial. Fertil Steril 91:2628–2631

Pabuccu R, Gomel V (2004) Reproductive outcome after hysteroscopic metroplasty in women with septate uterus and otherwise unexplained infertility. Fertil Steril 81:1675–1678

Pellerito JS, McCarthy SM, Doyle MB, Glickman MG, DeCherney AH (1992) Diagnosis of uterine anomalies: relative accuracy of MR imaging, endovaginal sonography, and hysterosalpingography. Radiology 183:795–800

Raga F, Bauset C, Remohi J, Bonilla-Musoles F, Simon C, Pellicer A (1997) Reproductive impact of congenital Mullerian anomalies. Hum Reprod 12:2277–2281

Rai R, Regan L (2006) Recurrent miscarriage. Lancet 368:601–611, Fertility and Sterility

Taylor E, Gomel V (2008) The uterus and fertility. Fertil Steril 89:1–16

Wu MH, Hsu CC, Huang KE (1997) Detection of congenital Mullerian duct anomalies using three-dimensional ultrasound. J Clin Ultrasound 25:487–492

Asherman Syndrome

4

Line Engelbrechtsen and Olav Istre

Contents

L. Engelbrechtsen, MD
Department of Gynecology and Obstetrics,
Rigshospitalet, Denmark
e-mail: line@sund.ku.dk

O. Istre, MD, PhD, DMSc (✉)
Head of Gynecology Aleris-Hamlet Hospital,
Scandinavia Professor in Minimal Invasive Gynecology,
University of Southern Denmark,
Fredriksberg, Denmark
e-mail: oistre@gmail.com

Asherman syndrome (AS) was first reported in 1894 by Heinrich Fritz, however it was not until 1948 that Joseph Asherman described the syndrome, frequency, and etiology based on a series of cases of intrauterine adhesions following curettage of a gravid uterus in 29 women with secondary amenorrhea (Asherman 1948; 1950).

4.1 Definition

Asherman syndrome is also known as uterine atresia, amenorrhea traumatica, endometrial sclerosis, and intrauterine adhesions or synechiae (Asherman 1950). AS arises due to trauma of the endometrium and produces partial or complete obliteration of the uterine cavity and/or cervical canal due to intrauterine adhesions (Asherman 1948; March 2011; Schenker and Margalioth 1982). Intrauterine adhesions are composed of fibrotic tissue and the extent of fibrosis can range from mild and superficial fibrosis in a small area of the uterine cavity to a severe fibrosis of a large area, extending deep into the myometrium and causing adhesion of the opposing surfaces in the uterine cavity. Fibrosis in the cervical canal can cause amenorrhea and retrograde menstruation.

AS can occur due to uterine and intrauterine surgery such as cesarean section, curettage, myomectomy involving the uterine cavity, endometrial ablation, and hysteroscopic removal of fibroids and polyps (Asherman 1950; March 1995, 2011; Yu et al. 2008a). However, intrauterine adhesions are also seen as a consequence of endometritis, congenital uterine abnormalities, and genetic predisposition. It is well known that the endometrium is more susceptible to trauma in a gravid uterus and the incidence of intrauterine adhesions following curettage for retained tissue is reported up to 40 % 3 months after curettage (Westendorp et al. 1998).

4.2   Symptoms

Trauma of the uterine cavity results in dysfunction of the endometrium which presents in conditions such as menstrual abnormalities (secondary amenorrhea and hypomenorrhea), dysmenorrhea, infertility, and recurrent pregnancy loss (March 2011). Symptoms have a broad clinical spectrum from asymptomatic in cases with mild adhesions to complain of severe pelvic pain and secondary amenorrhea in cases with retrograde menstruations due to fibrosis in the cervical canal.

In women with infertility or recurrent pregnancy loss, treatment is required for optimal conception possibilities. AS is furthermore, a cause of abnormal placentation in subsequent pregnancies due to defects in the decidua basalis (Nitabuchs layer) which in a gravid uterus can give rise to placenta previa and placenta accreta (Yu et al. 2008a; Jauniaux and Jurkovic 2012).

4.3   Prevalence

The prevalence of AS varies from 1.55 to 20 % (Schenker and Margalioth 1982; Westendorp et al. 1998; Dmowski and Greenblatt 1969; Friedler et al. 1993) according to population, mainly due to different diagnostic criteria, the number of abortions in the population, choice of management, awareness of clinicians, and incidence of infections (genital tuberculosis and puerperal infections) (Schenker and Margalioth 1982). It is well known that the endometrium is more susceptible to trauma in a gravid uterus and the incidence of intrauterine adhesions

following curettage for retained tissue is reported up to 40 % 3 months after curettage (Westendorp et al. 1998).

4.4   Diagnosis

AS should be suspected in any woman presenting with menstrual abnormalities and/or infertility and a history of previous curettage or intrauterine surgery. Accurate diagnosis of AS is possible by imaging the uterine cavity by a number of modalities.

Hysterosalpingography (HSG) has been the most widespread tool in diagnosis of AS. HSG can reveal filling defects described as sharply outlined intrauterine structures in the uterine cavity, however in the worst cases, HSG cannot be performed due to ostial occlusion. HSG has a high false positive rate and cannot reveal endometrial fibrosis, furthermore fibroids and polyps can be mistaken for intrauterine adhesions by the appearance at HSG. HSG has a sensitivity of 75 % and a positive predictive value of 50 % (Soares et al. 2000).

Transvaginal ultrasound is easily performed and can reveal an echo dense pattern with difficult visualization of the endometrium interrupted by cyst-like areas (Yu et al. 2008a). The diagnostic accuracy of ultrasound, however, allows visualization of the uterine cavity in cases where HSG and hysteroscopy cannot be performed due to obstruction of the cervix (Soares et al. 2000).

3D ultrasound and intrauterine saline infusion (3D-SHG) is another diagnostic tool for diagnosis of AS. 3D-SHG combined with 3D power Doppler has a sensitivity of 91.1 % and specificity of 98.5 % for detection of all kinds of intrauterine adhesions (Makris et al. 2007).

Magnetic resonance imaging (MRI) can be helpful as a supplementary diagnostic tool, especially when the adhesions involve the endocervix (Bacelar et al. 1995).

Despite the abovementioned diagnostic tools, hysteroscopy remains the golden standard in the assessment and diagnosis of AS. Hysteroscopy venables direct vision of the extent of lesions and adhesions and provides thorough planning of removal of adhesions by the surgeon (Figs. 4.1 and 4.2).

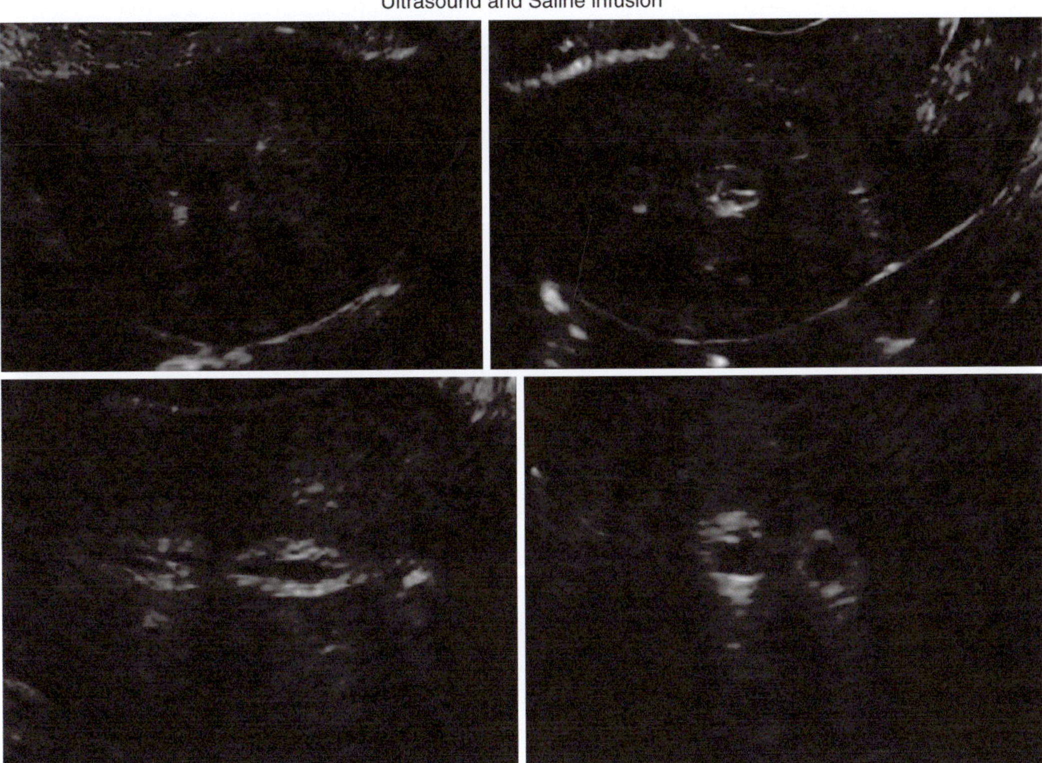

Fig. 4.1 Ultrasound and saline infusion revealing filling defects in a patient with AS

4.5 Classification

Since the description of AS was made in 1948, several attempts have been made to classify the extent of adhesions and lesions in patients with AS.

To date, several classification schemes are available for classification of the extent of Asherman disease. One of the most widely used is developed on behalf of the American Fertility Society and provides a classification of AS based on extent of the disease, menstrual pattern, and the morphological feature of the adhesions. Both hysteroscopy and HSG could be used for this kind of scoring system (Table 4.1).

More recently, a classification scheme published in 2000 by Nasr et al. illustrated an innovative way to classify AS (Table 4.2). This scoring system includes not only the menstrual symptoms but also the obstetric history of the woman (Nasr et al. 2000). According to this group, clinical history plays a more important role than the extent of the adhesions. The classification scheme provides good correlation in women with mild or severe disease, but not in those with moderate adhesions.

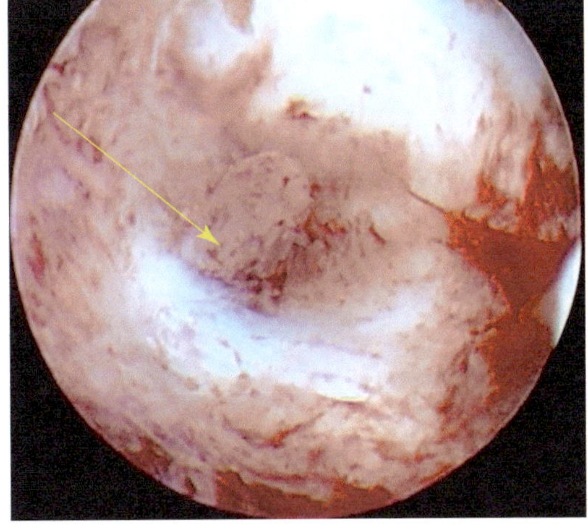

Fig. 4.2 Dense adhesion in the inner cervical area

Table 4.1 The American Fertility Society classification system for intrauterine adhesions

Classification		Score
Extent of cavity involved	<1/3	1
	1/3–2/3	2
	>2/3	4
Type of adhesion	Filmy	1
	Filmy and dense	2
	Dense	4
Menstrual pattern	Normal	0
	Hypomenorrhea	2
	Amenorrhea	4
Prognostic classification	Stage 1 (Mild): 1–4	
	Stage 2 (Moderate): 5–8	
	Stage 3 (Severe): 9–12	

Table 4.2 Clinico-hysteroscopic classification system for intrauterine adhesions

Hysteroscopic findings		Score
Isthmic fibrosis		2
Filmy adhesions	>50 % of the cavity	1
	<50 % of the cavity	2
Dense adhesions	Single band	2
	Multiple bands	4
Tubal ostium	Both visualized	0
	One visualized	2
	None visualized	4
Tubular cavity	Sound less than 6	10
Menstrual pattern		
	Normal	0
	Hypomenorrhea	4
	Amenorrhea	8
Reproductive performance		
	Good obstetric history	0
	Recurrent pregnancy loss	2
	Infertility	4
Stages	Mild	0–4
	Moderate	5–10
	Severe	11–22

4.6 Management

Treatment of AS should only be considered when there are signs or symptoms of pain, menstrual abnormalities, infertility, or recurrent pregnancy loss. The primary goal of intervention is to restore the volume and shape of the uterine cavity; to facilitate communication between fallopian tubes, uterine cavity, and cervical canal; and to restore reproductive function.

The management strategy of AS is based on four steps:

1. Surgical procedures
2. Prevention of the formation of re-adhesions
3. Restoring a normal endometrium
4. Postoperative assessment

4.6.1 Surgical Procedures

4.6.1.1 Hysteroscopic Adhesiolysis

Removal of adhesions can be performed by hysteroscopic adhesiolysis which is the current treatment of choice for AS (Pabuccu et al. 1997; Roy et al. 2010; Yu et al. 2008b). During hysteroscopy adhesions can be classified and adhesiolysis can be performed under direct vision. The procedure is minimally invasive. Adhesiolysis can be performed with the touch of the endoscope in cases of thin filmy adhesions or with the help of hysteroscopic scissors or cutting modalities as laser and diathermy in case of more dense adhesions.

Hysteroscopic adhesiolysis can be technically difficult even in the hands of a trained surgeon. The procedure is associated with risk of perforation of the uterus, especially in cases on cervical fibrosis. Approximately 2.5 % undergoing adhesiolysis experience perforation of the uterus; however, in severe cases the rate is as high as 10 % (Pabuccu et al. 1997).

In cases with extensive adhesions, one approach is to start with the wire loop of the smaller resectoscope and gradually remove the scarring tissue in the cervix until you reach the cavity. On this stage the loop is replaced by the knife, cold or warm, and then it is possible to open up the cavity.

In severe cases, in has been reported that concomitant laparoscopy may help the surgeon to avoid perforations, but simultaneous laparoscopy cannot prevent perforations of the uterine wall. Yet concomitant laparoscopy enables detection of perforations immediately and the prevention of trauma to other pelvic organs (Fig. 4.3).

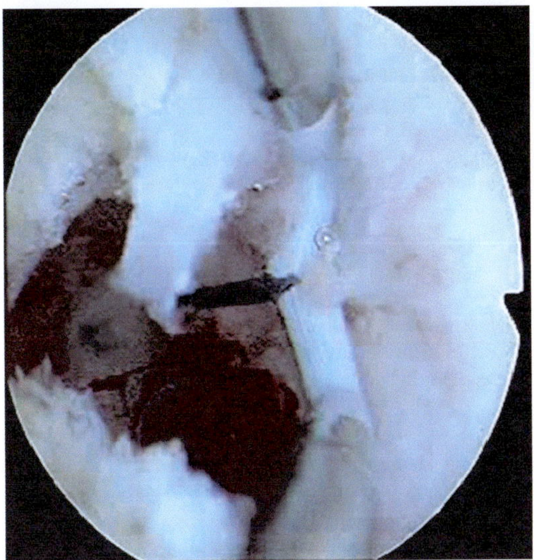

Fig. 4.3 Surgical treatment with resectoscopic needle

4.6.1.2 Myometrial Scoring Technique

Myometrial scoring technique is used in cases with dense adhesions and reduction of the size of the uterine cavity. The technique is used to restore the size of the cavity and to uncover functional endometrium by making six to eight longitudinal incisions into the myometrium, of which two to three are lateral incisions from the fundus to isthmus on both sides and two to three transverse incisions in the fundus. In the end of the procedure the cervical canal is dilated up to Hegar 12–18 in order to reduce the risk of cervical stenosis postoperatively (Protopapas et al. 1998).

4.6.2 Prevention of Reformation of Adhesions

Different techniques have been developed for the purpose of preventing reformation of adhesions following hysteroscopy.

Insertions of intrauterine devices (IUD), such as the loop IUD, have shown promising results in preventing reformation of adhesions. The loop IUD is placed in the uterus following hysteroscopy and is recommended to stay typically 1–3 months.

Intrauterine balloons have also been used to prevent adhesions, and the balloon is placed in uterus and is typically removed after 7 days. Balloons used have been Foley catheters as well as heart-shaped balloons.

Another technique for prevention of reformation of adhesions is installation of hyaluronic acid gel in the uterus following hysteroscopy. A recent study by Lin et al. compared the effect of cobber IUD, a heart-shaped balloon and hyaluronic acid in the prevention of reformation of adhesions in patients who had undergone hysteroscopic surgery for AS. The study demonstrated that treatment with balloon and IUD significantly decreases the extent of reformation of adhesions compared to the use of hyaluronic acid and no treatment following hysteroscopy. No difference in the extent of adhesions was found between patients who were treated with hyaluronic acid or the control group who received no postoperatively treatment (Lin et al. 2013).

Treatment with estrogen has shown good results preventing formation of adhesions following hysteroscopic surgery for AS. Use of per oral estrogen gives better fertility and menstrual outcome when given in combination with ancillary treatment (IUD, balloon, or hyaluronic acid). Estrogen therapy is favorable regardless of stage of AS and is typically given 4–6 weeks postoperatively (Johary et al. 2014).

4.6.3 Restoring a Normal Endometrium

Endometrium in AS can be sparse and fibrotic. Hysteroscopic treatment enables adhesiolysis and reformation size and function of uterine cavity. Yet, in order to reestablish a functioning endometrium and enable subsequent pregnancies, the standard treatment recommended to promote endometrial growth and reepithelialization of scarred surfaces is typically oral estradiol 2 mg daily for 30–60 days and medroxyprogesterone acetate 10 mg for the last 5 days of the estrogen therapy (Johary et al. 2014).

Restoration of a functioning endometrium by stem cells is a potential future treatment; however, the research and knowledge on treatment of AS with stem cells is still in its infancy.

4.6.4 Postoperative Assessment

Management of moderate and severe AS poses a challenge and repeat surgery is necessary in some cases, however does not always produce the desired outcome.

Postoperatively assessment of the effect of treatment is mainly reflected by the patient's symptoms. Ultrasound and repeat hysteroscopy can give an assessment of the uterine cavity, though reformation of adhesions is not always related to a poor outcome.

In those patients who succeed in achieving pregnancy, a thorough antenatal follow-up is necessary due to increased risk of abnormal placentation (March 2011).

4.6.5 Reproductive Outcome After Treatment

Infertility and recurrent pregnancy loss due to AS can be treated with good outcomes. A recent study by Roy et al. reported conception rates of 58 % in mild AS, 30 % in moderate AS, and 33.3 % in severe cases of AS following hysteroscopic adhesiolysis. Furthermore, the live birth rate reported was 86.1 %, the miscarriage rate 11.1 %, and the cumulative pregnancy rate showed that 97.2 % of the patients conceived within 24 months postoperatively (Roy et al. 2010).

References

Asherman JG (1948) Amenorrhoea traumatica (atretica). J Obstet Gynaecol Br Emp 55(1):23–30

Asherman JG (1950) Traumatic intra-uterine adhesions. J Obstet Gynaecol Br Emp 57(6):892–896

Bacelar AC, Wilcock D, Powell M, Worthington BS (1995) The value of MRI in the assessment of traumatic intra-uterine adhesions (Asherman's syndrome). Clin Radiol 50(2):80–83

Dmowski WP, Greenblatt RB (1969) Asherman's syndrome and risk of placenta accreta. Obstet Gynecol 34(2):288–299

Friedler S, Margalioth EJ, Kafka I, Yaffe H (1993) Incidence of post-abortion intra-uterine adhesions evaluated by hysteroscopy–a prospective study. Hum Reprod 8(3):442–444

Jauniaux E, Jurkovic D (2012) Placenta accreta: pathogenesis of a 20th century iatrogenic uterine disease. Placenta 33(4):244–251

Johary J, Xue M, Zhu X, Xu D, Velu PP (2014) Efficacy of estrogen therapy in patients with intrauterine adhesions: systematic review. J Minim Invasive Gynecol 21(1):44–54

Lin X, Wei M, Li TC, Huang Q, Huang D, Zhou F et al (2013) A comparison of intrauterine balloon, intrauterine contraceptive device and hyaluronic acid gel in the prevention of adhesion reformation following hysteroscopic surgery for Asherman syndrome: a cohort study. Eur J Obstet Gynecol Reprod Biol 170(2):512–516

Makris N, Kalmantis K, Skartados N, Papadimitriou A, Mantzaris G, Antsaklis A (2007) Three-dimensional hysterosonography versus hysteroscopy for the detection of intracavitary uterine abnormalities. Int J Gynaecol Obstet 97(1):6–9

March CM (1995) Intrauterine adhesions. Obstet Gynecol Clin North Am 22(3):491–505

March CM (2011) Asherman's syndrome. Semin Reprod Med 29(2):83–94

Nasr AL, Al-Inany HG, Thabet SM, Aboulghar M (2000) A clinicohysteroscopic scoring system of intrauterine adhesions. Gynecol Obstet Invest 50(3):178–181

Pabuccu R, Atay V, Orhon E, Urman B, Ergun A (1997) Hysteroscopic treatment of intrauterine adhesions is safe and effective in the restoration of normal menstruation and fertility. Fertil Steril 68(6):1141–1143

Protopapas A, Shushan A, Magos A (1998) Myometrial scoring: a new technique for the management of severe Asherman's syndrome. Fertil Steril 69(5):860–864

Roy KK, Baruah J, Sharma JB, Kumar S, Kachawa G, Singh N (2010) Reproductive outcome following hysteroscopic adhesiolysis in patients with infertility due to Asherman's syndrome. Arch Gynecol Obstet 281(2):355–361

Schenker JG, Margalioth EJ (1982) Intrauterine adhesions: an updated appraisal. Fertil Steril 37(5):593–610

Soares SR, Barbosa dos Reis MM, Camargos AF (2000) Diagnostic accuracy of sonohysterography, transvaginal sonography, and hysterosalpingography in patients with uterine cavity diseases. Fertil Steril 73(2):406–411

Westendorp IC, Ankum WM, Mol BW, Vonk J (1998) Prevalence of Asherman's syndrome after secondary removal of placental remnants or a repeat curettage for incomplete abortion. Hum Reprod 13(12):3347–3350

Yu D, Wong YM, Cheong Y, Xia E, Li TC (2008a) Asherman syndrome–one century later. Fertil Steril 89(4):759–779

Yu D, Li TC, Xia E, Huang X, Liu Y, Peng X (2008b) Factors affecting reproductive outcome of hysteroscopic adhesiolysis for Asherman's syndrome. Fertil Steril 89(3):715–722

Hysteroscopic Sterilization

5

Andreas L. Thurkow

Contents

A.L. Thurkow
St. Lucas Andreas Hospital,
J. Tooropstraat 164, Amsterdam
1061 AE, The Netherlands

DC Klinieken Lairesse,
Valeriusplein 11, Amsterdam
1075 BG, The Netherlands

MC Amstelveen,
Burg. Haspelslaan 131, Amstelveen
1181 NC, The Netherlands
e-mail: thurkow@me.com

5.1   Introduction and History

Female sterilization is the most frequently used method of permanent birth control: it is estimated that worldwide around 180 million couples rely on this form of contraception (EngenderHealth 2002). In the Netherlands around 9,000 women are sterilized each year (Prismant and Health Care and Advise Institute 2004).

In order to achieve this, from 1930 onwards the fallopian tubes have most commonly been ligated through a (mini) laparotomy, in the 1960s it became possible to do so via laparoscopic route and this method developed into the standard technique (Hyams 1934; Steptoe 1971), although the first laparoscopic sterilization has been described as early as 1936 (Bosch 1936).

Although it is a reliable method of contraception, in the CREST Study, a large multicenter, prospective cohort study in the US, the pregnancy rate after laparoscopic sterilization has shown to be higher than previously reported (Peterson et al. 1996).

In rare cases laparoscopy is known to potentially cause serious complications (Jansen et al. 1997).

In the Netherlands, 54 % of all female sterilizations were performed hysteroscopically in 2010 (Fig. 5.1; Vleugels 2014).

Even before the introduction of the hysteroscope in the nineteenth century attempts have been undertaken to ensure a permanent contraception by manipulating the uterus or the

O. Istre (ed.), *Minimally Invasive Gynecological Surgery*,
DOI 10.1007/978-3-662-44059-9_5, © Springer-Verlag Berlin Heidelberg 2015

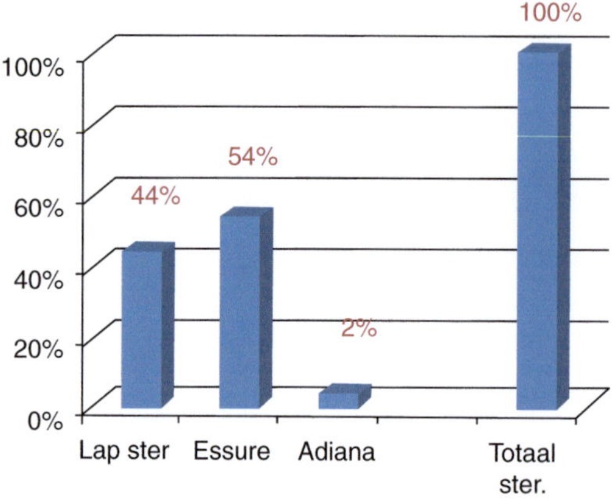

Fig. 5.1 Distribution of methods of sterilization in the Netherlands in 2010 (By courtesy of Michel Vleugels, MD, PhD, personal communication)

fallopian tubes transcervically through a vaginal route in the extent that passage is obstructed (van der Leij 1997). Initially chemical agents or electrothermical instruments were introduced blindly, with tactile feedback only, the effect of which was disappointing. In 1927 for the first time an electrocautery method with hysteroscopic guidance was tested albeit with the same mediocre results. Later attempts with electro-, cryo-, or Nd-YAG laser coagulation were equally unsuccessful in achieving bilateral occlusion (in 15 % up to a maximum of 60 % of cases) (Fig. 5.2a, b; van der Leij 1997; Wamsteker 1977; Cooper 1992; Lindemann and Mohr 1974).

In developing countries experiments with quinacrine pellets in the uterine cavity have been

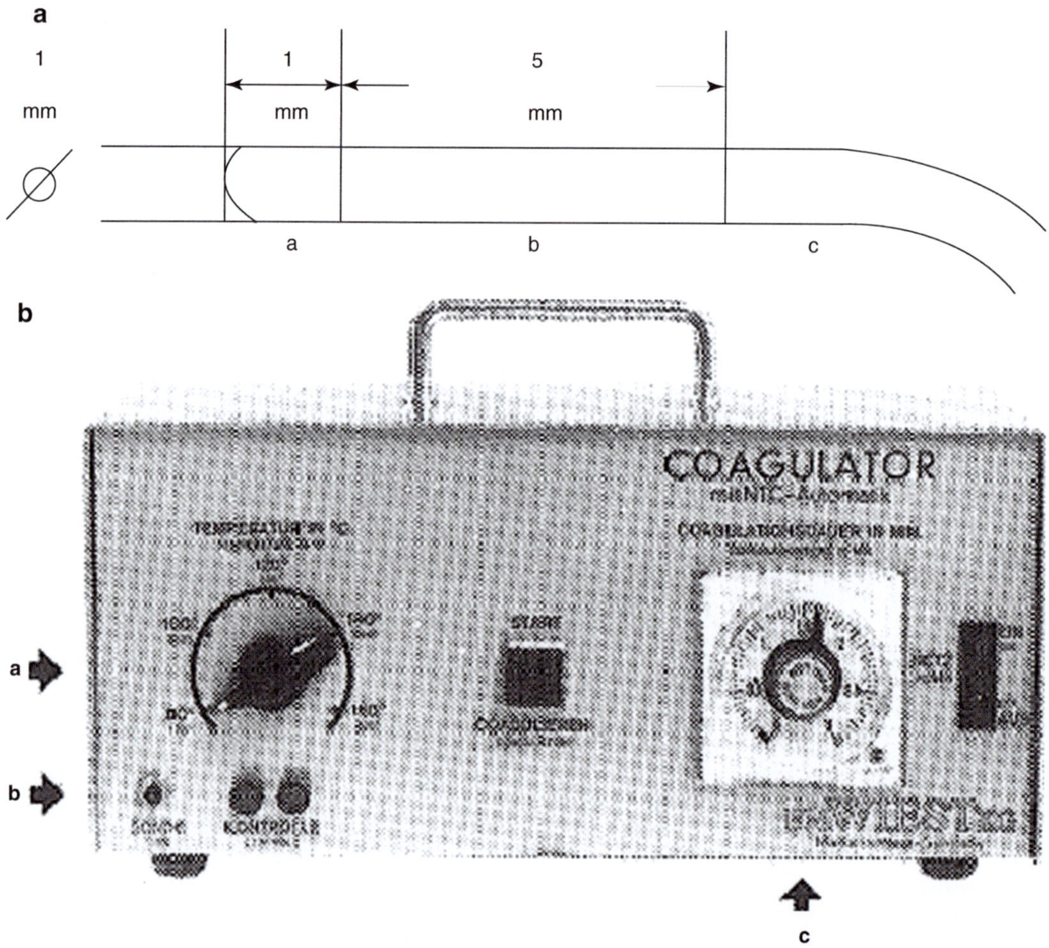

Fig. 5.2 (**a**) Distal tip of the coagulation probe; (*a*) insulated tip, (*b*) coagulation electrode, (*c*) flexible conduction cable. (**b**) Thermacoagulator (Wiest KG); (*a*) Temperature regulator, (*b*) connection for thermocoagulator probe, (*c*) timer (**a, b** Hyst ster Wamsteker: diss Wamsteker)

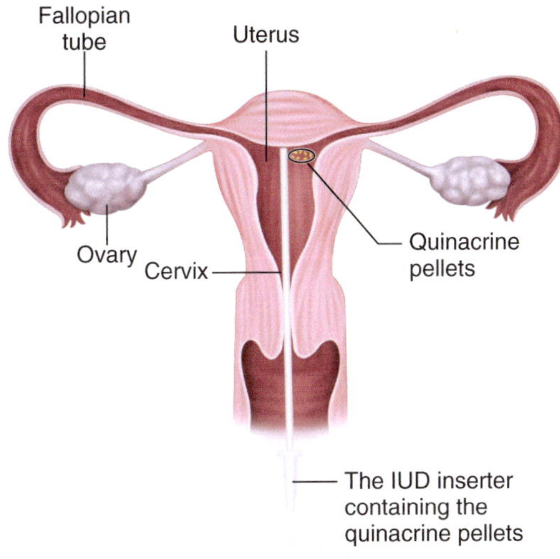

Fig. 5.3 Insertion of Quinacrine pellets (Quinacrine: http://www.google.nl/imgres?q=quinacrine&um=1&hl=n l&sa=N&biw=1584&bih=885&tbm=isch&tbnid=xZEEL s2hDhkDBM:&imgrefurl=http://panindigan.tripod.com/ quinacrine02.html&docid=aFzYbVavfE6b0M&imgurl=h ttp://panindigan.tripod.com/images/quinacrine01.gif&w= 300&h=256&ei=luBtULHjHKmc0AWFoICwCw&zoom =1&iact=rc&dur=458&sig=107070023854473941503& page=1&tbnh=156&tbnw=195&start=0&ndsp=28&ved= 1t:429,r:6,s:0,i:89&tx=96&ty=58)

performed with reasonable success, where the blind insertion has the advantage of low cost (Fig. 5.3). Serious side effects have not been seen, and the mutagen effects however are still under investigation (van der Leij 1997).

Since hysteroscopy found its way as a routine diagnostic and interventional technique in the 1970s and 1980s of the last century even more methods have been tested, among which are several types of intratubal occlusion devices (Fig. 5.4). All of these initial methods have been abandoned, either due to complications or to lack of effectiveness or both (Cooper 1992; Thatcher 1988; Brundin 1991; Hamou et al. 1984).

From 2003 to 2006 Chiroxia Ltd. (Dublin, Ireland) investigated the hysteroscopic application of a cyanoacrylate-based liquid polymer implant, in which the author of this article performed the study on explanted uteri (Figs. 5.5 and 5.6). Although the initial results were promising the investors withdrew their support and the project was discontinued.

5.2 Ovabloc

In 1988 Ovabloc®, a new hysteroscopic sterilization technique was introduced on the Dutch market after preclinical and clinical studies had been performed since 1967 (Loffer 1984; Reed and Erb 1979).

To date it is estimated that around 2,000 procedures have taken place in the Netherlands.

It is a formed-in-place silicone polymer that causes bilateral occlusion in 95 % of cases (Loffer 1984; Ligt-Veneman et al. 1999).

Through a double catheter system the two component fluid siloxane mixture with a high viscosity is injected in the fallopian tubes, which cures within minutes and hereby causes occlusion of the tubal lumen (Fig. 5.7). A specially designed siloxane obturator tip, which is preattached on the inner catheter, forms a complex with the intraluminal plug and causes sealing in the uterotubal junction.

Failures are caused by (among others) tubal spasm, intracavitary pathology, perforation and inability to position the catheter tip in correct alignment with the tubal lumen.

Especially the latter makes the procedure quite skill dependent.

Although the exact prediction of failure is not possible, some risk factors can be identified, among which are suspicion of intrauterine pathology and nulliparity (van der Leij and Lammes 1996).

After completion of the procedure a pelvic X-ray is made to ensure the integrity and correct position of the plug and the amount of ampullary filling (Fig. 5.8). If the thickness of the plug is insufficient (e.g. due to intracavitary reflux of the material) intrauterine expulsion may occur. The X-ray is then repeated after 3 months to rule out expulsion, which is stated to take place in 3–4 % of cases, usually within the first months after placement (Loffer 1984; van der Leij and Lammes 1996). The use of ultrasound for this second control may well be equivalent since assessment of correct tubal placement is the main goal at this stage and the intramural part of the plug as well as the intrauterine tip is usually easily visualized sonographically.

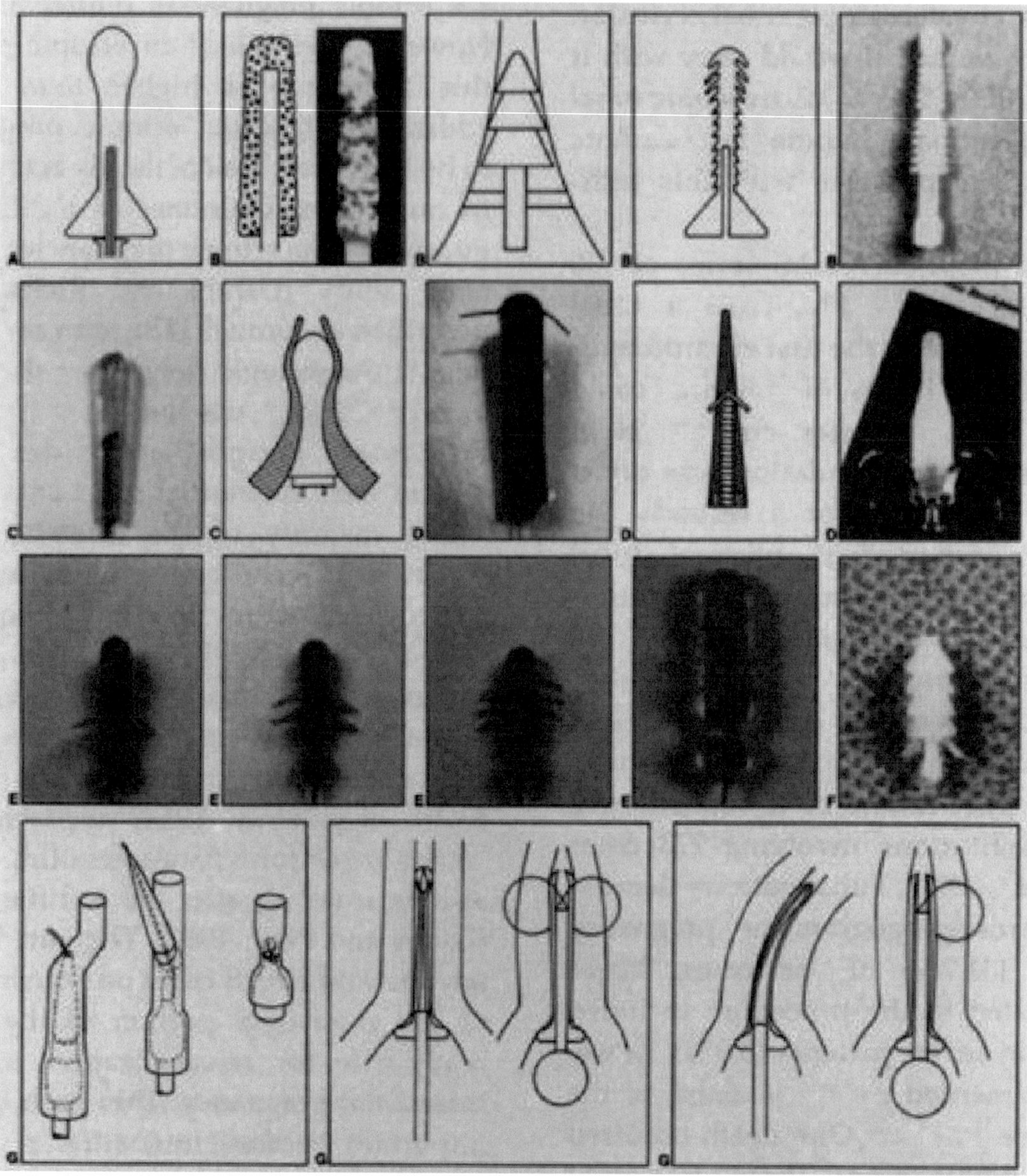

Fig. 5.4 Various experimental intratubal devices (Various devices: http://www.expert-reviews.com/doi/abs/10.1586/17434440.2.5.623)

As soon as correct position of both plugs has been established the patient can be allowed to rely on Ovabloc as the sole method of contraception.

According to a multicenter 3 years follow-up study in 398 patients the cumulative pregnancy rate is 0.99 % (Pearl Index 0.13/100 woman-years), which is comparable with the laparo-scopic alternative (Ligt-Veneman et al. 1999; Peterson et al. 1996).

The use of Ovabloc declined after the introduction of Essure and has virtually disappeared from the market after the introduction of Adiana.

The system is CE marked, but not FDA approved.

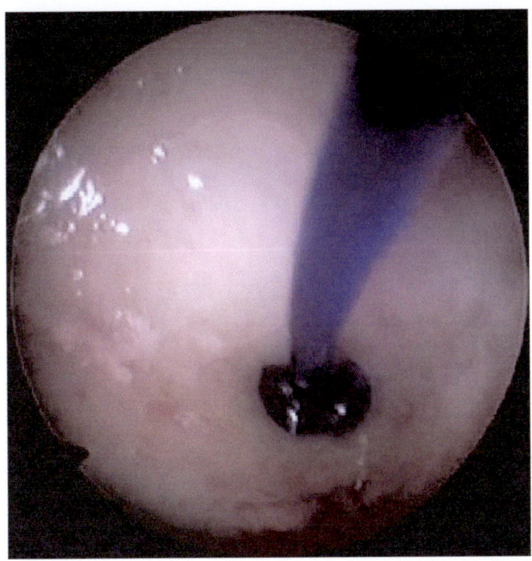

Fig. 5.5 Instillation of liquid Chiroxia obstructing material in explanted uterus (Recording of personal explant study)

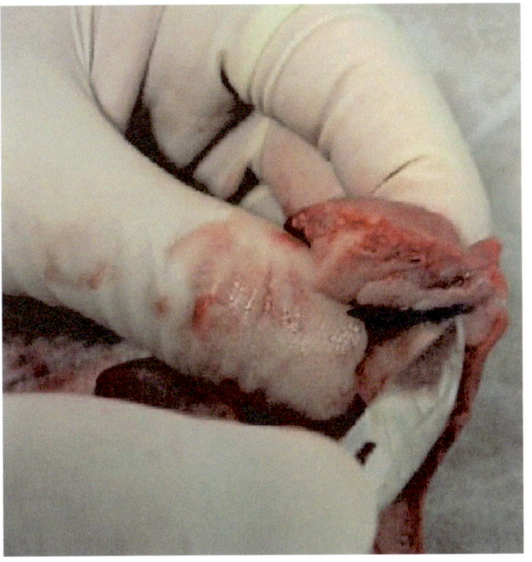

Fig. 5.6 Extremely firm adhesion of solidified Chiroxia material in intramural tubal lumen of explanted uterus (By courtesy of Chiroxia Ltd.)

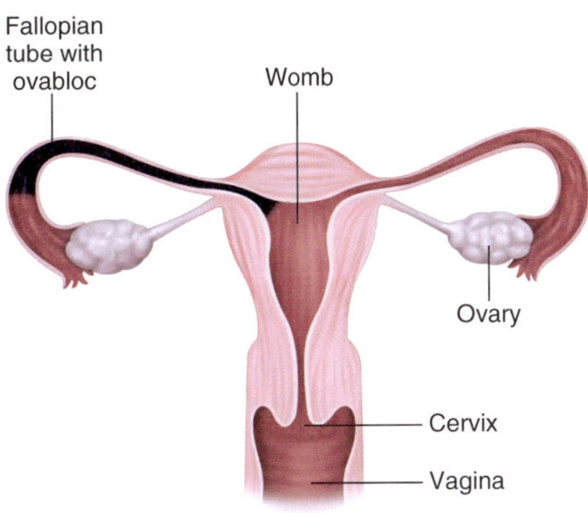

Fig. 5.7 Ovabloc material injected into right tubal lumen (Ovabloc: http://www.ovabloc.nl/ovabloc/the_treatment, Ovabloc cure: http://web.squ.edu.om/med-Lib/MED_ CD/E_CDs/Endoscopic%20Surgery%20for%20 Gynecologists/Published/Book_Content/Chapters_51-57/ Chapter_57/c57p03/c57p03.html)

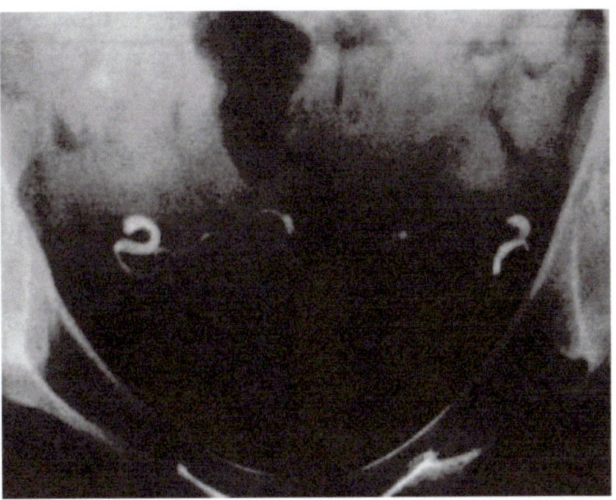

Fig. 5.8 X-ray confirmation test after Ovabloc sterilization showing two adequate plugs (Ovabloc X ray: http:// web.squ.edu.om/med-Lib/MED_CD/E_CDs/ Endoscopic%20Surgery%20for%20Gynecologists/ Published/Book_Content/Chapters_51-57/Chapter_57/ c57p03/c57p03.html)

A new version of this device with the same material has recently been developed (Ovalastic). Only scarse clinical data are available yet, the only procedures having been performed either by the author or under his supervision. Basically the procedure has not changed, the ease of use however has made a significant step forward in comparison with the original Ovabloc procedure. A clinical study is in preparation.

5.3 Essure

In November 2001 the European Health Office approved (CE mark) the use of another method of hysteroscopic sterilization which was

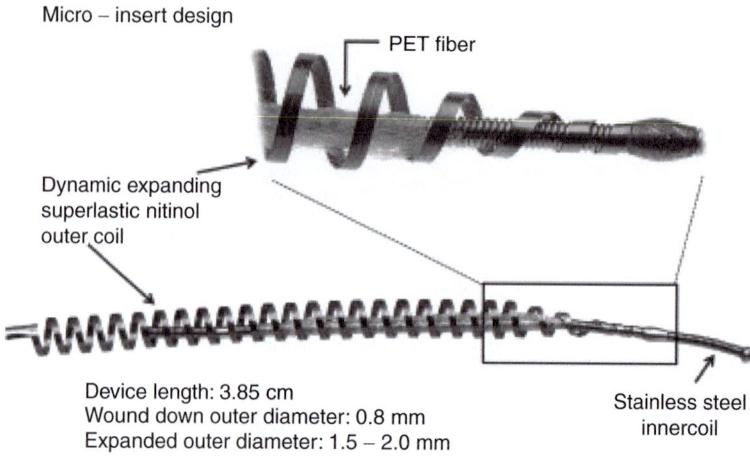

Fig. 5.9 Essure device with magnification view showing inner and outer coil with PET fibers (Essure micro: http://download.journals. elsevierhealth.com/pdfs/ journals/1553-4650/ PIIS1553465009001150.pdf)

launched on the Dutch market in 2003: the Essure® system. The FDA PMA approval followed in November 2002.

The Essure® micro-insert (Conceptus Inc., sold to Bayer AG. In 2013), initially called STOP, is a dynamically expanding micro-coil with polyethylene terephthalate (PET) fibers wound in and around the inner coil (Fig. 5.9). It is placed through a 5 Fr working channel of a hysteroscope in the intramural section of the fallopian tube, in which it anchors itself by expansion of the coil. The PET fibers subsequently cause a fibrotic reaction, which renders an additional anchoring and obstructing effect (Fig. 5.10a, b).

For an experienced hysteroscopist the technique is simple and fast. The mean procedure time is less than 15 min, partly due to the fact that most cases can be completed without anesthesia by vaginoscopic approach (Bettocchi and Selvaggi 1997).

In 92 % of cases bilateral occlusion is achieved, but in experienced hands rates up to 98.5 % can be attained (Belotte et al. 2011; Povedano et al. 2012). After 3 years of follow-up an effectiveness of 99.8 % has been shown in a multicenter pivotal study of 518 patients (Cooper et al. 2003).

Complications that have been encountered are rare perforations with no clinical symptoms, with the exception of two recent reports of bowel obstruction (Derks and Stael 2011; Belotte et al. 2011).

More than 600,000 procedures have been performed worldwide to date with a rapid increase.

The current confirmation test required by the FDA is HSG (Fig. 5.11), but received CE mark

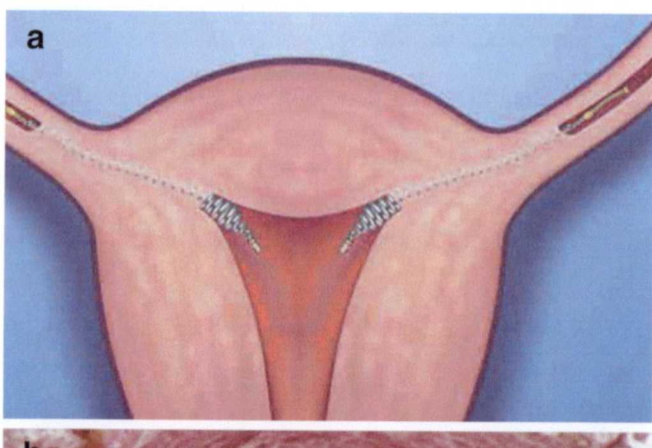

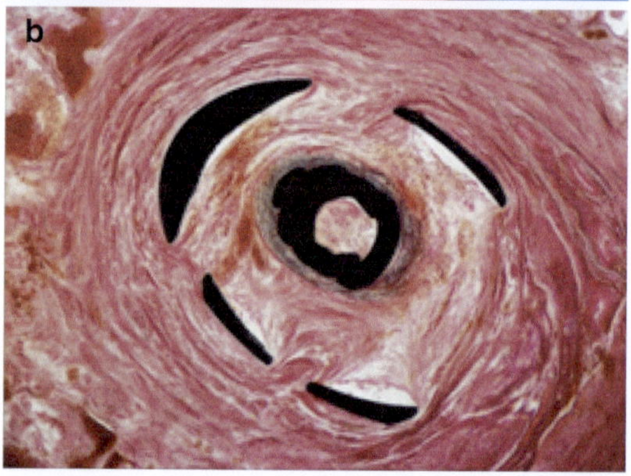

Fig. 5.10 (**a**) Frontal view of uterus with two correctly placed Essure devices after ingrowth of fibrous tissue (Essure sterilization1: http://www.women-health-info. com/88-Sterilization.html). (**b**) Transection of tubal lumen with Essure and ingrowth of fibrous tissue (Essure fibrosis: http://essuremd.com/Home/AboutEssure/FAQs/ tabid/285/Default.aspx, http://ginemartin.blogspot. nl/2011/08/obstruccion-de-trompas-metodo-essure.html)

for the use of transvaginal ultrasound in the European market in 2011 (Fig. 5.12), after studies showing the reliability of this modality (Veersema et al. 2011).

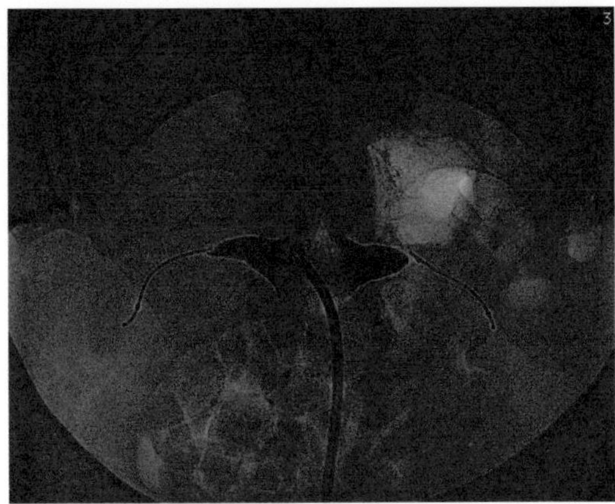

Fig. 5.11 HSG confirmation test after Essure showing two correctly placed devices blocking the tubes (Own picture, made at the St Lucas Andreas Hospital)

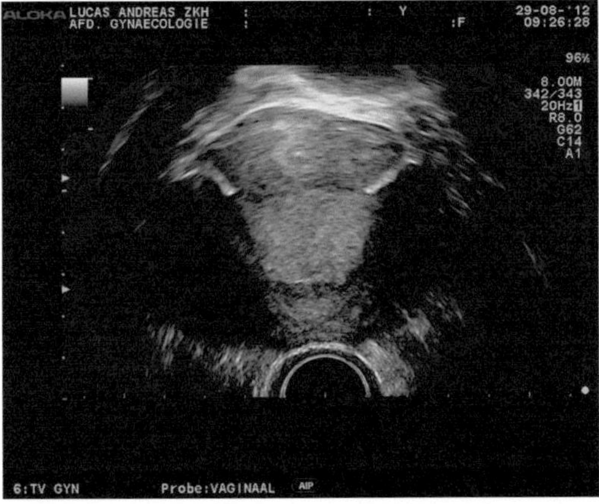

Fig. 5.12 Essure confirmation test with transversal vaginal ultrasound showing correct position of both devices in intramural portion of the tubal lumen (Own picture, made at the St Lucas Andreas Hospital)

A multicenter phase 4 study has started in the same year with the goal to obtain FDA approval for this change of the standard confirmation method.

5.4 Adiana

In 2009 another hysteroscopic sterilization system, Adiana ®, received CE marking and was approved by the FDA later in the same year.

The device consists of a 1.5 × 3.5 mm silicone matrix that is introduced in the intramural portion of the fallopian tube after superficial radiofrequency coagulation of the tubal mucosa (3 W during 60 s for each side) to stimulate fibrotic tissue ingrowth into the matrix (Fig. 5.13a–d). The system includes a dedicated generator that controls the correct positioning and delivers the energy for the coagulation (Fig. 5.13e).

Although the device is visible on transvaginal ultrasound (Fig. 5.14), the confirmation test required is a HSG after 3 months to ensure blockage of the fallopian tubes.

The initial version of the matrix was not radiopaque, in 2011 a radiopaque version was introduced in the European market, which added significantly to the reliability of the confirmation test (Fig. 5.15).

As with Essure any hysteroscope with a 5 Fr working channel can be used to perform the procedure.

The 3-year pregnancy prevention effectiveness rate is 98.4 % (Anderson and Vancaillie 2009).

Twenty nine thousand five hundred procedures have been performed worldwide, until the Hologic company decided to withdraw the product from the market in May 2012.

5.5 New Developments

Several alternative methods are in the pipeline and may be introduced in the future.

Among these are the Altaseal device (Altascience Ltd.), the ZRO Operculum (Fig. 5.16), and the Daisyclip device (Invectus Biomedical Inc., sold to Hologic Inc. in 2012). It is not clear what the current status of the latter devices is, as far as known to the author neither has been subjected to clinical studies yet. The former is a high grade stainless steel instant blocking device of the fallopian tube that does not depend on tissue ingrowth and therefore might have the advantage of immediate closure (Fig. 5.17). The perihysterectomy pilot study performed by the author of this article has been promising in this respect and further multicenter studies are been performed or in preparation.

Yet other devices are bound to be developed, in view of the interest for minimal invasive sterilization options, specially in the developing countries, where the current devices have not yet shown a large penetration in the market due to the present-day costs of the material.

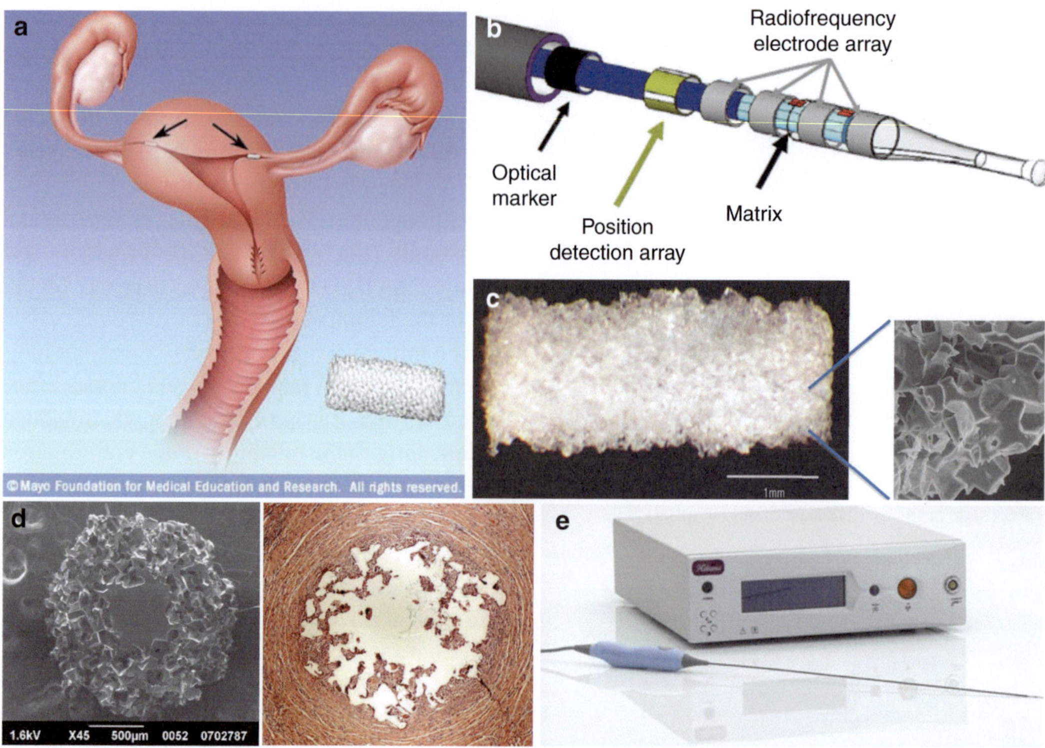

Fig. 5.13 (**a**) Adiana in the intramural portion of the tubal lumen; close up of the device (http://www.mayoclinic.com/health/medical/IM04341). (**b**) Magnification view of the distal tip of the Adiana device showing the matrix, radiofrequency electrode array, position detection array, and optical marker (Adiana: http://www.histeroscopia.es/Adiana.htm). (**c**) Microscopic and electron microscopic view of Adiana matrix. (**d**) Scanning electron micrographic cross dissection of Adiana matrix; Human tissue specimen H&E stain (10× magnification) showing ingrowth in matrix (**c**, **d** Adiana: Hologic Inc). (**e**) Adiana inserter and device with proprietary generator (Adiana Generator: http://www.google.nl/imgres?q=adiana&um=1&hl=nl&sa=N&biw=1584&bih=885&tbm=isch&tbnid=W693f0oyf0gYqM:&imgrefurl=http://medgadget.com/2009/07/minimally_invasive_adiana_contraception_device_gets_us_approval.html&docid=Sym6bk0qh5I6_M&imgurl=http://cdn.medgadget.com/img/f34f34ghu6.jpg&w=468&h=218&ei=8PNtUPvSBcXT0QXnqoHACQ&zoom=1&iact=rc&dur=459&sig=107070023854473941503&page=1&tbnh=121&tbnw=259&start=0&ndsp=25&ved=1t:429,r:13,s:0,i:112&tx=120&ty=60)

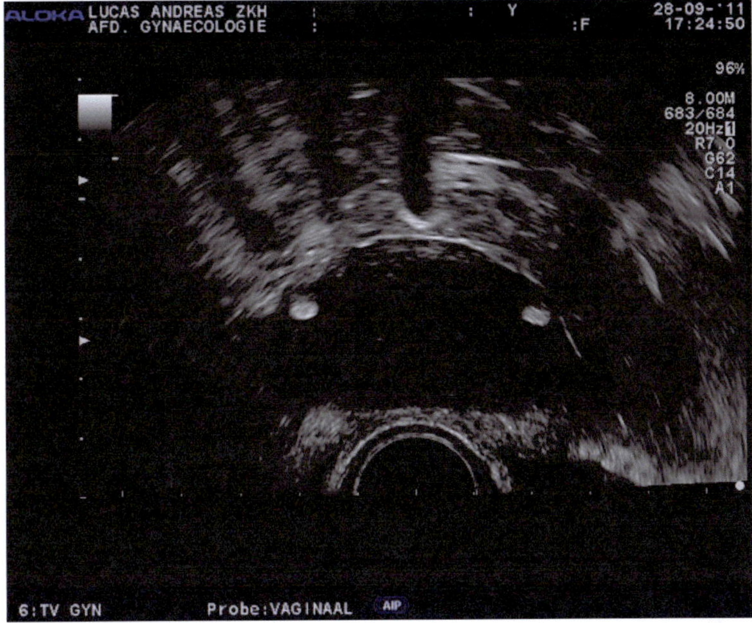

Fig. 5.14 Adiana devices as seen on transversal transvaginal ultrasound (Own picture, made at the St Lucas Andreas Hospital)

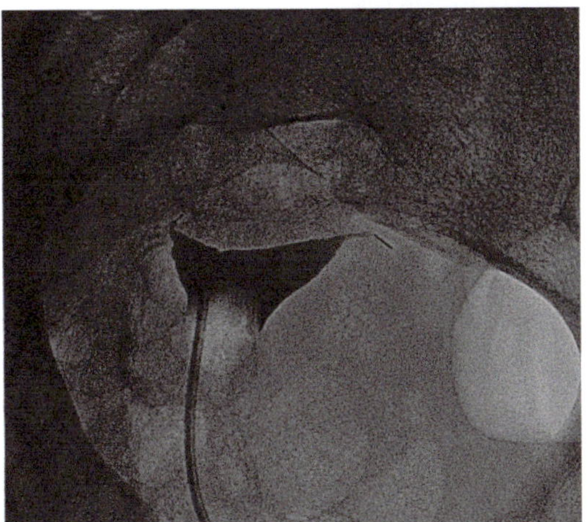

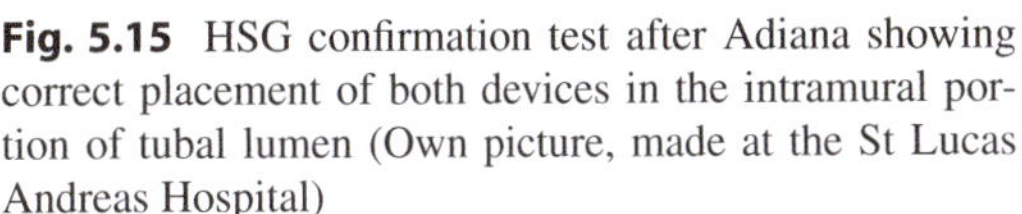

Fig. 5.15 HSG confirmation test after Adiana showing correct placement of both devices in the intramural portion of tubal lumen (Own picture, made at the St Lucas Andreas Hospital)

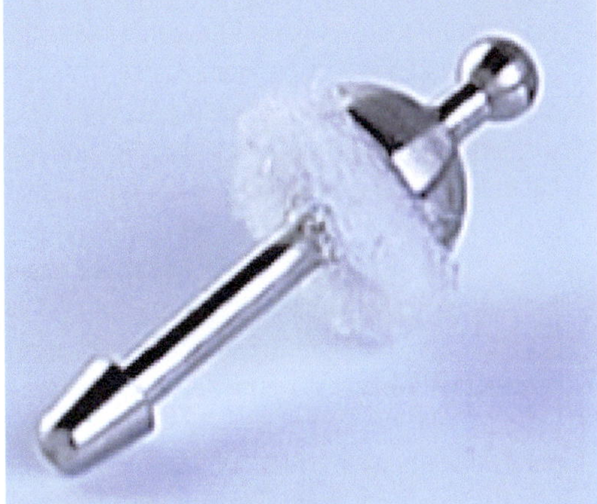

Fig. 5.16 ZRO Operculum intratubal device (Operculum: http://www.operculum.net/products.html)

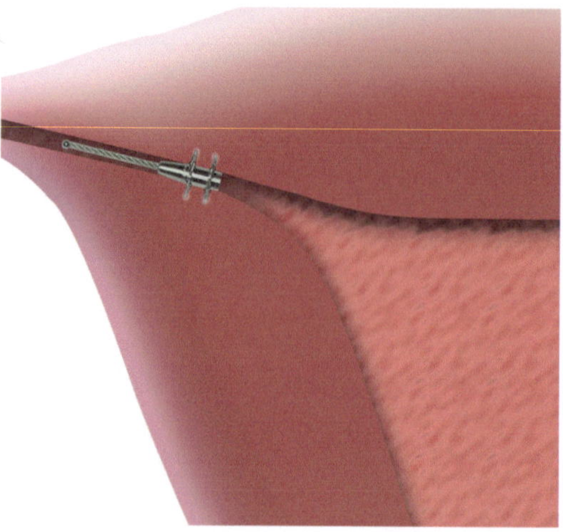

Fig. 5.17 Altaseal device anchored into intramural portion of right tubal lumen (By courtesy of Altascience Ltd.)

Conclusion

Hysteroscopic sterilization is an elegant alternative for laparoscopic sterilization with the advantage of preventing incisions and general anesthesia and ensuring faster recovery. In women with a (relative) contraindication for laparoscopy (obesity, intra-abdominal adhesions, hemorrhagic diathesis, cardiopulmonary disease) these features probably form a clear indication for hysteroscopic approach.

The only still standing indication for laparoscopic sterilization seems to exist for those patients who desire not to have to return for a control visit, as long as this remains to be required for hysteroscopic methods.

Author's Disclosures of Potential Conflicts of Interest The author is a trainer for Bayer AG (formerly Conceptus Inc.) for Essure sterilization and for Urogyn BV for Ovalastic procedures and has been trainer in the past for Ovabloc and Adiana and is principal investigator in the Altaseal Study for Altascience, Dublin, Ireland. He has been investigator for Chiroxia in the past.

No other potential conflicts of interest exist.

References

Anderson TL, Vancaillie TG (2009) Adiana system for transcervical sterilization: 3-year efficacy results. J Minim Invasive Gynecol 16(6):S38

Belotte J, Shavell VI, Awonuga AO, Diamond MP, Berman JM, Yancy AF (2011) Small bowel obstruction subsequent to Essure microinsert sterilization: a case report. Fertil Steril 96(1):4–6

Bettocchi S, Selvaggi L (1997) A vaginoscopic approach to reduce the pain of office hysteroscopy. J Am Assoc Gynecol Laparosc 4(2):255–258

Bosch PF (1936) Laparoskopische sterilization. Schweizerische Zeitschrift fur Krankenhaus und Anstaltswesen 6:62 [German]

Brundin J (1991) Transcervical sterilization in the human female by hysteroscopic application of hydrogelic occlusive devices into the intramural parts of the fallopian tubes: 10 years experience of the P-block. Eur J Gynecol Reprod Biol 39(1):41–49

Cooper JM (1992) Hysteroscopic sterilization. Clin Obstet Gynecol 35(2):282–298

Cooper JM, Carignan CS, Cher D, Kerin JF (2003) Microinsert nonincisional hysteroscopic sterilization. Obstet Gynecol 102(1):59–67

Derks R, Stael A (2011) Ileus after Essure sterilization. Medisch Contact 35 (Sept):2058 [Dutch]

EngenderHealth (2002) Contraceptive sterilization: global issues and trends. EngenderHealth, New York

Hamou J, Gasparri F, Scarselli GF, Mencaglia L, Perino A, Quartararo P et al (1984) Hysteroscopic reversible tubal sterilization. Acta Eur Fertil 15(2):123–129

Hyams MN (1934) Sterilization of the female by coagulation of the uterine cornu. Am J Obstet Gynecol 28:96

Jansen FW, Kapiteyn K, Trimbos-Kemper T, Hermans J, Trimbos JB (1997) Complications of laparoscopy: a prospective multicentre observational study. Br J Obstet Gynaecol 104(5):595–600

Levie M, Chudnoff SG (2011) A comparison of novice and experienced physicians performing hysteroscopic sterilization: an analysis of an FDA-mandated trial. Fertil Steril 96(3):643–648

Ligt-Veneman NG, Tinga DJ, Kragt H, Brandsma G, van der Leij G (1999) The efficacy of intratubal silicone in the Ovabloc hysteroscopic method of sterilization. Acta Obstet Gynecol Scand 78(9):824–825

Lindemann HJ, Mohr J (1974) Results of 274 transuterine tubal sterilizations by hysteroscopy (author's transl). Geburtshilfe Frauenheilkd 34(9):775–779

Loffer FD (1984) Hysteroscopic sterilization with the use of formed-in-place silicone plugs. Am J Obstet Gynecol 149(3):261–270

Peterson HB, Xia Z, Hughes JM, Wilcox LS, Tylor LR, Trussell J (1996) The risk of pregnancy after tubal sterilization: findings from the U.S. Collaborative Review of Sterilization. Am J Obstet Gynecol 174(4):1161–1168

Povedano B, Arjona JE, Velasco E, Monserrat JA, Lorente J, Castelo-Branco C (2012) Complications of hysteroscopic Essure(®) sterilisation: report on 4306 procedures performed in a single centre. BJOG 119(7):795–799

Prismant, Health Care and Advise Institute (2004) Landelijke LMR-informatie – Verrichtingen: destructie of afsluiting van tubae faloppii mbv endoscopie. Prismant, Health Care and Advise Institute, Utrecht. Ref Type: Report [Dutch]

Reed TP, Erb RA (1979) Hysteroscopic oviductal blocking with formed-in-place silicone rubber plugs II. Clinical studies. J Reprod Med 23(2): 69–72

Steptoe P (1971) Laparoscopic tubal sterilization–a British viewpoint. IPPF Med Bull 5(2):4

Thatcher SS (1988) Hysteroscopic sterilization. Obstet Gynecol Clin North Am 15(1):51–59

van der Leij G (1997) Hysteroscopic sterilization: study of the siloxane intratubal device application method. Dissertation, Universiteit van Amsterdam

van der Leij G, Lammes FB (1996) Office hysteroscopic tubal occlusion with siloxane intratubal devices (the Ovabloc method). Int J Gynaecol Obstet 53(3):253–260

Veersema S, Vleugels M, Koks C, Thurkow A, van der Vaart H, Brölmann H (2011) Confirmation of Essure placement using transvaginal ultrasound. J Minim Invasive Gynecol 18(2):164–168, Epub 1 Feb 2011

Vleugels M (2014) Personal communication, based on data collection for a review in press

Wamsteker K (1977) Hysteroscopie. Dissertation, Rijksuniversiteit Leiden

Endometrial Polyps

6

Marit Lieng

Contents

Abbreviations

3D	Three-dimensional
AUB	Abnormal uterine bleeding
BMI	Body mass index
CEUS	Contrast-enhanced ultrasonography
GF	Growth factors
GIS	Gel installation sonography
HT	Hormone therapy
IGF	Insulin-like growth factor
IVF	In vitro fertilization
SHBG	Sex-hormone-binding globulin
SIS	Saline infusion sonography
TCRP	Transcervical resection of endometrial polyps
TVUS	Transvaginal ultrasonography

6.1 Definition

Endometrial polyps are sessile or pedunculated smooth-margined masses merging from the endometrium and protruding into the uterine cavity (Fig. 6.1). Endometrial polyps are usually benign and occur over a wide age range. They may be diagnosed in asymptomatic women, but occur more frequently in women suffering from AUB (Anastasiadis et al. 2000; Clevenger-Hoeft et al. 1999; Peterson and Novak 1956; Reslova et al. 1999). Endometrial polyps are usually solitary, but may be multiple (Mazur and Kurman 2005). They vary in size, ranging from a few millimetres to large lesions

M. Lieng, MD, PhD
Department of Gynaecology,
Oslo University Hospital, Oslo, Norway

Institute of Clinical Medician,
University of Oslo, Oslo, Norway
e-mail: m.lieng@online.no

O. Istre (ed.), *Minimally Invasive Gynecological Surgery*,
DOI 10.1007/978-3-662-44059-9_6, © Springer-Verlag Berlin Heidelberg 2015

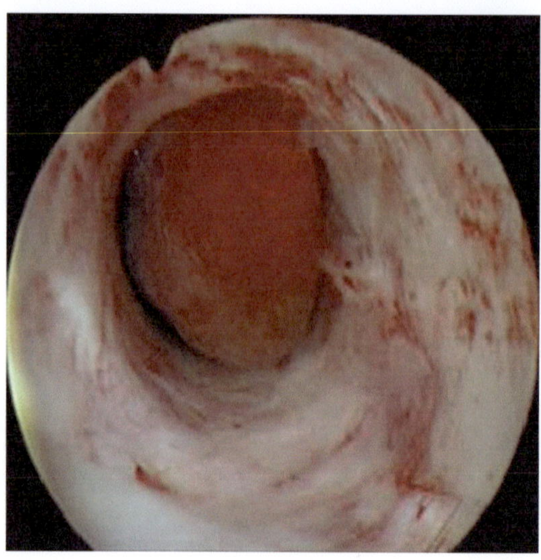

Fig. 6.1 Endometrial polyp as seen by hysteroscopy

that can fill the uterine cavity or prolapse through the endocervical canal.

6.2 Histological Features and Classification

The pathogenesis of endometrial polyps is not well understood, but they appear to originate from the endometrial basalis layer as focal overgrowths and consist of glands, stroma and thick-walled vessels (Mazur and Kurman 2005; Kurman 1982; Mutter et al. 2009). They may have a large flat base (sessile) or be attached to the endometrium by an elongated pedicle (pedunculated). Despite their diverse growth pattern, all endometrial polyps show typical histological features (Mazur and Kurman 2005; Kurman 1982; Mutter et al. 2009; Schlaen et al. 1988). In biopsy specimens, endometrial polyps typically present as larger, often polypoid shaped, tissue fragments with surface epithelium on three sides. The stroma of the polyp can be highly variable, but is often dense, and may include thick-walled vessels. The glands are irregular in shape and have a variable architecture.

Benign endometrial polyps can be classified, based on morphological features, into five morphological forms: proliferative/hyperplastic polyps, atrophic polyps, functional polyps, mixed endometrial–endocervical polyps, and adenomyomatous polyps (Mazur and Kurman 2005). The morphological patterns of benign endometrial polyps often overlap and have limited clinical significance for therapeutic decisions. Endometrial polyps are usually benign, but they may contain focal hyperplasia, focal complex hyperplasia, atypical hyperplasia, intraepithelial carcinoma or carcinoma (Peterson and Novak 1956; Mazur and Kurman 2005).

6.3 Prevalence

In textbooks of pathology, the prevalence of endometrial polyps is quoted to be approximately 25 % (Mazur and Kurman 2005; Kurman 1982; Mutter et al. 2009). The reported prevalence of endometrial polyps in women suffering from AUB varies between 10 and 40 % (Anastasiadis et al. 2000; Clevenger-Hoeft et al. 1999; Cohen 2004; Goldstein et al. 1997; Nagele et al. 1996a; van Bogaert 1988). The prevalence appears to increase by age during the reproductive years, but it is not clear whether it subsequently peaks or decreases after menopause (Anastasiadis et al. 2000; Clevenger-Hoeft et al. 1999; Peterson and Novak 1956; Reslova et al. 1999; van Bogaert 1988). Endometrial polyps are more common in women suffering from AUB, compared to women without such symptoms (Clevenger-Hoeft et al. 1999). Consequently, the large variation in reported prevalence of polyps may, among other factors, be explained by heterogeneous study populations in terms of age and eventual presence of symptoms. Furthermore, varying definitions and diagnostic methods, and difficulties in establishment of the histological diagnosis may contribute to the large variation in the reported prevalence of endometrial polyps (Mazur and Kurman 2005; van Bogaert 1988; Dreisler et al. 2009a).

The prevalence of endometrial polyps in asymptomatic women has been sparsely studied. In asymptomatic premenopausal women, the reported prevalence of endometrial polyps varies between 1 and 11 % (Clevenger-Hoeft et al. 1999;

Dreisler et al. 2009a; Cooper et al. 1983; DeWaay et al. 2002). In asymptomatic women aged 45–50 years, the prevalence is reported to be 12 %, and in two studies evaluating asymptomatic postmenopausal women, the prevalence of endometrial polyps was found to be 12 and 17 % respectively (Dreisler et al. 2009a; Fay et al. 1999; Lieng et al. 2009).

6.4 Pathophysiology

Although endometrial polyps occur relatively often, the knowledge of the aetiology and pathogenesis of such polyps is limited. Endometrial polyps are believed to develop as a consequence of focal stromal and glandular overgrowth caused by prolonged oestrogen exposure (Schlaen et al. 1988; Lopes et al. 2007; Ryan et al. 2005; Sant'Ana de Almeida et al. 2004). The balance between mitotic activity and apoptosis is considered to regulate normal endometrial development during the menstrual cycle, and disturbances of these physiological processes have been proposed to occur in endometrial polyps (Stewart et al. 1999). Oestrogen and progesterone act, via their receptors, as modulators of proliferation and differentiation in the normal endometrium (Inceboz et al. 2006). Both oestrogen and progesterone receptors have been identified in the glandular epithelium of endometrial polyps in both post- and premenopausal women, but the receptor expression appears to be disorderly compared with normal endometrium (Lopes et al. 2007; Ryan et al. 2005; Mittal et al. 1996; McGurgan et al. 2006a).

Furthermore, demonstrations of increased levels of Ki61, a marker of cell proliferation, and Bcl-2, an inhibitor of apoptosis, indicate that loss of usual control mechanisms for growth may be of importance in development of endometrial polyps (Inceboz et al. 2006; McGurgan et al. 2006a; Maia et al. 2004a; Mertens et al. 2002; Taylor et al. 2003). This loss of proapoptotic mechanisms may be related to unopposed hyperestrogenism, because Bcl-2 expression increases in response to oestrogen (Mertens et al. 2002; Dahmoun et al. 1999). Oestrogen may conse-

quently have a role in the development of endometrial polyps either by direct stimulation of localized proliferation, or by stimulation of proliferation via activation of Ki67 or inhibition of apoptosis via Bcl-2 (Inceboz et al. 2006). Available data also indicate that unopposed hyperestrogenism can lead to an abnormal increase of certain growth factors (GF) and growth factor receptors within the endometrium, which may stimulate endometrial polyp growth (Maia et al. 2001). Cytogenic abnormalities following altered gene expressions have been identified in endometrial polyp tissue (Bol et al. 1996; Nogueira et al. 2006; Vanni et al. 1993). However, any effect of these findings in the development of endometrial polyps is not known, and the studies are small and need to be confirmed in future studies including a larger number of endometrial polyps.

6.5 Associated Factors

Increasing age appears to be the best-documented risk indicator for endometrial polyps (Anastasiadis et al. 2000; Clevenger-Hoeft et al. 1999; Reslova et al. 1999; Nagele et al. 1996a; van Bogaert 1988; Dreisler et al. 2009a; Nappi et al. 2009; Vilodre et al. 1997). Some authors report that the peak prevalence of endometrial polyps occurs during the last decade of the fertile years (Clevenger-Hoeft et al. 1999; van Bogaert 1988), while others report menopause as a risk indicator for the development of endometrial polyps (Anastasiadis et al. 2000; Reslova et al. 1999; Nagele et al. 1996a; Dreisler et al. 2009a; Vilodre et al. 1997). In two reports using age-adjusted regression models, menopause was not found to be associated with a higher prevalence of endometrial polyps (Nappi et al. 2009; Dreisler et al. 2009b).

Endometrial polyps have been reported to occur more often in women with obesity, hypertension, fibroids, endometriosis, or cervical polyps (Clevenger-Hoeft et al. 1999; Peterson and Novak 1956; Reslova et al. 1999; Vilodre et al. 1997; Dreisler et al. 2009b; Onalan et al. 2009; Oguz et al. 2005; Coeman et al. 1993; Kim et al. 2003;

McBean et al. 1996). The results of two prospective trials including 245 and 375 women, respectively, indicate an association of obesity and endometrial polyps (Reslova et al. 1999; Oguz et al. 2005). This association was also reported in a retrospective study including 230 women undergoing in vitro fertilization (IVF), where $BMI \geq 30$ kg/m^2 was found to be an independent risk factor for the development of endometrial polyps (Onalan et al. 2009). Obesity is characterized by decreased sex-hormone-binding globulin (SHBG) levels, increased aromatization of androgens to oestrogens in adipose tissue and high levels of unopposed oestrogen in the circulation (Onalan et al. 2009). This relative hyperestrogenism may explain the development of endometrial polyps in obese women. Both obesity and hypertension are conditions related to an abnormal increase in serum and endometrial tissue of growth factors such as free insulin-like GF (IGF)-1, which might be of importance for the development of endometrial polyps (Maia et al. 2001). But reports regarding obesity as an associated factor with endometrial polyps are not consistent.

Similarly, a relationship between hypertension and development of endometrial polyps has been suggested (Reslova et al. 1999). However, no association between hypertension and development of endometrial polyps was found in the two studies using logistic regression models for adjustments for age and overweight (Nappi et al. 2009; Dreisler et al. 2009b).

Endometrial polyps are furthermore reported to occur more often in women with fibroids, cervical polyps, and endometriosis (Clevenger-Hoeft et al. 1999; Peterson and Novak 1956; Vilodre et al. 1997; Coeman et al. 1993; Kim et al. 2003; McBean et al. 1996). Most of these studies are retrospective and include relatively few patients. The pathogeneses of any associations between endometrial polyps and fibroids, cervical polyps and endometriosis appears not to be considered, but it might be related to oestrogen influence.

Tibolon appears to increase the risk of endometrial polyp development (Perez-Medina et al. 2003). Data regarding an eventual relationship between hormone therapy (HT) and endometrial polyps are contradicting, as some studies report higher prevalence of endometrial polyps in women using HT (Dreisler et al. 2009b; Maia et al. 1996), whereas others do not (Akkad et al. 1995; Bakour et al. 2002; Elliott et al. 2003; Orvieto et al. 1999). In an experimental study, Maja et al. found that HT may cause endometrial polyp involution by decreasing proliferation and stimulating apoptosis (Maia et al. 2004b). In accordance with this finding, Perrone et al. reported a lower prevalence of endometrial polyps in women using HT compared to a control group (Perrone et al. 2002). Endometrial polyp formation has been reported to be dependent on the type and dosage of HT (Oguz et al. 2005; Iatrakis et al. 2006). Furthermore, a progestogen with high antipestrogenic activity, as well as use of oral contraceptive pills may have a protective effect on the development of endometrial polyps (Dreisler et al. 2009b; Oguz et al. 2005). An eventual protective effect of levonorgesterel-releasing intrauterine devices on the development of endometrial polyps seems not to have been evaluated.

Tamoxifen has in previous studies shown a consistent relationship with the development of endometrial polyps (Reslova et al. 1999; Cohen 2004; Bakour et al. 2002; Chalas et al. 2005; De Muylder et al. 1991; Kedar et al. 1994). Tamoxifen appears to have a significant effect on hormone receptor expression and markers of apoptosis in endometrial polyps, which support the hypothesis stating that tamoxifen promotes polyp growth by inhibiting apoptosis (McGurgan et al. 2006b). This hypothesis is furthermore substantiated by the report by Gardener et al., indicating that the levonorgestrel-releasing intrauterine system has a protective action against the uterine effects of tamoxifen (Gardner et al. 2000).

6.6 Symptoms and Clinical Consequences

The majority of endometrial polyps are probably asymptomatic (Ryan et al. 2005). Most symptomatic women with endometrial polyps present with different forms of AUB (intermenstrual bleeding, menorrhagia, metrorrhagia, postmenopausal bleeding), and endometrial polyps are found in about 10–40 % of women suffering from such symptoms (Anastasiadis et al. 2000; Clevenger-Hoeft et al. 1999; Goldstein et al. 1997; van Bogaert 1988). It is not known why endometrial polyps may cause AUB, but it is believed that abbreviations in hormone receptor expression within polyps may lead to an abnormal response to the hormonal environment, causing tissue breakdown and bleeding (Ryan et al. 2005). Although different forms of AUB constitute the dominating symptom in women with endometrial polyps, women with such polyps also may present with dysmenorrhoea, vaginal discharge or endometritis caused by extension of large polyps into the endocervix by dilatation of the internal cervical os (Mazur and Kurman 2005; Ryan et al. 2005).

In a large prospective trial evaluating 1,000 infertile women scheduled for IVF, the prevalence of endometrial polyps was found to be 32 % (Hinckley and Milki 2004). The high prevalence of endometrial polyps in infertile women suggests a causative relationship between the presence of endometrial polyps and infertility (Hinckley and Milki 2004; Frydman et al. 1987; Seinera et al. 1988; Syrop and Sahakian 1992). However, a causal relationship between endometrial polyps and infertility appears to have been confirmed in only one prospective randomized trial (Perez-Medina et al. 2005). In this trial allocating women with endometrial polyps to hysteroscopic polypectomy or diagnostic hysteroscopy prior to intrauterine insemination, women in the resection group had a significant higher chance of becoming pregnant. The results of a retrospective trial also indicate that hysteroscopic polypectomy may enhance fertility in women with endometrial polyps compared with infertile women with normal cavity (Varasteh et al. 1999). On the other hand, endometrial polyps did not appear to impair implantation outcome during IVF in two other retrospective studies (Isikoglu et al. 2006; Lass et al. 1999). A trend towards increased early pregnancy loss among women with endometrial polyps was reported in one of these studies (Lass et al. 1999).

The knowledge regarding the natural history and clinical consequences of endometrial polyps without treatment is limited. Only two studies have prospectively followed a cohort of women with endometrial polyps to investigate the spontaneous polyp regression rate (DeWaay et al. 2002; Lieng et al. 2009). The follow up-period was 2.5 and 1 year, and the spontaneous regression rate was reported to be 0.6 and 0.3, respectively. In both studies, polyps that regressed tended to be smaller compared to polyps that persisted during the follow-up period. Because of small study samples, these results must be interpreted with care.

6.7 Malignancy

Although the knowledge regarding the malignant potential of endometrial polyps is limited, polyps are believed to be a risk indicator for the development of premalignant and malignant tissue changes (Savelli et al. 2003). Both atypical hyperplasia and endometrial carcinoma may originate from endometrial polyps. The most common subtypes of endometrial carcinoma in malignant endometrial polyps appear to be endometroid carcinoma and serous papillary carcinoma (Farrell et al. 2005; Giordano et al. 2007). Most commonly, endometrial carcinoma arising in endometrial polyps is an early carcinoma with good prognosis, except for papillary serous carcinoma, which can be associated with omental involvement, despite low stage of malignant development in the uterus (Giordano et al. 2007).

There appears to be only one controlled study evaluating an association of endometrial polyps with premalignant and malignant pathology (Bakour et al. 2000). In this prospective study including 248 women with AUB, hyperplasia was found to be more frequent among women with endometrial polyps compared to women without polyps (7/62 vs 8/186), but no such differences between the two study groups were found for malignancy (2/62 vs 6/162).

The results of numerous previous case series evaluating histological diagnosis of resected polyps indicate that atypia and malignancy occur within 0.3–23.8 % and 0.8–3.2 % of endometrial polyps respectively (Anastasiadis et al. 2000; Orvieto et al. 1999; Savelli et al. 2003; Bakour et al. 2000; Antunes et al. 2007; Ben-Arie et al. 2004; Ferrazzi et al. 2009; Machtinger et al. 2005; Papadia et al. 2007; Shushan et al. 2004; Lieng et al. 2007). Most authors seem to agree that the prevalence of malignancy in endometrial polyps varies by age and menopausal status. According to the available evidence, the risk of malignancy in premenopausal women appears to be low. Gynaecological symptoms have also been identified as a possible risk indicator of malignancy within endometrial polyps (Antunes et al. 2007; Ferrazzi et al. 2009; Shushan et al. 2004; Lieng et al. 2007). However, previous reports evaluating the prevalence of malignancy within endometrial polyps in symptomatic as well as asymptomatic women are not consistent. Polyp size has been reported to be a risk indicator for malignant endometrial polyps (Ben-Arie et al. 2004; Ferrazzi et al. 2009), among others by the authors of a large retrospective multicenter study including both asymptomatic and symptomatic postmenopausal women with endometrial polyps (Ferrazzi et al. 2009).

Although the reports are not consistent, other known risk factors for endometrial carcinoma, such as obesity, diabetes mellitus and hypertension have also been reported to increase the risk of malignancy within endometrial polyps (Anastasiadis et al. 2000; Savelli et al. 2003; Bernstein et al. 1999). Furthermore, tamoxifen appears to increase the risk of atypical hyperplasia and malignancy in endometrial polyps (Cohen 2004; Kedar et al. 1994; Bernstein et al. 1999).

The reported prevalence of atypia and malignancy within endometrial polyps consequently varies according to the population studied, and the relatively large variation in reported prevalence probably reflects that the populations in the different studies are heterogeneous in terms of age and symptoms. Furthermore, the definition of a malignant endometrial polyp varies in previous publications, as some define the malignant tissue changes as a malignant polyp only if the stalk and surrounding endometrium are free of cancer, while others do not require this as an assumption (Ferrazzi et al. 2009). Varying definitions of the histopathological diagnosis may consequently contribute to the relatively large variation of reported prevalence of malignancy within endometrial polyps.

6.8 Diagnosis

Previously, endometrial polyps were diagnosed by histological examination of specimens retrieved by curettage and hysterectomy from women suffering from AUB. The technical advancement of ultrasound, including high-frequency vaginal transducers, has enabled an improved view of the endometrium. This has led to a new era in the diagnostics of focal intracavitary processes.

In women with postmenopausal bleeding, measurements of the bilayer endometrial thickness have been documented effective for exclusion of malignancy, but it appear to have poor discriminative ability for detecting or excluding endometrial polyps (Gupta et al. 2002; Timmermans et al. 2008). In premenopausal women with AUB, diverging results have been reported regarding the diagnostic value of endometrial thickness measurements for the detection of focal intracavitary processes, including endometrial polyps (Goldstein et al. 1997; Dijkhuizen et al. 1996; Dueholm et al. 2001; Schwarzler et al. 1998; Vercellini et al. 1997). Despite the widespread use of TVUS during general gynaecological examinations, the diagnostic value of endometrial thickness measurements in asymptomatic women has been sparsely investigated. In a study including 375 asymptomatic women aged 20–74 years, measurement of endometrial thickness by TVUS was found of little use as a diagnostic tool for the detection of focal intracavitary processes, but more efficacious in excluding focal intrauterine pathology, especially in postmenopausal women (Dreisler et al. 2009c). Sonographic examination using artificial uterine cavity distension, such as saline infusion sonography (SIS) or gel installation sonography (GIS), appears to improve the diagnostic accuracy of TVUS in case of abnormal or

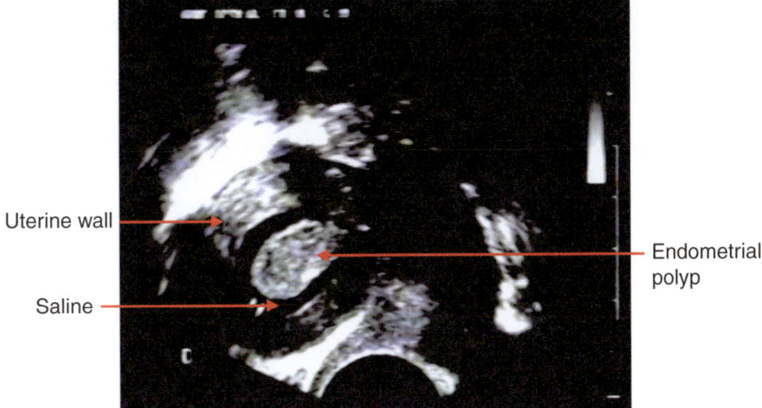

Fig. 6.2 Endometrial polyp protruding into the uterine cavity as seen during saline infusion sonography

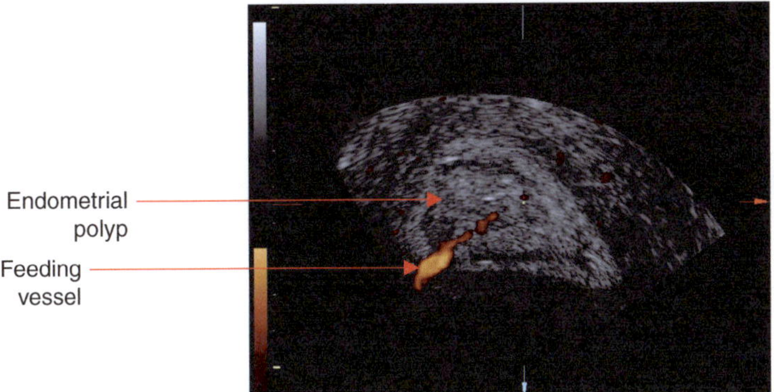

Fig. 6.3 Power Doppler sonogram showing the feeding vessel characteristic of endometrial polyps

inclusive findings and has a high sensitivity and specificity for the detection of intrauterine pathology (Fig. 6.2) (Anastasiadis et al. 2000; Syrop and Sahakian 1992; van Roessel et al. 1987; Parsons and Lense 1993; de Kroon et al. 2003; Jansen et al. 2006; Guven et al. 2004). Hysteroscopy and SIS appear to be equivalent diagnostic tools for the detection of endometrial polyps and intrauterine myomas in the evaluation of both premenopausal and postmenopausal women with AUB (van Roessel et al. 1987; Parsons and Lense 1993; Dijkhuizen et al. 2000; Pasqualotto et al. 2000; Widrich et al. 1996).

Demonstration of the feeding vessel of the endometrial polyp by transvaginal colour or power Doppler examination may be of diagnostic importance in discrimination of endometrial lesions with different vascular patterns, such as polyps and fibroids (Fig. 6.3) (Krampl et al. 2001; Exalto et al. 2007; Fleischer and Shappell 2003).

Neither ultrasonography nor hysteroscopic features have been proved successful in distinguishing benign from malignant endometrial polyps (Shushan et al. 2004; Jakab et al. 2005; Timmerman et al. 2003; Bettocchi et al. 2004a). Previous studies suggest that evaluation of tissue vascularization by power or colour flow Doppler imaging may be useful in the prediction of malignant endometrial changes, due to the increased blood flow in malignant lesions (Epstein et al. 2001; Fernandez-Parra et al. 2006). Low Doppler resistance of the feeding vessel of endometrial polyps has been reported to be predictive of atypia and malignancy (Aleem et al. 1995; Lieng et al. 2008).

Techniques such as three-dimensional (3D) ultrasonography, power Doppler angiography and contrast-enhanced ultrasonography (CEUS) appear to improve the quality and accuracy of Doppler examinations and provide a relatively new and more comprehensive assessment of tumour vascularization, compared to the two-dimensional colour or power Doppler. Such new techniques may prove to be useful for prediction of atypia or malignancy in intrauterine lesions such as endometrial polyps, in the future. However, this needs further investigation.

Accordingly, histopathology is still required to exclude atypia and malignancy within endometrial polyps. The diagnostic accuracy of blind endometrial sampling obtained by an endometrial suction curette is low in the presence of endometrial polyps (Maia et al. 1996; Carter et al. 1994; Perez-Medina et al. 2002; Merce et al. 2007; Raine-Fenning et al. 2003). A device for SIS-based guided biopsies has been developed, but the diagnostic accuracy of this method has not been evaluated in comparative studies (Sidhu et al. 2006). As curettage misses the endometrial polyps in many cases, hysteroscopy combined with histopathological examination of retrieved specimens is still the gold standard for exclusion of malignancy in endometrial polyps (Bokor et al. 2001; Testa et al. 2005).

6.9   Treatment

Treatment of endometrial polyps is performed in order to exclude premalignant and/or malignant tissue changes, relieve symptoms (AUB) or improve fertility outcomes in infertile women.

Endometrial polyps were previously treated by curettage or hysterectomy (Elpek et al. 1998). The results of previous studies indicate that about 10 % of polyps remain in situ after curettage (Hann et al. 2003; Svirsky et al. 2008). More recently, Bonvolonta et al. found, by control hysteroscopy after curettage, that the polyp was fully removed in only 2 out of 25 women (Tanriverdi et al. 2004). As opposed to curettage, hysteroscopy allows, under visional control, the complete removal of the polyp. Due to the considerable limitation of curettage, transcervical (hysteroscopic) resection of endometrial polyps (TCRP) is today regarded as the optimal treatment of endometrial polyps (de Kroon and Jansen 2006; Smith and Schulman 1985; Gimpelson and Rappold 1988). The procedure is most often performed in an inpatient setting

under general anaesthesia (Chavez et al. 2002). However, it appears that at least smaller endometrial polyps may be resected in an office setting without significant discomfort to the women (Englund et al. 1957).

TCRP carries a relative low risk of complications (Nagele et al. 1996a; de Kroon and Jansen 2006; Word et al. 1958; Bonavolonta et al. 1994). Complications during hysteroscopic polyp resection are most often related to fluid overload or hyponatremia, or are encountered during cervical dilatation (Bonavolonta et al. 1994; Cravello et al. 2000). Complications during cervical dilatation occur mainly in nulliparous or postmenopausal women and include cervical tears, creation of false passages and uterine perforation. However, the risk of complications during dilatation may be reduced by ensuring adequate preoperative cervical priming (Bonavolonta et al. 1994; Gebauer et al. 2001).

Despite the widespread use of TCRP, the efficacy of the procedure has been scarcely evaluated (Preutthipan and Herabutya 2005). The results of previous studies indicate that the procedure is effective in terms of relieving symptoms (de Kroon and Jansen 2006; Gimpelson and Rappold 1988; Clark et al. 2002). The effect appears to be better in women suffering from intermenstrual bleedings/spotting compared to women with heavy bleeding (Lieng et al. 2010a). However, the risk of persistence or recurrence of AUB in premenopausal women after treatment appears to be relatively high (Bettocchi et al. 2004b; Propst et al. 2000).

Hysterectomy is a major procedure and is nowadays considered too comprehensive for the treatment of isolated benign intrauterine lesions. Hysterectomy is consequently confined to polyps with premalignant or malignant changes. If histological evaluation following TCRP reveals atypical complex hyperplasia or carcinoma in endometrial polyps, a subsequent hysterectomy should be performed, even if the malignant or premalignant tissue changes appear confined to the polyp in the initial sampling (Bradley 2002).

The large range of prevalence of premalignant and/or malignant tissue changes within endometrial polyps as well as the scarcity of evidence supporting transcervical resection of polyps in order to relieve symptoms or improve fertility outcomes limits the strength of clinical recommendations. Although TCRP is a relatively safe procedure with a low risk of major complications, it should be performed on indication in order to reduce both surgical-related morbidity and costs. An individual approach is mandatory in the management of women with endometrial polyps and the woman's opinion regarding treatment or not also has to be taken into account. An expectant approach may be reasonable in asymptomatic premenopausal women, as the malignant potential appears to be low. In infertile women, resection of endometrial polyps appears to improve fertility outcome. Premenopausal women with endometrial polyps suffering from intermenstrual bleedings seem to have a favourable outcome of TCRP in terms of symptom relief. However, removal of endometrial polyps in women suffering from heavy bleeding appears to be less effective, and appropriate additional treatment such as the levonorgesterel intrauterine device or a concomitant endometrial resection in order to reduce periodic blood loss should be considered. In asymptomatic postmenopausal women, treatment needs to be individualised based on polyp size, malignancy risk indicators, general condition as well as women's concerns regarding malignancy. If the woman wants to have malignancy ruled out by histopathological examination, if the polyp is large or if other risk indicators for malignancy such as use of tamoxifen or obesity are present, TCRP should be recommended. Symptomatic postmenopausal women carry the highest risk of malignancy and should consequently have the polyp resected for curative as well as diagnostic reasons (Lieng et al. 2010b; Abbott et al. 2012).

References

Abbott J, Jansen FW, Lieng M, Tulandi T (2012) AAGL practice report: practice guidelines for the diagnosis and management of endometrial polyps. J Minim Invasive Gynecol 19:3–10

Akkad AA, Habiba MA, Ismail N, Abrams K, Al-Azzawi F (1995) Abnormal uterine bleeding on hormone replacement: the importance of intrauterine structural abnormalities. Obstet Gynecol 86:330–334

Aleem F, Predanic M, Calame R, Moukhtar M, Pennisi J (1995) Transvaginal color and pulsed Doppler sonography of the endometrium: a possible role in reducing the number of dilatation and curettage procedures. J Ultrasound Med 14:139–145

Anastasiadis PG, Koutlaki NG, Skaphida PG, Galazios GC, Tsikouras PN, Liberis VA (2000) Endometrial polyps: prevalence, detection, and malignant potential in women with abnormal uterine bleeding. Eur J Gynaecol Oncol 21:180–183

Antunes A Jr, Costa-Paiva L, Arthuso M, Costa JV, Pinto-Neto AM (2007) Endometrial polyps in pre- and postmenopausal women: factors associated with malignancy. Maturitas 57:415–421

Bakour SH, Khan KS, Gupta JK (2000) The risk of premalignant and malignant pathology in endometrial polyps. Acta Obstet Gynecol Scand 79:317–320

Bakour SH, Gupta JK, Khan KS (2002) Risk factors associated with endometrial polyps in abnormal uterine bleeding. Int J Gynaecol Obstet 76:165–168

Ben-Arie A, Goldchmit C, Laviv Y et al (2004) The malignant potential of endometrial polyps. Eur J Obstet Gynecol Reprod Biol 115:206–210

Bernstein L, Deapen D, Cerhan JR et al (1999) Tamoxifen therapy for breast cancer and endometrial cancer risk. J Natl Cancer Inst 91:1654–1662

Bettocchi S, Nappi L, Ceci O, Selvaggi L (2004a) Office hysteroscopy. Obstet Gynecol Clin North Am 31: 641–654

Bettocchi S, Ceci O, Nappi L, Di VR, Masciopinto V, Pansini V et al (2004b) Operative office hysteroscopy without anesthesia: analysis of 4863 cases performed with mechanical instruments. J Am Assoc Gynecol Laparosc 11:59–61

Bokor D, Chambers JB, Rees PJ, Mant TG, Luzzani F, Spinazzi A (2001) Clinical safety of SonoVue, a new contrast agent for ultrasound imaging, in healthy volunteers and in patients with chronic obstructive pulmonary disease. Invest Radiol 36:104–109

Bol S, Wanschura S, Thode B et al (1996) An endometrial polyp with a rearrangement of HMGI-C underlying a complex cytogenetic rearrangement involving chromosomes 2 and 12. Cancer Genet Cytogenet 90:88–90

Bonavolonta G, Rossetti A, Cannella PL, Campo S, Garcea N (1994) Curettage vs. hysteroscopic resection. Minerva Ginecol 46:1–3

Bradley LD (2002) Complications in hysteroscopy: prevention, treatment and legal risk. Curr Opin Obstet Gynecol 14:409–415

Carter J, Saltzman A, Hartenbach E, Fowler J, Carson L, Twiggs LB (1994) Flow characteristics in benign and malignant gynecologic tumors using transvaginal color flow Doppler. Obstet Gynecol 83:125–130

Chalas E, Costantino JP, Wickerham DL, Wolmark N, Lewis GC, Bergman C et al (2005) Benign gynecologic conditions among participants in the Breast Cancer Prevention Trial. Am J Obstet Gynecol 192: 1230–1237

Chavez NF, Garner EO, Khan W et al (2002) Does the introduction of new technology change population demographics? Minimally invasive technologies and endometrial polyps. Gynecol Obstet Invest 54:217–220

Clark TJ, Khan KS, Gupta JK (2002) Current practice for the treatment of benign intrauterine polyps: a national questionnaire survey of consultant gynaecologists in UK. Eur J Obstet Gynecol Reprod Biol 103:65–67

Clevenger-Hoeft M, Syrop CH, Stovall DW, Van Voorhis BJ (1999) Sonohysterography in premenopausal women with and without abnormal bleeding. Obstet Gynecol 94:516–520

Coeman D, Van BY, Vanderick G, De Muylder X, De Muylder E, Campo R (1993) Hysteroscopic findings in patients with a cervical polyp. Am J Obstet Gynecol 169:1563–1565

Cohen I (2004) Endometrial pathologies associated with postmenopausal tamoxifen treatment. Gynecol Oncol 94:256–266

Cooper JM, Houck RM, Rigberg HS (1983) The incidence of intrauterine abnormalities found at hysteroscopy in patients undergoing elective hysteroscopic sterilization. J Reprod Med 28:659–661

Cravello L, Stolla V, Bretelle F, Roger V, Blanc B (2000) Hysteroscopic resection of endometrial polyps: a study of 195 cases. Eur J Obstet Gynecol Reprod Biol 93:131–134

Dahmoun M, Boman K, Cajander S, Westin P, Backstrom T (1999) Apoptosis, proliferation, and sex hormone receptors in superficial parts of human endometrium at the end of the secretory phase. J Clin Endocrinol Metab 84:1737–1743

de Kroon CD, Jansen FW (2006) Saline infusion sonography in women with abnormal uterine bleeding: an update of recent findings. Curr Opin Obstet Gynecol 18:653–657

de Kroon CD, de Bock GH, Dieben SW, Jansen FW (2003) Saline contrast hysterosonography in abnormal uterine bleeding: a systematic review and meta-analysis. Br J Obstet Gynaecol 110:938–947

De Muylder X, Neven P, De Somer M, Van Belle Y, Vanderick G, De Muylder E (1991) Endometrial lesions in patients undergoing tamoxifen therapy. Int J Gynaecol Obstet 36:127–130

DeWaay DJ, Syrop CH, Nygaard IE, Davis WA, Van Voorhis BJ (2002) Natural history of uterine polyps and leiomyomata. Obstet Gynecol 100:3–7

Dijkhuizen FP, Brolmann HA, Potters AE, Bongers MY, Heinz AP (1996) The accuracy of transvaginal ultrasonography in the diagnosis of endometrial abnormalities. Obstet Gynecol 87:345–349

Dijkhuizen FP, De Vries LD, Mol BW et al (2000) Comparison of transvaginal ultrasonography and saline infusion sonography for the detection of intracavitary abnormalities in premenopausal women. Ultrasound Obstet Gynecol 15:372–376

Dreisler E, Stampe SS, Ibsen PH, Lose G (2009a) Prevalence of endometrial polyps and abnormal uterine bleeding in a Danish population aged 20–74 years. Ultrasound Obstet Gynecol 33:102–108

Dreisler E, Sorensen SS, Lose G (2009b) Endometrial polyps and associated factors in Danish women aged 36–74 years. Am J Obstet Gynecol 200:147.e1–6

Dreisler E, Sorensen SS, Ibsen PH, Lose G (2009c) Value of endometrial thickness measurement for diagnosing focal intrauterine pathology in women without abnormal uterine bleeding. Ultrasound Obstet Gynecol 33:344–348

Dueholm M, Jensen ML, Laursen H, Kracht P (2001) Can the endometrial thickness as measured by transvaginal sonography be used to exclude polyps or hyperplasia in pre-menopausal patients with abnormal uterine bleeding? Acta Obstet Gynecol Scand 80:645–651

Elliott J, Connor ME, Lashen H (2003) The value of outpatient hysteroscopy in diagnosing endometrial pathology in postmenopausal women with and without hormone replacement therapy. Acta Obstet Gynecol Scand 82:1112–1119

Elpek G, Uner M, Elpek GO, Sedele M, Karaveli S (1998) The diagnostic accuracy of the Pipelle endometrial sampler in the presence of endometrial polyps. J Obstet Gynaecol 18:274–275

Englund S, Ingelman-Sundberg A, Westin B (1957) Hysteroscopy in diagnosis and treatment of uterine bleeding. Gynaecologia 143:217–222

Epstein E, Ramirez A, Skoog L, Valentin L (2001) Transvaginal sonography, saline contrast sonohysterography and hysteroscopy for the investigation of women with postmenopausal bleeding and endometrium>5 mm. Ultrasound Obstet Gynecol 18:157–162

Exalto N, Stappers C, van Raamsdonk LA, Emanuel MH (2007) Gel instillation sonohysterography: first experience with a new technique. Fertil Steril 87:152–155

Farrell R, Scurry J, Otton G, Hacker NF (2005) Clinicopathologic review of malignant polyps in stage 1A carcinoma of the endometrium. Gynecol Oncol 98:254–262

Fay TN, Khanem N, Hosking D (1999) Out-patient hysteroscopy in asymptomatic postmenopausal women. Climacteric 2:263–267

Fernandez-Parra J, Rodriguez OA, Lopez CS, Parrilla FF, Montoya VF (2006) Hysteroscopic evaluation of endometrial polyps. Int J Gynaecol Obstet 95:144–148

Ferrazzi E, Zupi E, Leone FP et al (2009) How often are endometrial polyps malignant in asymptomatic postmenopausal women? A multicenter study. Am J Obstet Gynecol 200:235–236

Fleischer AC, Shappell HW (2003) Color Doppler sonohysterography of endometrial polyps and submucosal fibroids. J Ultrasound Med 22:601–604

Frydman R, Eibschitz I, Fernandez H, Hamou J (1987) Uterine evaluation by microhysteroscopy in IVF candidates. Hum Reprod 2:481–485

Gardner FJ, Konje JC, Abrams KR et al (2000) Endometrial protection from tamoxifen-stimulated changes by a levonorgestrel-releasing intrauterine system: a randomised controlled trial. Lancet 356:1711–1717

Gebauer G, Hafner A, Siebzehnrubl E, Lang N (2001) Role of hysteroscopy in detection and extraction of endometrial polyps: results of a prospective study. Am J Obstet Gynecol 184:59–63

Gimpelson RJ, Rappold HO (1988) A comparative study between panoramic hysteroscopy with directed biopsies and dilatation and curettage. A review of 276 cases. Am J Obstet Gynecol 158:489–492

Giordano G, Gnetti L, Merisio C, Melpignano M (2007) Postmenopausal status, hypertension and obesity as risk factors for malignant transformation in endometrial polyps. Maturitas 56:190–197

Goldstein SR, Zeltser I, Horan CK, Snyder JR, Schwartz LB (1997) Ultrasonography-based triage for perimenopausal patients with abnormal uterine bleeding. Am J Obstet Gynecol 177:102–108

Gupta JK, Chien PF, Voit D, Clark TJ, Khan KS (2002) Ultrasonographic endometrial thickness for diagnosing endometrial pathology in women with postmenopausal bleeding: a meta-analysis. Acta Obstet Gynecol Scand 81:799–816

Guven MA, Bese T, Demirkiran F (2004) Comparison of hydrosonography and transvaginal ultrasonography in the detection of intracavitary pathologies in women with abnormal uterine bleeding. Int J Gynecol Cancer 14:57–63

Hann LE, Kim CM, Gonen M, Barakat R, Choi PH, Bach AM (2003) Sonohysterography compared with endometrial biopsy for evaluation of the endometrium in tamoxifen-treated women. J Ultrasound Med 22:1173–1179

Hinckley MD, Milki AA (2004) 1000 office-based hysteroscopies prior to in vitro fertilization: feasibility and findings. JSLS 8:103–107

Iatrakis G, Zervoudis S, Antoniou E, Tsionis C, Pavlou A, Kourounis G et al (2006) Is dosage of hormone replacement therapy related with endometrial polyp formation? Eur J Gynaecol Oncol 27:393–394

Inceboz US, Nese N, Uyar Y et al (2006) Hormone receptor expressions and proliferation markers in postmenopausal endometrial polyps. Gynecol Obstet Invest 61:24–28

Isikoglu M, Berkkanoglu M, Senturk Z, Coetzee K, Ozgur K (2006) Endometrial polyps smaller than 1.5 cm do not affect ICSI outcome. Reprod Biomed Online 12:199–204

Jakab A, Ovari L, Juhasz B, Birinyi L, Bacsko G, Toth Z (2005) Detection of feeding artery improves the ultrasound diagnosis of endometrial polyps in asymptomatic patients. Eur J Obstet Gynecol Reprod Biol 119:103–107

Jansen FW, de Kroon CD, van Dongen H, Grooters C, Louwe L, Trimbos-Kemper T (2006) Diagnostic hysteroscopy and saline infusion sonography: prediction of intrauterine polyps and myomas. J Minim Invasive Gynecol 13:320–324

Kedar RP, Bourne TH, Powles TJ, Collins WP, Ashley SE, Cosgrove DO et al (1994) Effects of tamoxifen on uterus and ovaries of postmenopausal women in a randomised breast cancer prevention trial. Lancet 343:1318–1321

Kim MR, Kim YA, Jo MY, Hwang KJ, Ryu HS (2003) High frequency of endometrial polyps in endometriosis. J Am Assoc Gynecol Laparosc 10:46–48

Krampl E, Bourne T, Hurlen-Solbakken H, Istre O (2001) Transvaginal ultrasonography sonohysterography and operative hysteroscopy for the evaluation of abnormal uterine bleeding. Acta Obstet Gynecol Scand 80:616–622

Kurman RJ (1982) Benign diseases of the endometrium. In: Blaustein A (ed) Pathology of the female genital tract, 2nd edn. Springer, New York/Heidelberg/Berlin, pp 279–310

Lass A, Williams G, Abusheikha N, Brinsden P (1999) The effect of endometrial polyps on outcomes of in vitro fertilization (IVF) cycles. J Assist Reprod Genet 16:410–415

Lieng M, Qvigstad E, Sandvik L, Jørgensen H, Langebrekke A, Istre O (2007) Hysteroscopic resection of symptomatic and asymptomatic endometrial polyps. J Minim Invasive Gynecol 14(2):189–194

Lieng M, Qvigstad E, Dahl GF, Istre O (2008) Flow differences between endometrial polyps and endometrial cancer: a prospective study using contrasted transvaginal color flow Doppler and three-dimensional power Doppler. Ultrasound Obstet Gynecol 32:935–940

Lieng M, Istre O, Sandvik L, Qvigstad E (2009) Prevalence, 1-year regression rate, and clinical significance of asymptomatic endometrial polyps: a cross-sectional study. J Minim Invasive Gynecol 16(4):465–471

Lieng M, Istre O, Sandvik L, Engh V, Qvigstad E (2010a) Clinical effectiveness of transcervical polyp resection in women with endometrial polyps: a randomised controlled trial. J Minim Invasive Gynecol 17:351–357

Lieng M, Istre O, Qvigstad E (2010b) Treatment of endometrial polyps A systematic review. Acta Obstet Gynecol Scand 89:992–1002

Lopes RG, Baracat EC, de Albuquerque Neto LC et al (2007) Analysis of estrogen- and progesterone-receptor expression in endometrial polyps. J Minim Invasive Gynecol 14:300–303

Machtinger R, Korach J, Padoa A et al (2005) Transvaginal ultrasound and diagnostic hysteroscopy as a predictor of endometrial polyps: risk factors for premalignancy and malignancy. Int J Gynecol Cancer 15:325–328

Maia H Jr, Barbosa IC, Marques D, Calmon LC, Ladipo OA, Coutinho EM (1996) Hysteroscopy and transvaginal sonography in menopausal women receiving hormone replacement therapy. J Am Assoc Gynecol Laparosc 4:13–18

Maia H, Maltez A, Athayde C, Coutinho EM (2001) Proliferation profile of endometrial polyps in postmenopausal women. Maturitas 40:273–281

Maia H Jr, Maltez A, Studart E, Athayde C, Coutinho EM (2004a) Ki-67, Bcl-2 and p53 expression in endometrial polyps and in the normal endometrium during the menstrual cycle. BJOG 111:1242–1247

Maia H Jr, Maltez A, Studard E, Athayde C, Coutinho EM (2004b) Effect of previous hormone replacement therapy on endometrial polyps during menopause. Gynecol Endocrinol 18:299–304

Mazur MT, Kurman RJ (2005) Polyps. In: Mazur MT, Kurman RJ (eds) Diagnosis of endometrial biopsies and curettings. A practical approach, 2nd edn. Springer Science and Business Media Inc., New York, pp 163–177

McBean JH, Gibson M, Brumsted JR (1996) The association of intrauterine filling defects on hysterosalpingogram with endometriosis. Fertil Steril 66:522–526

McGurgan P, Taylor LJ, Duffy SR, O'Donovan PJ (2006a) Are endometrial polyps from premenopausal women similar to post-menopausal women? An immunohistochemical comparison of endometrial polyps from pre- and post-menopausal women. Maturitas 54:277–284

McGurgan P, Taylor LJ, Duffy SR, O'Donovan PJ (2006b) Does tamoxifen therapy affect the hormone receptor expression and cell proliferation indices of endometrial polyps? An immunohistochemical comparison of endometrial polyps from postmenopausal women exposed and not exposed to tamoxifen. Maturitas 54:252–259

Merce LT, Alcazar JL, Lopez C, Iglesias E et al (2007) Clinical usefulness of 3-dimensional sonography and power Doppler angiography for diagnosis of endometrial carcinoma. J Ultrasound Med 26:1279–1287

Mertens HJ, Heineman MJ, Evers JL (2002) The expression of apoptosis-related proteins Bcl-2 and Ki67 in endometrium of ovulatory menstrual cycles. Gynecol Obstet Invest 53:224–230

Mittal K, Schwartz L, Goswami S, Demopoulos R (1996) Estrogen and progesterone receptor expression in endometrial polyps. Int J Gynecol Pathol 15:345–348

Mutter GL, Nucci MR, Robboy SJ (2009) Endometritis, metaplasias, polyps and miscellaneous changes. In: Robboy SJ, Mutter GL, Prat J, Bentley RC, Russell P, Anderson MC (eds) Robboy's pathology of the female reproductive tract, 2nd edn. Churchill Livingstone Elsevier, Edinburgh, pp 343–366

Nappi L, Indraccolo U, Di Spiezio SA, Gentile G, Palombino K, Castaldi MA et al (2009) Are diabetes, hypertension, and obesity independent risk factors for endometrial polyps? J Minim Invasive Gynecol 16:157–162

Nogueira AA, Sant'Ana de Almeida EC, Poli Neto OB, Zambelli Ramalho LN, Rosa e Silva JC, Candido dos Reis FJ (2006) Immunohistochemical expression of p63 in endometrial polyps: evidence that a basal cell immunophenotype is maintained. Menopause 13:826–830

Oguz S, Sargin A, Kelekci S, Aytan H, Tapisiz OL, Mollamahmutoglu L (2005) The role of hormone replacement therapy in endometrial polyp formation. Maturitas 50:231–236

Onalan R, Onalan G, Tonguc E, Ozdener T, Dogan M, Mollamahmutoglu L (2009) Body mass index is an independent risk factor for the development of endometrial polyps in patients undergoing in vitro fertilization. Fertil Steril 91:1056–1060

Orvieto R, Bar-Hava I, Dicker D, Bar J, Ben-Rafael Z, Neri A (1999) Endometrial polyps during menopause: characterization and significance. Acta Obstet Gynecol Scand 78:883–886

Papadia A, Gerbaldo D, Fulcheri E et al (2007) The risk of premalignant and malignant pathology in endometrial polyps: should every polyp be resected? Minerva Ginecol 59:117–124

Parsons AK, Lense JJ (1993) Sonohysterography for endometrial abnormalities: preliminary results. J Clin Ultrasound 21:87–95

Pasqualotto EB, Margossian H, Price LL, Bradley LD (2000) Accuracy of preoperative diagnostic tools and outcome of hysteroscopic management of menstrual dysfunction. J Am Assoc Gynecol Laparosc 7:201–209

Perez-Medina T, Bajo J, Huertas MA, Rubio A (2002) Predicting atypia inside endometrial polyps. J Ultrasound Med 21:125–128

Perez-Medina T, Bajo-Arenas J, Haya J et al (2003) Tibolone and risk of endometrial polyps: a prospective, comparative study with hormone therapy. Menopause 10:534–537

Perez-Medina T, Bajo-Arenas J, Salazar F et al (2005) Endometrial polyps and their implication in the pregnancy rates of patients undergoing intrauterine insemination: a prospective, randomized study. Hum Reprod 20:1632–1635

Perrone G, DeAngelis C, Critelli C, Capri O, Galoppi P, Santoro G et al (2002) Hysteroscopic findings in postmenopausal abnormal uterine bleeding: a comparison between HRT users and non-users. Maturitas 43:251–255

Peterson WF, Novak ER (1956) Endometrial polyps. Obstet Gynecol 8:40–49

Preutthipan S, Herabutya Y (2005) Hysteroscopic polypectomy in 240 premenopausal and postmenopausal women. Fertil Steril 83:705–709

Propst AM, Liberman RF, Harlow BL, Ginsburg ES (2000) Complications of hysteroscopic surgery: predicting patients at risk. Obstet Gynecol 96:517–520

Raine-Fenning NJ, Campbell BK, Clewes JS, Kendall NR, Johnson IR (2003) The reliability of virtual organ computer-aided analysis (VOCAL) for the semiquantification of ovarian, endometrial and subendometrial perfusion. Ultrasound Obstet Gynecol 22:633–639

Reslova T, Tosner J, Resl M, Kugler R, Vavrova I (1999) Endometrial polyps. A clinical study of 245 cases. Arch Gynecol Obstet 262:133–139

Ryan GL, Syrop CH, Van Voorhis BJ (2005) Role, epidemiology, and natural history of benign uterine mass lesions. Clin Obstet Gynecol 48:312–324

Sant'Ana de Almeida EC, Nogueira AA, Candido dos Reis FJ, Zambelli Ramalho LN, Zucoloto S (2004) Immunohistochemical expression of estrogen and progesterone receptors in endometrial polyps and adjacent endometrium in postmenopausal women. Maturitas 49:229–233

Savelli L, De IP, Santini D, Rosati F, Ghi T, Pignotti E et al (2003) Histopathologic features and risk factors for benignity, hyperplasia, and cancer in endometrial polyps. Am J Obstet Gynecol 188:927–931

Schlaen I, Bergeron C, Ferenczy A, Wong P, Naves A, Bertoli R (1988) Endometrial polyps: a study of 204 cases. Surg Pathol 262:133–139

Schwarzler P, Concin H, Bosch H, Berlinger A, Wohlgenannt K, Collins WP et al (1998) An evaluation of sonohysterography and diagnostic hysteroscopy for the assessment of intrauterine pathology. Ultrasound Obstet Gynecol 11:337–342

Seinera P, Maccario S, Visentin L, DiGregorio A (1988) Hysteroscopy in an IVF-ER program. Clinical experience with 360 infertile patients. Acta Obstet Gynecol Scand 67:135–137

Shushan A, Revel A, Rojansky N (2004) How often are endometrial polyps malignant? Gynecol Obstet Invest 58:212–215

Sidhu PS, Allan PL, Cattin F et al (2006) Diagnostic efficacy of SonoVue, a second generation contrast agent, in the assessment of extracranial carotid or peripheral arteries using colour and spectral Doppler ultrasound: a multicentre study. Br J Radiol 79:44–51

Smith JJ, Schulman H (1985) Current dilatation and curettage practice: a need for revision. Obstet Gynecol 65:516–518

Stewart CJ, Campbell-Brown M, Critchley HO, Farquharson MA (1999) Endometrial apoptosis in patients with dysfunctional uterine bleeding. Histopathology 34:99–105

Svirsky R, Smorgick N, Rozowski U et al (2008) Can we rely on blind endometrial biopsy for detection of focal intrauterine pathology? Am J Obstet Gynecol 199:115.e1–3

Syrop CH, Sahakian V (1992) Transvaginal sonographic detection of endometrial polyps with fluid contrast augmentation. Obstet Gynecol 79:1041–1043

Tanriverdi HA, Barut A, Gun BD, Kaya E (2004) Is pipelle biopsy really adequate for diagnosing endometrial disease? Med Sci Monit 10:CR271–CR274

Taylor LJ, Jackson TL, Reid JG, Duffy SR (2003) The differential expression of oestrogen receptors, progesterone receptors, Bcl-2 and Ki67 in endometrial polyps. Br J Obstet Gynaecol 110:794–798

Testa AC, Ferrandina G, Fruscella E et al (2005) The use of contrasted transvaginal sonography in the diagnosis of gynecologic diseases: a preliminary study. J Ultrasound Med 24:1267–1278

Timmerman D, Verguts J, Konstantinovic ML et al (2003) The pedicle artery sign based on sonography with color Doppler imaging can replace second-stage tests in women with abnormal vaginal bleeding. Ultrasound Obstet Gynecol 22:166–171

Timmermans A, Gerritse MB, Opmeer BC, Jansen FW, Mol BW, Veersema S (2008) Diagnostic accuracy of endometrial thickness to exclude polyps in women with postmenopausal bleeding. J Clin Ultrasound 36:286–290

van Bogaert LJ (1988) Clinicopathologic findings in endometrial polyps. Obstet Gynecol 71:771–773

Vanni R, Dal CP, Marras S, Moerman P, Andria M, Valdes E et al (1993) Endometrial polyp: another benign tumor characterized by 12q13-q15 changes. Cancer Genet Cytogenet 68:32–33

van Roessel J, Wamsteker K, Exalto N (1987) Sonographic investigation of the uterus during artificial uterine cavity distention. J Clin Ultrasound 15:439–450

Varasteh NN, Neuwirth RS, Levin B, Keltz MD (1999) Pregnancy rates after hysteroscopic polypectomy and myomectomy in infertile women. Obstet Gynecol 94:168–171

Vercellini P, Cortesi I, Oldani S, Moschetta M, De GO, Crosignani PG (1997) The role of transvaginal ultrasonography and outpatient diagnostic hysteroscopy in the evaluation of patients with menorrhagia. Hum Reprod 12:1768–1771

Vilodre LC, Bertat R, Petters R, Reis FM (1997) Cervical polyp as risk factor for hysteroscopically diagnosed endometrial polyps. Gynecol Obstet Invest 44:191–195

Widrich T, Bradley LD, Mitchinson AR, Collins RL (1996) Comparison of saline infusion sonography with office hysteroscopy for the evaluation of the endometrium. Am J Obstet Gynecol 174:1327–1334

Word B, Gravelee LC, Wideman GL (1958) The fallacy of simple uterine curettage. Obstet Gynecol 12:642–648

J.A.F. Huirne, M. BijdeVaate, L. Van der Voet,
M. Witmer, and H.A.M. Brölmann

Contents

J.A.F. Huirne (✉) • M. BijdeVaate • M. Witmer
H.A.M. Brölmann
Department Obstetrics and Gynaecology, VUMC,
Amsterdam, The Netherlands
e-mail: j.huirne@vumc.nl; huirne@planet.nl

L. Van der Voet
Department Obstetrics and Gynaecology,
Deventer Ziekenhuis, Deventer, The Netherlands

7.1   Introduction and Nomenclature

Incomplete healing of caesarean section (CS) scars may be associated with complications in later pregnancies, such as uterine rupture, abnormal adherent placenta. The first publications on CS scar defects in relation to bleeding symptoms date from 1975 (Stewart and Evans 1975). However, the relation of such defects with gynecological symptoms in non-pregnant state such as postmenstrual bleeding has only recently been proven in prospective cohort studies in a unselected population of women with a history of CS (BijdeVaate et al. 2011). Since then the number of publications describing CS scar defects is increasing. Different terminology in the assessment of CS scars has been used (Naji et al. 2012a). A hypoechoic triangular area at the site of previous CS scars observed using ultrasonography has been given the term "niche" (Fig. 7.1).

However, more shapes have been described (Figs. 7.2 and 7.3). A generally accepted definition for a niche is still under debate. Alternative terms for a niche are caesarean scar defect (Armstrong et al. 2003; Vikhareva Osser et al. 2009; Wang et al. 2009), deficient caesarean scar (Ofili-Yebovi et al. 2008), diverticulum (Surapaneni and Silberzweig 2008), pouch (Fabres et al. 2003), and isthmocele (Borges et al. 2010). Some of these terms are unfortunate as

O. Istre (ed.), *Minimally Invasive Gynecological Surgery*,
DOI 10.1007/978-3-662-44059-9_7, © Springer-Verlag Berlin Heidelberg 2015

they imply a relationship between the appearance of the niche and function, particularly in any future pregnancy. Until now there is no evidence yet to underline a relation with the appearance of the CS and its function. In this chapter, we will use the term "niche."

7.2 Prevalence of Niches and Diagnostic Methods

Various methods to detect and measure a niche have been described. In earlier publications, it was observed during hystesterosalpingraphy (Surapaneni and Silberzweig 2008). However, this method may be considered as less imprecise for

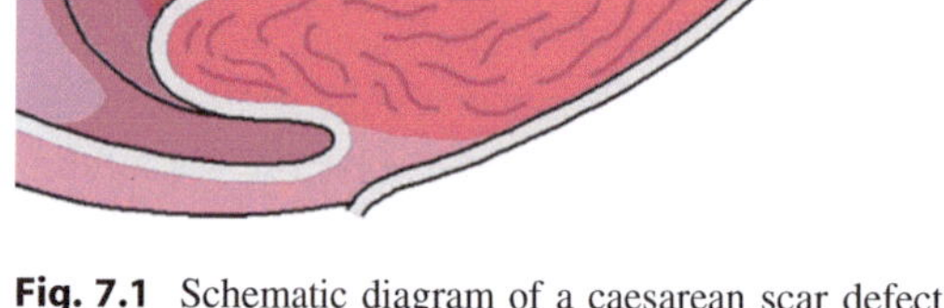

Fig. 7.1 Schematic diagram of a caesarean scar defect, also known as a niche

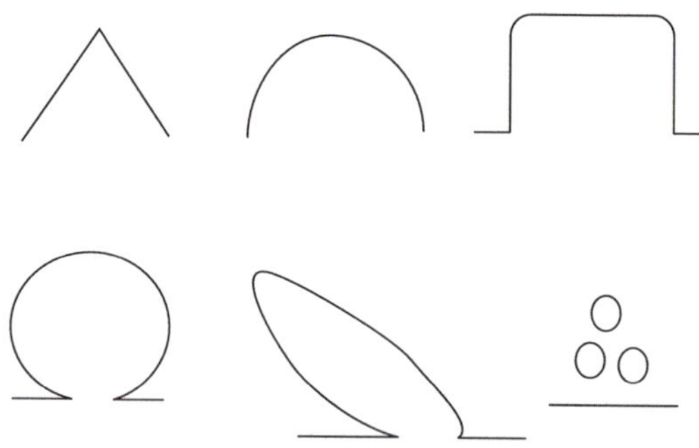

Fig. 7.3 Niche shape. Schematic diagram demonstrating classification used to assess niche shape: triangle, semi-circle, rectangle, circle, droplet and inclusion cysts (Published in Bij de Vaate et al. 2011)

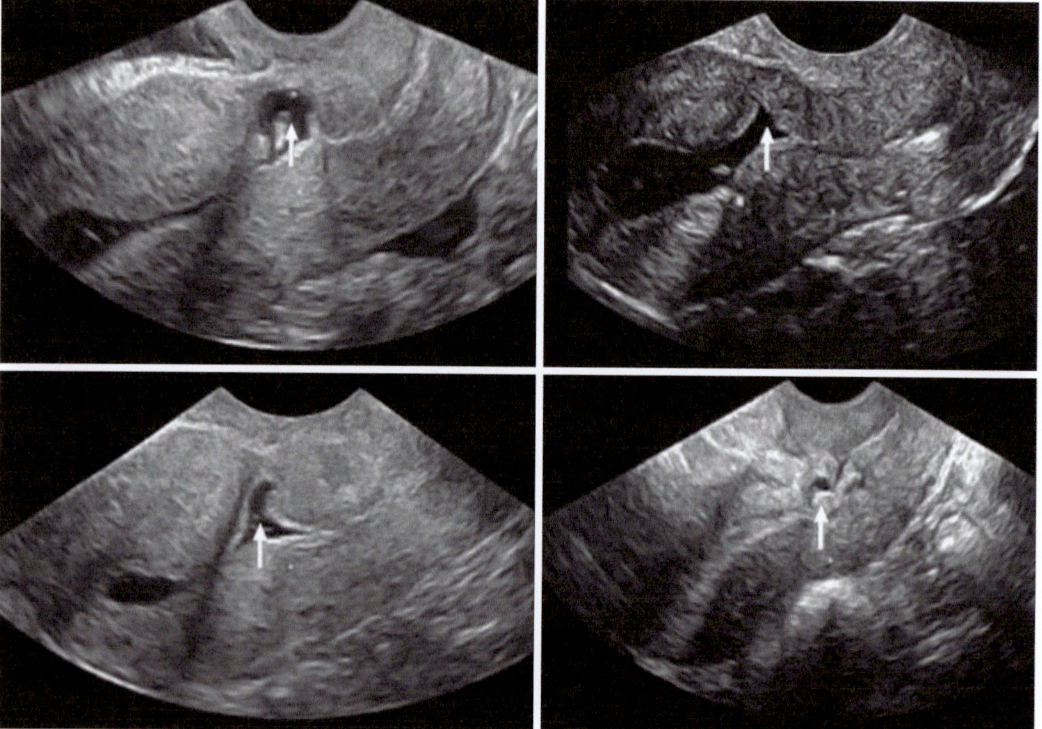

Fig. 7.2 Different niches on sonohysterography (Published in Bij de Vaate et al. 2011)

this objective and small niches may be missed. The most applied techniques are transvaginal sonography (TVS) (BijdeVaate et al. 2011; Vikhareva Osser et al. 2009; Armstrong et al. 2003) and sono-hysterography (SHG) (BijdeVaate et al. 2011; Vikhareva Osser et al. 2009; Regnard et al. 2004; Valenzano et al. 2006). The latter technique is proposed to be more accurate due to improved delineation of the borders of a niche in comparison with TVS (Vikhareva Osser 2010a). This is underlined by a larger proportion of patients with a niche after SHG in comparison to TVS. BijdeVaate et al. (2011) observed in 56 % of women a niche using SHG compared to 24 % using TVS 6–12 months after a CS in a prospective cohort study. This is in line with an other prospective cohort study, studying niches in women after a CS, reporting a niche in 84 % of women using SHG compared to 70 % using TVS (Vikhareva Osser 2010a). Using SHG, the prevalence of niches in relatively unselected women after CS varies between 56 and 84 % (BijdeVaate et al. 2011; Regnard et al. 2004; Valenzano 2006; Vikhareva Osser 2010a). Reported prevalence of niches in women after CS using hysteroscopy varies between 31 and 88 % (Borges et al. 2010; El-Mazny et al. 2011). Besides the applied diagnostic methods, the prevalence of niches is highly dependent on the population, the awareness of the observers and of course the applied definitions. Until now there is no agreement about the gold standard for the detection and measurement of a niche. Higher prevalence is expected in women undergoing examination because of symptoms such as bleeding disorders or fertility problems. CS scar assessment during pregnancy is a different topic and requires other techniques and definitions since a SHG is not possible to apply. Naji et al. studied CS scars during pregnancy using TVS and was able to detect CS scars with low inter- and intra-observer variability (Naji et al. 2012b).

7.3 Niche Shapes

Various niche shapes have been described using sonography (see Figs. 7.2 and 7.3). Most studies report on a triangular shape (Vikhareva Osser et al. 2009; Chen et al. 1990). Using sonohysterography, the semicircular and triangular shapes were reported to be most prominent (BijdeVaate et al. 2011). Another reported classification based on the direction of the external surface is inward protrusion (internal surface bulging toward the bladder), outward protrusion (external surface bulging toward the bladder) or inward retraction (external surface of the scar dimpling toward the myometrial layer). (Chen et al. 1990).

7.4 Predisposing Factors for Niches

As not all women with a history of CS develop a niche, it is a subject of interest to identify the risk factors for the development of a niche. Several publications tried to elucidate the main risk factors, however, most individual publications are of insufficient power to study all relevant risk factors. Different diagnostic methods were used to identify niches in a selected population of women with gynaecological symtoms and used definitions were not uniform and often not clearly defined. So far only two studies have studied risk factors in an unselected population after a CS (Armstrong et al. 2003; Vikhareva Osser 2010a). Three other studies were performed in a population of women who were assessed for a variety of gynecological symptoms (Monteagudo 2001; Wang et al. 2009; Ofili-Yebovi et al. 2008).

Cervical dilatation and station of the presenting fetal part below pelvic inlet at the time of CS were the only predictive factors in one prospective study including patients with only one previous CS using TVS or SHG (Vikhareva Osser 2010, 2). Prolonged labor and multiple caesarean sections were identified as risk factors for niches in an unselected population using TVS (Armstrong et al. 2003). Using TVS, multiple caesarean sections were also identified as predisposing factor for niches (Ofili-Yebovi et al. 2008) and for larger niches (Wang et al. 2009). Uterine retroflexion was also associated with niches Moeten er geen referenties bij aangezien er staat 'several'? (Vikhareva Osser et al. 2009) However, it is not clear if the retroflected position is a predisposing factor for the development of a niche or that retroflexion is caused by insufficient CS scar healing. Suturing technique should be considered as a predisposing factor as well. There are two small randomized trials and one prospective trial studying the effect of the suturing technique on the prevalence of a niche using ultrasound 4–6 weeks after the CS (Hayakawa et al. 2006; Hamar et al. 2007; Yazicioglu et al. 2006). There was no difference in myometrial thickness between one-layer or two-layer closure (Hamar et al. 2007), but there were less niches identified after double-layer closure compared to single layer (Hayakawa et al. 2006) or to split-level closure without inclusion of the endometrial layer (Yazicioglu et al. 2006).

7.5 Related Symptoms

Several complications of a scar defect have been reported, including niche pregnancies (BijdeVaate et al. 2010), malplacentation (Naji et al. 2013a), and perforated intrauterine devices (Voet et al. 2009). Recently, it has been shown that the thickness of the residual myometrium is an independent prognostic factor for success rate after trial of labor (Naji et al. 2013). However, the exact risk of niches on uterine ruptures has to be elucidated.

The relation between a niche and gynecological symptoms in non-pregnant patients has been acknowledged only recently. An association between a niche and prolonged menstrual bleeding and postmenstrual spotting has been reported in several studies (BijdeVaate et al. 2011; Fabres et al. 2003; Regnard et al. 2004; Thurmond et al. 1999; Wang et al. 2009; Borges et al. 2010). A niche is observed in almost 60 % of all women after a CS. The incidence of postmenstrual spotting is higher in these patients compared to those without a niche (OR 3.1 [95 % CI, 1.5–6.3]) (BijdeVaate et al. 2011). An association between the size of the niche and postmenstrual spotting is reported in three studies (Wang et al. 2009; Bij de Vaate et al. 2011; Uppal et al. 2011). Whilst a larger niche volume was demonstrated in women with postmenstrual spotting, there was no relation with the shape of the niche (BijdeVaate

et al. 2011). In another study (Wang et al. 2009), scar defects were significantly wider in women with postmenstrual spotting, dysmenorrhea or chronic pelvic pain. In the third study, the incidence of postmenstrual spotting or prolonged menstrual bleeding was higher with an increase of the diameter of the niche (Uppal et al. 2011). Niche-related menstrual bleeding disorders do often not respond to hormonal therapies and are associated with cyclic pain (Gubbini et al. 2008) and may be responsible for a substantial part of gynecological consultations and interventions. Other reported symptoms in women with a niche were dysmenorrhea (53.1 %), chronic pelvic pain (36.9 %), and dyspareunia (18.3 %) (Wang et al. 2009).

7.6 Etiology of Niche-Related Bleeding Disorders

It has been assumed that abnormal uterine bleeding may be due to the retention of menstrual blood in the niche, which is intermittently expelled after the majority of the menstruation has ceased, causing postmenstrual spotting and pain (Thurmond et al. 1999; Fabres et al. 2005). The presence of fibrotic tissue below the niche may impair the drainage of menstrual flow (Fabres et al. 2003). Additional new formed fragile vessels in the niche may also attribute to the accumulation of in situ produced blood (Morris 1995).

7.7 Treatment Modalities

Since the recent acknowledged association between CS-related niches and bleeding disorders, several innovative surgical therapies have been developed. The effectiveness of surgical interventions for the treatment of niche-related uterine bleeding disorders has been reported in a limited number of studies. Most studies include case reports or small prospective or retrospective case series. Surgical treatment includes hysteroscopic resection (Chang et al. 2009; Fabres et al. 2005; Gubbini et al. 2008, 2011; Wang et al. 2011),

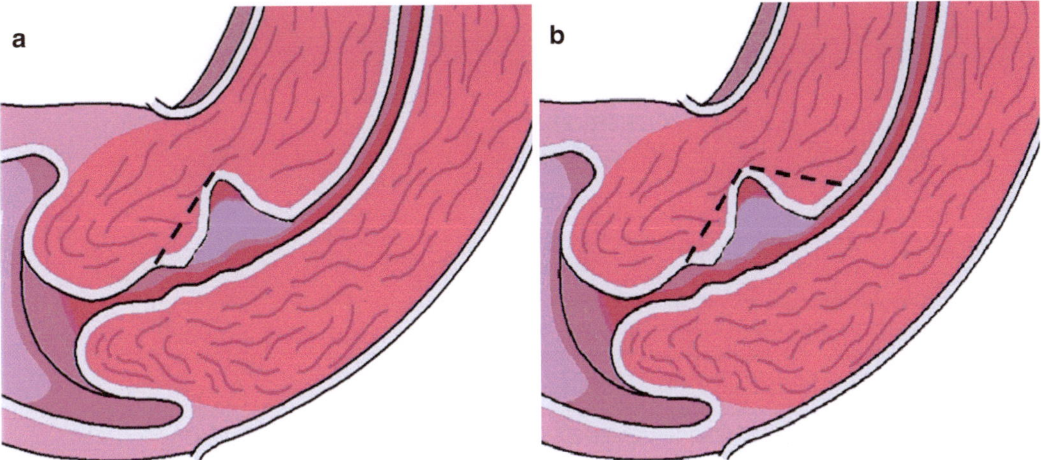

Fig. 7.4 Technique of hysteroscopic resection: (**a**) resection of distal part of the niche, (**b**) resection of both distal and proximal part (**b** was published in Gubbini et al. 2008)

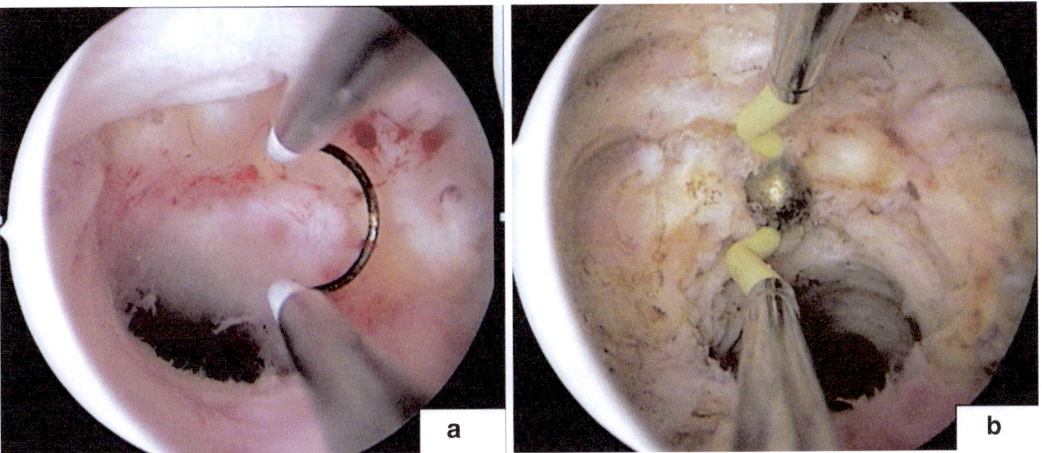

Fig. 7.5 (**a**) Resectoscope for resection of the distal part of the niche. (**b**) Coagulation of the niche bottom with a rollerball (Published in Gubbini et al. 2008)

laparoscopic (Donnez et al. 2008; Klemm et al. 2005) or vaginal repair (Klemm et al. 2005).

7.8   Hysteroscopic Niche Resection

The least invasive surgical therapy, which can be performed in day care, is the hysteroscopic resection of the niche. The proposed theory behind this treatment is to improve outflow of menstrual blood and to prevent in situ produced hemorrhage by the fragile vessels in the niche itself.

7.8.1   Technique

The hysteroscopic resection was all done by a monopolar resectoscoop varying between 9 and 12 mm. In most studies, the distal part of the niche was resected with (Fabres et al. 2005; Chang et al. 2009) or without coagulation of the bottom of the niche (Fernandez et al. 1996) (see Fig. 7.4). In some studies both the distal and the proximal part of the niche were resected (see Fig. 7.4b) in combination with coagulation of the bottom with a rollerball (see Figs. 7.4b and 7.5) (Wang et al. 2009; Gubbini et al. 2008, 2011). Given the

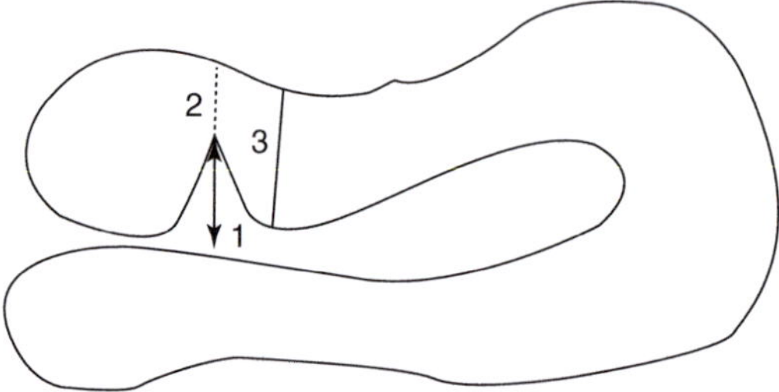

Fig. 7.6 Schematic diagram on the measurement of niches. Niche characteristics: niche depth (*1*), thickness of the residual myometrium (*2*), total thickness of adjacent myometrium (*3*), (Published in Bij de Vaate et al. 2011)

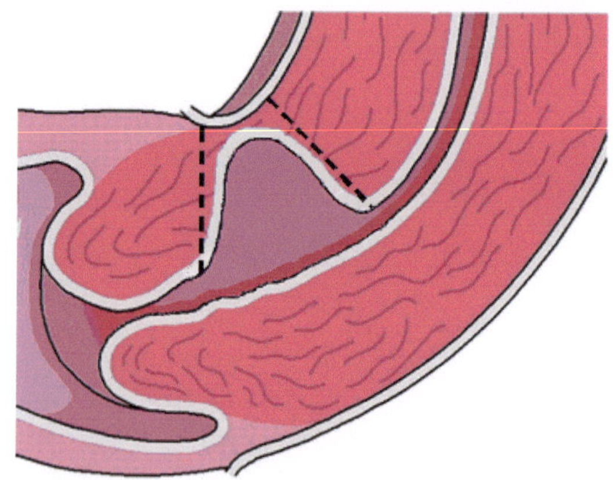

Fig. 7.7 Part that is removed during a laparoscopic or vaginal niche resection

potential risk on perforation or bladder injury a certain distance between the niche and bladder is required, also known as residual myometrium, presented as 2 in Fig. 7.6. Minimal required residual myometrium thickness varies among the different studies between 2 and 2.5 mm (Wang et al. 2009; Gubbini et al. 2008, 2011).

7.8.2 Effectiveness of Hysteroscopic Niche Resection

So far only three prospective cohort, one case–control study and four retrospective cohort studies are published on hysteroscopic resections. Apart from one case–control study (Florio et al. 2011), which compared hysteroscopic resection with medical therapy, all studies were single-arm studies. The populations varied, all had an observed niche, however the niche was not always clearly defined and the minimal required thickness of the residual myometrium was only reported in one study, in which it had to be at least 2.5 mm (Chang et al. 2009). Symptoms of the patients varied, these included postmenstrual spotting in four studies (Wang et al. 2009; Gubbini et al. 2008; Chang et al. 2009; Fernandez et al. 1996). Reported success rates were as high as 60–84 % (Wang et al. 2009; Gubbini et al. 2008, 2011; Chang et al. 2009). The three prospective studies included a total of 61 patients receiving a hysteroscopic intervention. Mean reported reduction of postmenstrual spotting varied between 3 and 3.4 days (Gubbini

et al. 2008, 2011; Chang et al. 2009). One retrospective case–control study reported better outcomes of the hysteroscopic niche resection in comparison to applied hormonal therapies (Florio et al. 2011).

Complications were not reported. However exact methodology, follow-up or used (validated) tools to measure outcomes are mostly not reported. In theory, several complications could be expected. In case of a very thin residual myometrium, one should be aware of perforation and bladder injuries. Therefore, some studies propose preoperative installation of methylene blue dye in the bladder to enable the identification of any bladder injury in case of an unintended perforation.

7.9 Laparoscopic or Vaginal Niche Repair

Large niches with thin residual myometrium are less suitable for hysteroscopic resection. In these cases, surgical resection of the entire CS scar and suturing is proposed in case of severe symptoms. Such a niche repair or uterine reconstruction can be performed either by a laparoscopic (Donnez et al. 2008; Kostov et al. 2009; Klemm et al. 2005), robot-assisted (Yalcinkaya et al. 2011), or a vaginal (Khoshnow et al. 2010; Klemm et al. 2005) approach (Fig. 7.7).

7.9.1 Effectiveness of Laparoscopic or Vaginal Niche Repair

There is only limited evidence for good results. So far only small case series reported on niche reconstruction in non-pregnant patients. In total only 14 patients underwent a laparoscopic repair (Donnez et al. 2008; Kostov et al. 2009; Klemm et al. 2005), 2 patients a robot-assisted (Yalcinkaya et al. 2011), and 4 patients a vaginal repair (Kostov et al. 2009; Hoorenbeeck 2002; Klemm et al. 2005). Indications for niche repair were diverse, these included women with secondary infertility, pelvic pain or metrorrhage, abnormal uterine bleeding, postmenstrual spotting, and previous cesarean scar pregnancy. Although an association between a niche and symptoms was presumed in these studies, one may still question if a niche is responsible for these symptoms. Outcome parameters in the reported publications were symptom reduction or MRI or hysteroscopic appearance of the niche. However, structural evaluation of clearly defined outcome parameters or follow-up was mostly not described. Although these techniques seem to be promising, more prospective studies are required with sufficient sample sizes and structural follow-up for the evaluation of the efficacy. In addition, long-term follow-up is required to draw conclusion on implications of these techniques on later pregnancies.

Conclusion

Niches are frequently seen after caesarean sections and are related to postmenstrual spotting and potentially associated with menstrual pain (therapies). Related postmenstrual spotting can be treated by hysteroscopic resection or more invasive niche reconstructions by an abdominal, laparoscopic or vaginal approach. Type of treatment depends on symptomatology and on the measured residual myometrium, given the risk on perforation or bladder injury during hysteroscopic resection in case it is less than 2.5 mm. More studies are needed to study the effect of niches on fertility and pregnancy outcome, to elucidate etiology of niches and related symptoms and to study the effect of current applied therapies on symptoms and later pregnancies.

References

Armstrong V, Hansen WF, Van Voorhis BJ, Syrop CH (2003) Detection of cesarean scars by transvaginal ultrasound. Obstet Gynecol 101(1):61–65

BijdeVaate AJ, Brolmann HA, van der Slikke JW, Wouters MG, Schats R, Huirne JA (2010) Therapeutic options of caesarean scar pregnancy: case series and literature review. J Clin Ultrasound 38(2):75–84

BijdeVaate AJ, Brolmann HA, van der Voet LF, van der Slikke JW, Veersema S, Huirne JA (2011) Ultrasound evaluation of the cesarean scar: relation between a niche and postmenstrual spotting. Ultrasound Obstet Gynecol 37(1):93–99

Borges LM, Scapinelli A, de Baptista Depes D, Lippi UG, Coelho Lopes RG (2010) Findings in patients with postmenstrual spotting with prior cesarean section. J Minim Invasive Gynecol 17(3):361–364

Chang Y, Tsai EM, Long CY, Lee CL, Kay N (2009) Resectoscopic treatment combined with sonohysterographic evaluation of women with postmenstrual bleeding as a result of previous cesarean delivery scar defects. Am J Obstet Gynecol 200(4):370 e1–4

Chen HY, Chen SJ, Hsieh FJ (1990) Observation of cesarean section scar by transvaginal ultrasonography. Ultrasound Med Biol 16(5):443–447

Donnez O, Jadoul P, Squifflet J, Donnez J (2008) Laparoscopic repair of wide and deep uterine scar dehiscence after cesarean section. Fertil Steril 89(4): 974–980

El-Mazny A, Abou-Salem N, El-Khayat W, Farouk A (2011) Diagnostic correlation between sonohysterography and hysteroscopy in the assessment of uterine cavity after cesarean section. Middle East Fertil Soc J 16(1):72–76

Fabres C, Aviles G, De La Jara C, Escalona J, Munoz JF, Mackenna A et al (2003) The cesarean delivery scar pouch: clinical implications and diagnostic correlation between transvaginal sonography and hysteroscopy. J Ultrasound Med 22(7):695–700; 01–2

Fabres C, Arriagada P, Fernandez C, Mackenna A, Zegers F, Fernandez E (2005) Surgical treatment and follow-up of women with intermenstrual bleeding due to cesarean section scar defect. J Minim Invasive Gynecol 12(1):25–28

Fernandez E, Fernandez C, Fabres C, Alam V (1996) Hysteroscopic correction of cesarean section scars in women with abnormal uterine bleeding. J Am Assoc Gynecol Laparosc 3:S13

Florio P, Gubbini G, Marra E, Dores D, Nascetti D, Bruni L, Battista R, Moncini I, Filippeschi M, Petraglia F (2011) A retrospective case-control study comparing hysteroscopic resection versus hormonal modulation in treating menstrual disorders due to isthmocele. Gynaecol Endocrinol 27(6):434–438

Gubbini G, Casadio P, Marra E (2008) Resectoscopic correction of the "isthmocele" in women with postmenstrual abnormal uterine bleeding and secondary infertility. J Minim Invasive Gynecol 15(2):172–175

Gubbini G, Centini G, Nascetti D, Marra E, Moncini I, Bruni L, Petraglia F, Florio P (2011) Surgical hysteroscopic treatment of cesarean-induced isthmocele in restoring fertility: prospective study. J Minim Invasive Gynecol 18(2):234–237

Hamar BD, Saber SB, Cackovic M, Magloire LK, Pettker CM, Abdel-Razeq SS, Rosenberg VA, Buhimschi IA, Buhimschi CS (2007) Ultrasound evaluation of the uterine scar after cesarean delivery: a randomized controlled trial of one- and two-layer closure. Obstet Gynecol 110(4):808–813

Hayakawa H, Itakura A, Mitsui T, Okada M, Suzuki M, Tamakoshi K, Kikkawa F (2006) Methods for myometrium closure and other factors impacting effects on cesarean section scars of the uterine segment detected by the ultrasonography. Acta Obstet Gynecol Scand 85(4):429–434

Khoshnow Q, Pardey J, Uppal T (2010) Transvaginal repair of caesarean scar dehiscence. Aust N Z J Obstet Gynaecol 50(1):94–95

Klemm P, Koehler C, Mangler M, Schneider U, Schneider A (2005) Laparoscopic and vaginal repair of uterine scar dehiscence following cesarean section as detected by ultrasound. J Perinat Med 33(4):324–331

Kostov P, Huber AW, Raio L, Mueller MD (2009) Uterine scar dehiscence repair in rendezvous technique. Gynaecol Surg 6(Suppl 1) (S65)

Monteagudo A, Carreno C, Timor-Tritsch IE (2001) Saline infusion sonohysterography in nonpregnant women with previous caesarean delivery: the "niche" in the scar. J Ultrasound Med 20:1105–15

Morris H (1995) Surgical pathology of the lower uterine segment caesarean section scar: is the scar a source of clinical symptoms? Int J Gynecol Pathol 14(1):16–20

Naji O, Abdallah Y, Bij De Vaate AJ, Smith A, Pexsters A, Stalder C, McIndoe A, Ghaem-Maghami S, Lees C, Brölmann HA, Huirne JA, Timmerman D, Bourne T (2012a) Standardized approach for imaging and measuring cesarean section scars using ultrasonography. Ultrasound Obstet Gynecol 39:252–259. doi:10.1002/uog.12334

Naji O, Daemen A, Smith A, Abdallah Y, Bradburn E, Giggens R, Chan D, Stalder C, Ghaem-Maghami S, Timmerman D, Bourne T (2012b) Does the presence of a caesarean section scar influence the site of placental implantation and subsequent migration in future pregnancies: a prospective case-control study. Ultrasound Obstet Gynecol 40:557–561. doi:10.1002/uog.11133

Naji O, Wynants L, Smith A, Abdallah Y, Stalder C, Sayasneh A, McIndoe A, Ghaem-Maghami S, Van Huffel S, Van Calster B, Timmerman D, Bourne T (2013) Predicting successful vaginal birth after Cesarean section using a model based on Cesarean scar features examined by transvaginal sonography. Ultrasound Obstet Gynecol 41(6):672-8. doi: 10.1002/uog.12423.

Naji O, Daemen A, Smith A, Abdallah Y, Saso S, Stalder C, Sayasneh A, McIndoe A, Ghaem-Maghami S, Timmerman D, Bourne T (2013a) Changes in cesarean section scar dimensions during pregnancy: a prospective longitudinal study. Ultrasound Obstet Gynecol 41:556–562

Ofili-Yebovi D, Ben-Nagi J, Sawyer E, Yazbek J, Lee C, Gonzalez J et al (2008) Deficient lower-segment cesarean section scars: prevalence and risk factors. Ultrasound Obstet Gynecol 31(1):72–77

Regnard C, Nosbusch M, Fellemans C, Benali N, van Rysselberghe M, Barlow P et al (2004) Cesarean section scar evaluation by saline contrast sonohysterography. Ultrasound Obstet Gynecol 23(3): 289–292

Stewart KS, Evans TW (1975) Recurrent bleeding from the lower segment scar–a late complication of caesarean section. Br J Obstet Gynaecol 82(8): 682–686

Surapaneni K, Silberzweig JE (2008) Cesarean section scar diverticulum: appearance on hysterosalpingography. AJR Am J Roentgenol 190(4):870–874

Thurmond AS, Harvey WJ, Smith SA (1999) Cesarean section scar as a cause of abnormal vaginal bleeding: diagnosis by sonohysterography. J Ultrasound Med 18(1):13–16; quiz 17–8

Uppal T, Lanzarone V, Mongelli M (2011) Sonographically detected caesarean section scar defects and menstrual irregularity. J Obstet Gynaecol 31(5):413–416

Valenzano MM, Mistrangelo E, Lijoi D, Fortunato T, Lantieri PB, Risso D, Costantini S, Ragni N (2006) Transvaginal sonohysterographic evaluation of uterine malformations. Eur J Obstet Gynecol Reprod Biol 124: 246–249

Vikhareva Osser O, Valentin L (2010a) Risk factors for incomplete healing of the uterine incision after caesarean section. BJOG 117(9):1119–1126

Vikhareva Osser O, Jokubkiene L, Valentin L (2009) High prevalence of defects in cesarean section scars at transvaginal ultrasound examination. Ultrasound Obstet Gynecol 34(1):90–97

Vikhareva Osser O, Jokubkiene L, Valentin L (2010) Cesarean section scar defects: agreement between transvaginal sonographic findings with and without saline contrast enhancement. Ultrasound Obstet Gynecol 35(1):75–83

Voet LF van der, Graziosi GCM, Veersema S, BijDeVaate M, Huirne J, Brolmann HAM (2009) Perforation of an intra uterine device in a cesarean section scar. Gynecol Surg 6(Suppl. 1) (S106)

Wang CB, Chiu WW, Lee CY, Sun YL, Lin YH, Tseng CJ (2009) Cesarean scar defect: correlation between cesarean section number, defect size, clinical symptoms and uterine position. Ultrasound Obstet Gynecol 34(1):85–89

Wang CJ, Huang HJ, Chao A, Lin YP, Pan YJ, Horng SG (2011) Challenges in the transvaginal management of abnormal uterine bleeding secondary to cesarean section scar defect. Eur J Obstet Gynecol Reprod Biol 154(2):218–222

Yalcinkaya TM, Akar ME, Kammire LD, Johnston-MacAnnay EB, Mertz HL (2011) Robotic-assisted laparoscopic repair of symptomatic caesarean section defect:a report of two cases. J Reprod Med 56(5–6):265–270

Yazicioglu F, Gökdogan A, Kelekci S, Aygün M, Savan K (2006) Incomplete healing of the uterine incision after caesarean section: is it preventable? Eur J Obstet Gynecol Reprod Biol 124(1):32–36

Adenomyosis

8

Lydia Garcia and Keith Isaacson

Contents

L. Garcia, MD (✉) • K. Isaacson, MD
Department of Minimally Invasive Gynecological
Surgery, Newton Wellesley Hospital, 2014 Washington St,
Newton, MA 02462, USA
e-mail: lyds9906@gmail.com

8.1 Epidemiology and Risk Factors

The true incidence of adenomyosis has not been accurately determined since the diagnosis can only be confirmed with histology, usually after hysterectomy. The prevalence of adenomyosis reported in the literature ranges widely from 5 to 70 % (Azzi 1989; Bergholt et al. 2001; Bird et al. 1972). The discrepancy may be due to the lack of a uniform diagnostic criterion. Adenomyosis is confirmed by the microscopic presence of endometrial tissue in the myometrium (Fig. 8.1). However, the depth of invasion of these endometrial implants for classification is variable in different studies. One study defines adenomyosis as endometrial glands within the myometrium greater than one low power field from the basalis layer, while another definition states that the foci need to be deeper than 25 % of myometrial thickness (Bergeron et al. 2006; Ferenczy 1998). While there is a large variation in the definition for diagnosis, most studies use the cut off of endometrial glands 25 mm below the basalis layer (Bergholt et al. 2001; Farquhar and Bronsens 2006; Uduwela et al. 2000). With this criterion, the mean frequency of adenomyosis at the time of hysterectomy is approximately 20–30 % (Azzi 1989; Parazzini et al. 1997; Vercellini et al. 1995).

While the exact etiology of adenomyosis is unknown, several risk factors have been identified in clinical series. Seventy to eighty percent

O. Istre (ed.), *Minimally Invasive Gynecological Surgery*,
DOI 10.1007/978-3-662-44059-9_8, © Springer-Verlag Berlin Heidelberg 2015

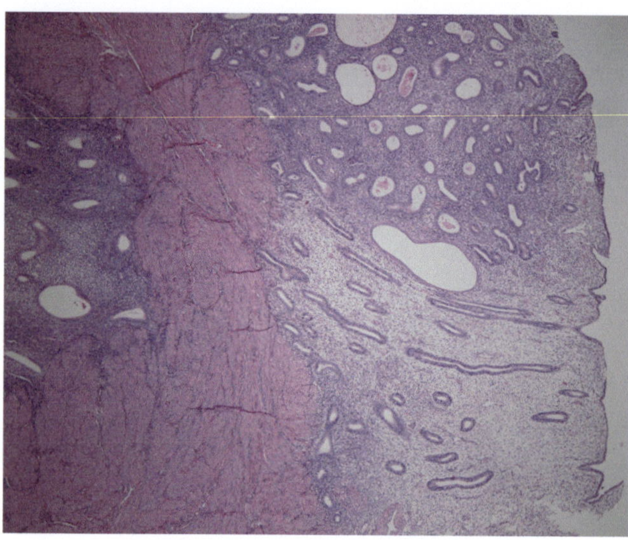

Fig. 8.1 Histological findings of adenomyosis with foci of endometrial glands and stroma found deep within the myometrium

of adenomyosis is reported in women in their fourth and fifth decades, but it is unclear if age is indeed a risk factor or a confounding factor (Azzi 1989). The higher prevalence in older women may be due to higher rates of hysterectomy later in life. It may, however, also be due to longer exposure to hormones that over time may stimulate endometriotic glands to invaginate into the myometrial wall (Garcia and Isaacson 2011).

Multiparous women also have higher rates of adenomyosis (Bergholt et al. 2001; Levgur et al. 2005; Parazzini et al. 1997; Vercellini et al. 1995; Taran et al. 2010). The frequency of adenomyosis has been linked directly to the number of pregnancies (Vercellini et al. 1995). The invasive nature of the trophoblast into the myometrium at the time of implantation may weaken the myometrium to allow active endometrial tissue to grow into the injured lining (Ferenczy 1998; Garcia and Isaacson 2011). In addition, the increase in hormones during pregnancy may also help stimulate the invagination of endometrial implants (Levgur et al. 2005).

Pelvic surgery, like pregnancy, can also weaken the myometrium through trauma with instrumentation during dilation and curettage, transmural surgery, or cesarean section (Ferenczy 1998). However, it remains unclear if prior uterine surgery is a risk factor since only a small series of cases show that pregnancy termination and dilation and curettage have an association with adenomyosis, while other studies show no statistical relationship between this disorder with cesarean section or myomectomy (Bergholt et al. 2001; Harris and Daniel 1985; Levgur et al. 2005; Parazzini et al. 1997; Taran et al. 2010).

8.2 Clinical Manifestations and Pathophysiology

Not all women with adenomyotic uteri are symptomatic but up to 75 % of women present with either menorrhagia, dysmenorrhea, or both (Benson and Sneeden 1958; Bergholt et al. 2001). Menorrhagia is likely caused by adenomyotic foci interfering with the normal musculature of the myometrium, preventing adequate contractions and permitting greater blood loss (Ferenczy 1998; Azzi 1989). Dysmenorrhea is likely a result of uterine irritability stimulated from the increase blood and from edema of the adenomyotic foci within the myometrium (Azzi 1989). Symptoms of chronic pelvic pain and dyspareunia are also common in women with adenomyosis. The pathophysiology of these symptoms is unclear. There is, however, high prevalence of adenomyosis in 70 % of women with endometriosis, which may contribute to these symptoms (Kunz et al. 2005). It is unclear if adenomyosis

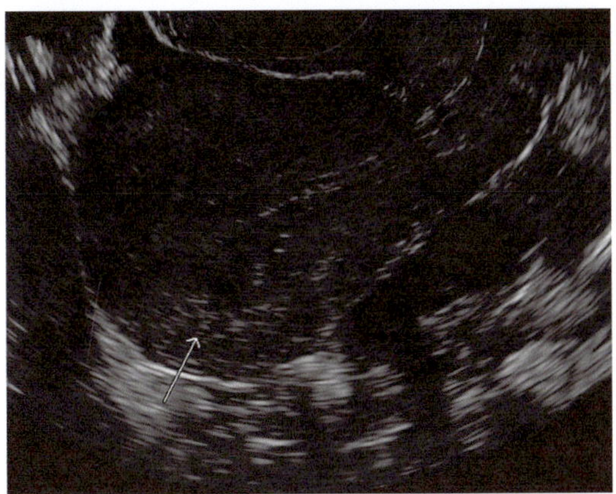

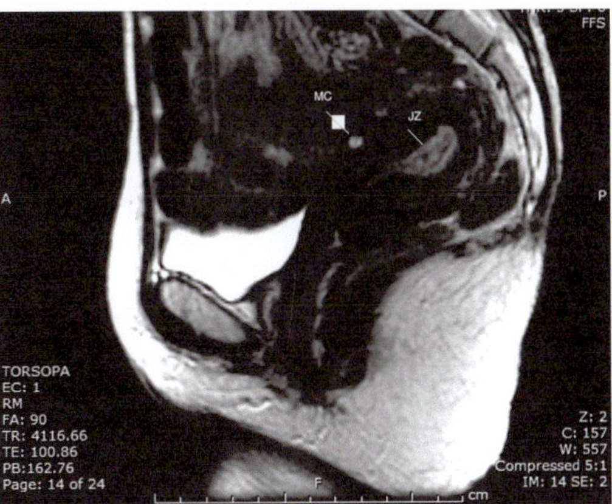

Fig. 8.2 Sagittal transvaginal sonography shows an asymmetric uterus with thickened posterior myometrial wall. The "*Arrow* show decreased echogencity and heterogeneity consistent with diffuse adenomyosis in the posterior wall of the uterus"

Fig. 8.3 Sagittal T2 weighted MRI images demonstrate ill defined 6.0×6.8 cm heterogeneous, hyperintense foci extending from the junctional zone (*JZ*) anteriorly measuring 21.94 mm (greater than 12 mm) suggesting adenomyosis. Myometrial cysts can be seen anteriorly (*MC*)

plays a role in reproductive outcomes, but some studies hypothesize that adenomyotic foci may interfere with implantation or impede sperm function through immune responses causing infertility (Devlieger et al. 2003; Ota et al. 1998).

8.3 Diagnostic Procedures

As described earlier (e.g. see Sect. 8.1), the diagnosis of adenomyosis is usually made from tissue specimens collected at the time of hysterectomy. Currently, the development of high quality, noninvasive imaging modalities has also been proven to be accurate in the diagnosis of adenomyosis as well. Findings of myometrial cysts, heterogeneous myometrial echotexture, and the visualization of the endometrial–myometrial interface (known as the junctional zone) have assisted with the differential diagnosis of adenomyosis using transvaginal ultrasound and magnetic resonance imaging (Bazot et al. 2001; Dueholm and Lundorf 2007; Felde et al. 1992; Reinhold et al. 1995) (Figs. 8.2 and 8.3).

In addition, advances in hysteroscopy and laparoscopy have provided minimally invasive techniques to assist in the diagnosis of adenomyosis. Hysteroscopy provides direct visualization into the uterine cavity and allows for the option

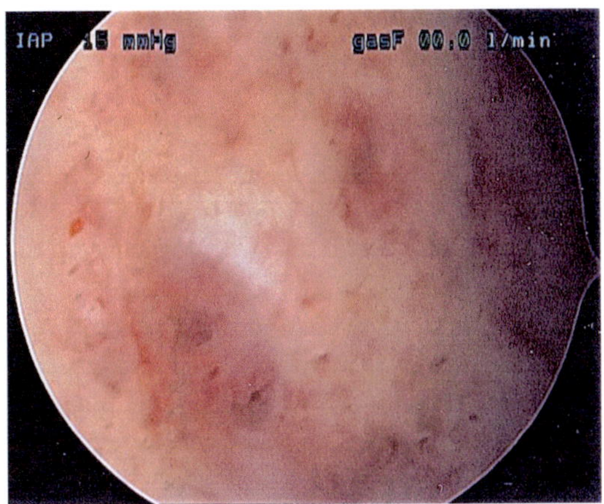

Fig. 8.4 Hysteroscopic image of adenomyosis with pathognomonic signs of pitting endometrial defects, cystic hemorrhagic lesions

of superficial myometrial biopsies for a histological diagnosis. Hysteroscopic findings of intramyometrial lacunae, an irregular endometrium with pitting defects, or cystic hemorrhagic lesions are all suggestive of adenomyosis (Fernandez et al. 2007; Molinas and Campo 2006) (Fig. 8.4). When adenomyosis cannot be seen, hysteroscopic myometrial biopsies can be performed at the posterior wall, where adenomyosis is most frequently found (Benson and Sneeden 1958; Emge 1962). In one study, hysteroscopic myometrial biopsies were performed using a 5 mm loop electrode in fifty women with normal appearing cavities as well as a history of menorrhagia. Of those 50 women, 33 (66 %) had adenomyosis present at a depth greater than 1 mm (McCausland 1992). However, the sensitivity of the biopsy depends on extent, depth, and location of disease (Garcia and Isaacson 2011). Laparoscopic myometrial biopsies can be performed as well but have a high risk of bleeding (Popp et al. 1993).

8.4 Treatment

Suppressive hormonal treatments are effective for reducing symptoms of menorrhagia and dysmenorrhea but these medications only temporarily induce regression of adenomyosis during the course of therapy. Continuous oral contraceptive pills, high dose progestins, the levonogestrol intrauterine device, danazol, and GnRH agonists have all been used as conservative treatment options, as an alternative for hysterectomy. The standard of treatment still remains hysterectomy for those women who have completed child bearing. As imaging and minimally invasive diagnostic methods have evolved, less aggressive surgical options have also been developed in place of hysterectomy (Levgur 2007). Interventional radiology techniques such as uterine artery embolization and magnetic resonance guided focused ultrasound surgery have been used to treat adenomyosis (Kim et al. 2007; Rabinovici et al. 2006). Other conservative surgical treatment options such as endometrial ablation and resection, adenomyotic muscle excision and reduction, and electrocoagulation have also been performed and will be discussed in further detail.

When considering surgery as a treatment option, it is important to try to determine the area and extent of disease (Farquhar and Bronsens 2006). Because adenomyosis tends to be a diffuse process with ectopic endometrium invading throughout the entire myometrium, hysterectomy still remains the gold standard of treatment. It is the only guaranteed treatment for adenomyosis. Less invasive approaches with vaginal and laparoscopic hysterectomy are preferable to abdominal hysterectomy because of lower morbidity and faster recovery. While vaginal hysterectomy is more cost effective than the laparoscopic approach, laparoscopy may be more beneficial to the patient.

Furuhashi et al. (1998) showed that women with adenomyosis had higher rates of bladder injury at the time of vaginal hysterectomy. The authors concluded that the reason for increased rate of injury was unknown but it was hypothesized that there may be greater difficulty in identifying the supravaginal septum and the vesicovaginal or vesicocervical planes without direct visualization. In addition to allowing direct visualization for dissection, laparoscopy has the advantage of detecting and removing endometriosis that is commonly found in patients with adenomyosis (Wood 1998). The laparoscopic approach may also be beneficial due to less postoperative pain in comparison to vaginal hysterectomy (Candiani et al. 2009; Ghezzi et al. 2010). A review of 70 articles regarding hysterectomy showed lower costs and shorter operating times with vaginal hysterectomy, but the rates of blood transfusions, unexplained fever, and bleeding were higher with vaginal rather than the laparoscopic approach (Wood et al. 1997).

Adenomyosis can also appear in focal forms of circumscribed nodular aggregates of smooth muscle, endometrial glands, and stroma called adenomyomas. When adenomyomas can be localized with ultrasound or MRI, attempts can be made to excise the lesion alone. This conservative surgical option is usually attempted in women who wish to maintain fertility. However, unlike myomectomies, it can be difficult to define margins and expose lesions, which can lead to postoperative sequale affecting fertility. With excision, scar formation can affect the gestational capability of uterus, putting women at higher risk for spontaneous miscarriages (38.8 %) and uterine rupture (Wood 1998; Wang et al. 2009). However, a small study showed that conservative treatment with adenomyoma excision (mean size of 55 mm) resulted in a 70 % pregnancy rate (49/71 patients) with relief of symptoms of menorrhagia and dysmenorrheal (Wang et al. 2009).

In addition, with an excisional procedure, lesions can be left behind causing patients to remain symptomatic or relapse due to the inability to clearly exposure margins in adenomyomas. Due to the low efficacy of excision of 50 %, medical therapy is often used in combination to help prevent relapses (Wang et al. 2009).

Excision of diffuse adenomyosis, also known as myometrial reduction, can be performed as well. A wedge defect is created in the myometrium and is repaired by metroplasty with laparoscopy or laparotomy (Levgur 2007). Only a small number of cases have been performed and the outcomes show low postoperative pregnancy rates likely due to scar tissue formation (Wood 1998; Fujishita et al. 2004; Nishida et al. 2010; Fedele et al. 1993). Similar to excision of adenomyomas, clinical improvement may only be temporary and there is high risk of recurrence due to poorly defined margins (Levgur 2007).

Laparoscopic myometrial electrocoagulation is another conservative treatment option that allows women to maintain their uterus this procedure is performed by the laparoscpic insertion of a unipolar or bipolar needle electrode into the affected myometrium. It can be used for both focal and diffuse adenomyosis, causing necrosis to the abnormal tissue. The procedure is not recommended for women who wish to conceive given that it can reduce the strength of the myometrium by replacing the adenomyotic foci with scar tissue and therefore has an increased risk of uterine rupture (Wood et al. 1994). Outcomes are inferior to surgical excision since the electrical conduction through the abnormal tissue may be incomplete and some foci of adenomyosis may be missed at the time of surgery (Levgur 2007). It can be performed concurrently with patients undergoing endometrial ablation/resection to improve rates of success (Wood 1998; Phillips et al. 1996).

The most common conservative surgical option performed for adenomyosis is endometrial ablation/resection. It can be performed with a YAG laser, rollerball resection, or with global ablation techniques including Novasure, ThermaChoice, or cryotherapy in women who no longer wish to conceive. However, success rates are dependent on the depth of invasion of adenomyotic foci into the uterine wall (McCausland and McCausland 1996). Resection is performed to a depth of 2–3 mm into the myometrium. Deeper resection has a higher risk of bleeding from the arteries that are situated approximately 5 mm deep to the myometrial surface. In patients with superficial adenomyosis (penetration less than 2 mm), endometrial resection has successful outcomes with no residual bleeding or postablation light cyclic periods that resolved with continuous progesterone therapy (McCausland and McCausland 1996). However, patients with deep adenomyosis (greater than a depth of 2 mm) have poor results with 33 % failure rate, which usually require hysterectomy (Raiga et al. 1994; McCausland and McCausland 1996). With deep adenomyosis, the ectopic deep endometrial glands can persist under the scar and eventually proliferate though the area of ablation or resection to cause recurrent bleeding. Repeat resection is usually unsuccessful for deep adenomyosis and these patients rarely respond to continuous progesterone therapy.

Global endometrial ablation has also been proven to successfully treat excessive bleeding in women with adenomyosis. However a retrospective review of women who underwent thermal balloon and radio frequency ablation showed 1.5 times increased risk of failures in women with findings of adenomyosis on ultrasound requiring the need for subsequent hysterectomy or repeat ablation (El Nashar et al. 2009).

8.5 Summary

Advances in endoscopic surgery have allowed for various diagnostic and therapeutic surgical options for adenomyosis other than hysterectomy. While hysterectomy still remains the gold standard treatment, minimally invasive procedures with hysteroscopy and laparoscopy can improve symptoms of dysmenorrhea and menorrhagia in young women. Laparoscopic treatments, such as adenomyotic muscle excision and reduction, and electrocoagulation, allow women to maintain their uterus but may have higher failure rates and compromise fertility due to scarring and incomplete excision. Hysteroscopic procedures such as ablation and resection are effective in improving symptoms of menorrhagia in women who have completed when adenomyotic foci are superficial (<2 mm). High failure rates are noted when deep adenomyosis is present.

References

Azzi R (1989) Adenomyosis: current perspectives. Obstet Gynecol Clin North Am 16:221–235

Bazot M, Cortez A, Darai E et al (2001) Ultrasound compared with magnetic resonance imaging for the diagnosis of adenomyosis: correlation with histopathology. Hum Reprod 16:2427–2433

Benson R, Sneeden V (1958) Adenomyosis: a reappraisal of symptomatology. Am J Obstet Gynecol 76:1044

Bergeron C, Amant F, Ferency A (2006) Pathology and physiology of adenomyosis. Best Pract Res Clin Obstet Gynaecol 20:511–521

Bergholt T, Eriksen L, Ferendt N et al (2001) Prevalence and risk factors of adenomyosis at hysterectomy. Hum Reprod 16:2418–2421

Bird C, McElin T, Manalo-Estrella P (1972) The elusive adenomyosis of the uterus revisited. Am J Obstet Gynecol 112:583–593

Candiani M, Izzo S, Bulfoni A et al (2009) Laparoscopic vs vaginal hysterectomy for benign pathology. Am J Obstet Gynecol 200:368.e1–7

Devlieger R, D'Hooghe T, Timmerman D (2003) Uterine adenomyosis in the infertility clinic. Hum Reprod Update 9:139–147

Dueholm M, Lundorf E (2007) Transvaginal ultrasound or MRI for diagnosis of adenomyosis. Curr Opin Obstet Gynecol 19:505–512

El Nashar S, Hopkins M, Creedon D (2009) Prediction of treatment outcomes after global endometrial ablation. Obstet Gynecol 113:97–106

Emge L (1962) The elusive adenomyosis of the uterus. Am J Obstet Gynecol 83:1541–1563

Farquhar C, Bronsens I (2006) Medical and surgical management of adenomyosis. Best Pract Res Clin Obstet Gynaecol 20:603–626

Fedele L, Bianchi S, Zanotti F et al (1993) Fertility after conservative surgery for adenomyomas. Hum Reprod 8:1708–1710

Felde L, Bianchi S, Dorta M et al (1992) Transvaginal ultrasonography in the diagnosis of diffuse adenomyosis. Fertil Steril 58:94–97

Ferenczy A (1998) Pathophysiology of adenomyosis. Hum Reprod Update 4:312–322

Fernandez C, Ricci P, Fernandez E (2007) Adenomyosis visualized during hysteroscopy. J Minim Invasive Gynecol 14:555–556

Fujishita A, Masuzaki H, Khan K et al (2004) Modified reduction surgery for adenomyosis. A preliminary report of the transverse H incision technique. Gynecol Obstet Invest 57:132–138

Furuhashi M, Miyabe Y, Katsumata Y et al (1998) Comparison of complications of vaginal hysterectomy in patients with leiomyomas and in patients with adenomyosis. Arch Gynecol Obstet 262:69–73

Garcia L, Isaacson K (2011) Adenomyosis: a review of the literature. J Minim Invasive Gynecol 18:428–437

Ghezzi F, Uccella S, Cromi A et al (2010) Postoperative pain after laparoscopic and vaginal hysterectomy for benign gynecologic disease: a randomized trial. Am J Obstet Gynecol 203:118.e1–8

Harris W, Daniel J (1985) Prior cesarean section: a risk factor for adenomyosis? J Reprod Med 30:173–175

Kim M, Kim S, Kim N (2007) Longer term results of uterine artery embolization for symptomatic adenomyosis. AJR Am J Roentgenol. 2007;188(1):176–181

Kunz G, Beil D, Huppert P et al (2005) Adenomyosis in endometriosis-prevalence and impact on fertility. Evidence from magnetic resonance imaging. Hum Reprod 20:2309–2316

Levgur M (2007) Therapeutic options for adenomyosis: a review. Arch Gynecol Obstet 276:1–15

Levgur M, Abdai MA, Tucker A (2005) Adenomyosis: symptoms, histology, and pregnancy terminations. Obstet Gynecol 95:688–691

McCausland A (1992) Hysteroscopic myometrial biopsy: its use in diagnosing adenomyosis and its clinical applications. Am J Obstet Gynecol 166:1619–1626

McCausland A, McCausland V (1996) Depth of endometrial penetration in adenomyosis helps determine outcome of rollerball ablation. Am J Obstet Gynecol 174:1786–1794

Molinas C, Campo R (2006) Office hysteroscopy and adenomyosis. Best Pract Res Clin Obstet Gynaecol 20:557–567

Nishida M, Takano K, Arai Y (2010) Conservative surgical management for diffuse uterine adenomyosis. Fertil Steril 94(2):715–719

Ota H, Igarshi S, Hatazawa J et al (1998) Is adenomyosis an immune disease? Hum Reprod 4:360–367

Parazzini F, Vercellini P, Pazza S et al (1997) Risk factors for adenomyosis. Hum Reprod 12:1275–1279

Phillips D, Nathanson H, Milim S et al (1996) Laparoscopic bipolar coagulation for the conservative treatment of adenomyomata. J Am Assoc Gynecol Laparosc 4:19–24

Popp L, Schwiedessen J, Gaetje R (1993) Myometrial biopsy in the diagnosis of adenomyosis uteri. Am J Obstet Gynecol 16(3):546–549

Rabinovici J, Inbar Y, Eylon S (2006) Pregnancy and live birth after focused ultrasound surgery for symptomatic focal adenomyosis: a case report. Hum Reprod 21:1255–1259

Raiga J, Bowen E, Glowaczower E et al (1994) Failure factors in endometrial resection. J Gynecol Obstet Biol Reprod 23:274–278

Reinhold C, Atrim M, Mehio A et al (1995) Diffuse uterine adenomyosis: morphologic criteria and diagnostic accuracy of endovaginal sonography. Radiology 1197:609–614

Taran F, Weaver A, Coddington C et al (2010) Characteristics indicating adenomyosis coexisting with leiomyomas: a case control study. Hum Reprod 25:1177–1182

Uduwela A, Perra M, Aiquig L et al (2000) Endometrial-myometrial interface: relationship to adenomyosis and changes in pregnancy. Obstet Gynecol Surv 55:390–400

Vercellini P, Parazzini F, Oldani S et al (1995) Adenomyosis at hysterectomy: a study on frequency distribution and patient characteristics. Hum Reprod 10:1160–1162

Wang P, Wei-Min L, Jong LF et al (2009) Comparison of surgery alone and combined surgical-medical treatment in the management of symptomatic uterine adenomyoma. Fertil Steril 92:876–885

Wood C (1998) Surgical and medical treatment of adenomyosis. Hum Reprod 4:323–336

Wood C, Maher P, Hill D (1994) Biopsy and conservative surgical treatment of adenomyosis. J Am Assoc Gynecol Laparosc 4:313–316

Wood C, Maher P, Hill D (1997) Bleeding associated with vaginal hysterectomy. Aust N Z J Obstet Gynaecol 37:457–461

Laparoscopic Hysterectomy: Surgical Approach

9

Sarah L. Cohen and Jon I. Einarsson

Contents

S.L. Cohen, MD, MPH (✉)
J.I. Einarsson, MD, MPH
Division of Minimally Invasive Gynecologic Surgery,
Brigham and Women's Hospital,
75 Francis Street, Boston, MA 02115, USA
e-mail: scohen20@partners.org,
slcohen47@gmail.com; jeinarsson@partners.org

9.1   Introduction

Since the first successful performance of hysterectomy in the nineteenth century (Langenbeck 1817; Burnham 1854), the procedure has been transformed by advances in surgical technique and technological innovations. Laparoscopic approach to hysterectomy was introduced in the late 1980s by Kurt Semm and Harry Reich (Semm 1991; Reich et al. 1989). As of 2005, national surveillance data from the United States shows that 14 % of hysterectomies were performed laparoscopically, 22 % vaginally, and 64 % abdominally (Jacoby et al. 2009). The laparoscopic approach has demonstrated benefits of decreased morbidity, shorter hospital stay, and quicker return to normal activities when compared to abdominal hysterectomy (Nieboer et al. 2009), with decreased postoperative pain and shorter length of hospitalization when compared to vaginal hysterectomy (Gendy et al. 2011).

As with all surgical procedures, the first steps to a successful operation involve careful preoperative planning, medical clearance, and informed consent. Specifically with regard to laparoscopic hysterectomy, the patient must be informed of the option to retain versus remove the cervix; issues surrounding concomitant removal of adnexal structures should also be discussed. Finally, appropriate preoperative antibiotic and venous thromboembolism prophylaxis should be administered. The routine use of mechanical bowel preparations is not recommended, though

O. Istre (ed.), *Minimally Invasive Gynecological Surgery*,
DOI 10.1007/978-3-662-44059-9_9, © Springer-Verlag Berlin Heidelberg 2015

antibiotic bowel preparation may be appropriate in select cases (Cohen and Einarsson 2011).

9.2 Choice of Equipment

A uterine manipulator system can be useful for mobilization of the uterus at the time of hysterectomy, though some surgeons prefer to achieve this with abdominal instrumentation such as a tenaculum or myoma screw. Additional advantages of a uterine manipulator include: excellent cephalad displacement at the time of colpotomy, enhanced delineation of the vaginal cuff, provision of a channel through which chromopertubation can be performed, and maintenance of pneumoperitoneum. Although many options for uterine manipulators exist, including disposable, partially reusable, and reusable devices, two of the more commonly utilized devices for laparoscopic hysterectomy are the RUMI® Uterine Manipulator (Cooper-Surgical, Trumbull, CT) and the VCare® Uterine Manipulator/Elevator (ConMed Endosurgery, Utica, NY). The VCare® device is a streamlined option which is relatively easy to insert. The RUMI® manipulator cervical cup provides excellent visualization of the vaginal fornices, particularly in cases of a long cervix, however is more cumbersome to employ (Einarsson and Suzuki 2009). Other versatile options include the MANGESHIKAR and CLERMONT-FERRAND Uterine Manipulators (both from Storz, Tuttlingen, Germany), along with reusable simpler designs that are commonly used for general laparoscopy.

Standard laparoscopic tools which are useful for laparoscopic hysterectomy include: blunt graspers, scissors, a suction/irrigation device, and one or more electrosurgical devices. Regarding electrosurgical devices, options exist for monopolar or bipolar tools, ultrasonic dissectors, and advanced bipolar vessel sealing/ligation devices. Monopolar devices, available in blade, hook, or scissor form, create cutting, fulgurating, and desiccating effects. Care must be taken when employing monopolar energy to avoid complications such as direct or capacitive coupling and insulation failure (Brill et al. 1998). Conventional bipolar devices, available in grasper form, are less prone to visceral injury but can cause char formation and lateral thermal spread on the target tissue (Brill 2008). Advanced vessel sealing/ligation devices include: LigaSure™ sealing device (Covidien, Boulder, CO), PlaskmaKinetics™ (PK) Sealer (Gyrus ACMI Medical, Maple Grove, MN), Harmonic® Scalpel (Ethicon Endo-Surgery, Somerville, NJ), EnSeal™ Vessel Fusion System (SurgRx, Inc., Palo Alto, CA), and the Thunderbeat integrated bipolar/ultrasonic device (Olympus, Center Valley, PA), among others. Surgeon preference dictates the selection of a particular electrosurgical device and should include consideration of cost related to using multiple disposable instruments.

9.3 Operative Technique

After induction of anesthesia, the patient is carefully positioned in a neurologically neutral fashion in dorsal lithotomy position with arms tucked at her sides. Antislip devices, such as egg crate foam or a vacuum-beanbag mattress, are helpful to limit cephalad movement of the patient when in Trendelenburg position. Abdominal access is obtained by surgeon's preferred technique and trocars are placed. For conventional multiport laparoscopy, an umbilical trocar and bilateral lower quadrant trocars are utilized. A fourth trocar may be placed to aid with laparoscopic suturing or advanced dissection; common locations for an additional trocar site include midline suprapubic or left upper quadrant.

After normalizing pelvic anatomy as necessary, the hysterectomy is begun by dividing the infundibulopelvic ligaments (if removing the ovaries) or utero-ovarian ligaments (if preserving the ovaries). By remaining close to the ovary when controlling these ligaments, one can avoid ascending uterine vasculature or retroperitoneal structures, respectively (Fig. 9.1). After transecting the round ligament, the broad ligament is opened to reveal anterior and posterior leaves (Fig. 9.2). The dissection continues along the peritoneal reflection of the vesicouterine peritoneum in order to mobilize the bladder caudally

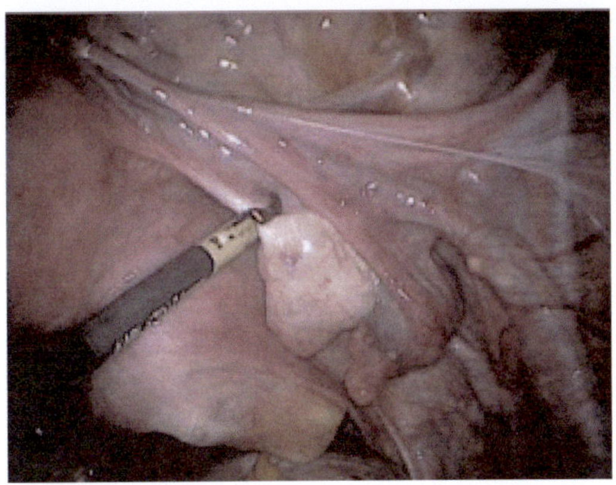

Fig. 9.1 Coagulation of ligament ovari proprium

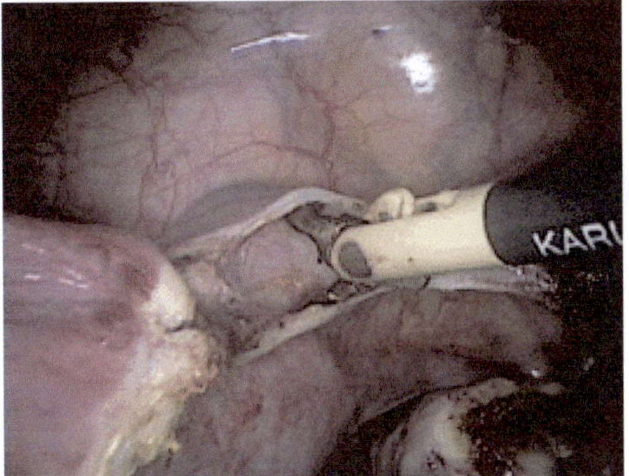

Fig. 9.2 Opening of ligamentar latum

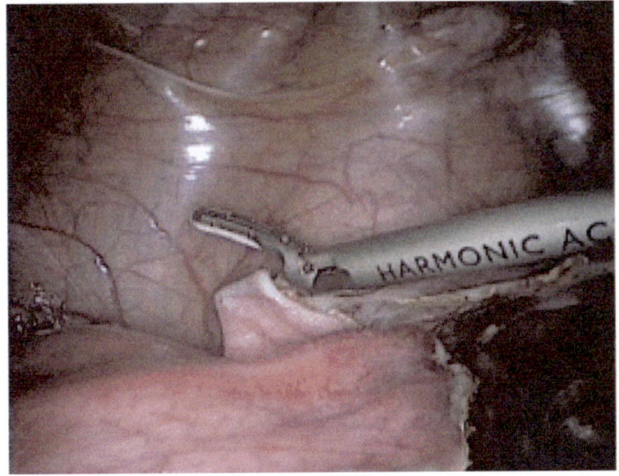

Fig. 9.3 Incision of bladder flap

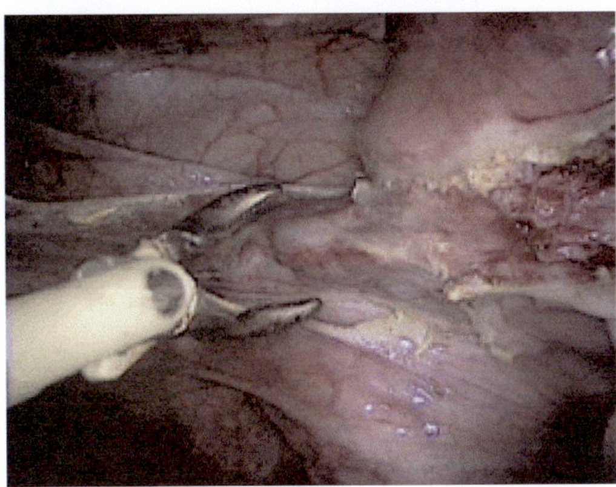

Fig. 9.4 Coagulation of uterine artery

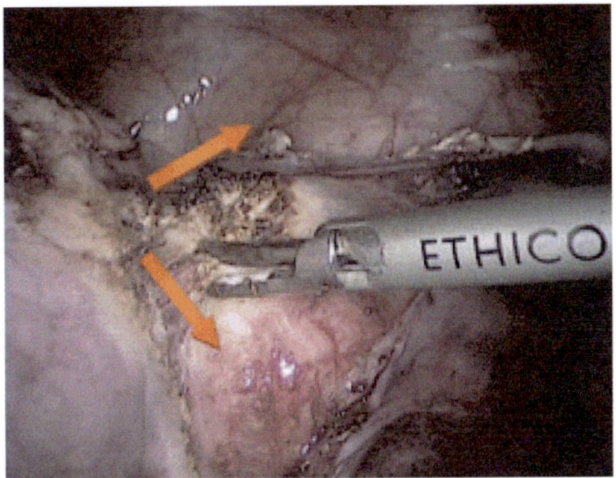

Fig. 9.5 Opening to vagina

(Fig. 9.3). The uterine vessels are then skeletonized, sealed, and incised at the level of the internal cervical os; the uterus should be mobilized cephalad during this step to increase distance from the ureter (Fig. 9.4).

When performing a supracervical hysterectomy, the uterus is separated from the cervix at the level of the internal cervical os with either a monopolar device (such as a spatula, scissor, hook, or loop) or harmonic scalpel. After transection of the uterine corpus, the endocervical canal may be desiccated in an attempt to decrease the occurrence of postoperative cyclic spotting. Specimen removal is then achieved with a mechanical tissue morcellation device or via minilaparotomy. Care should be taken whenever performing morcellation to do so in a contained fashion to avoid inadvertent spread of tissue within the abdomen.

In the case of total laparoscopic hysterectomy, the uterine vascular pedicle is further lateralized

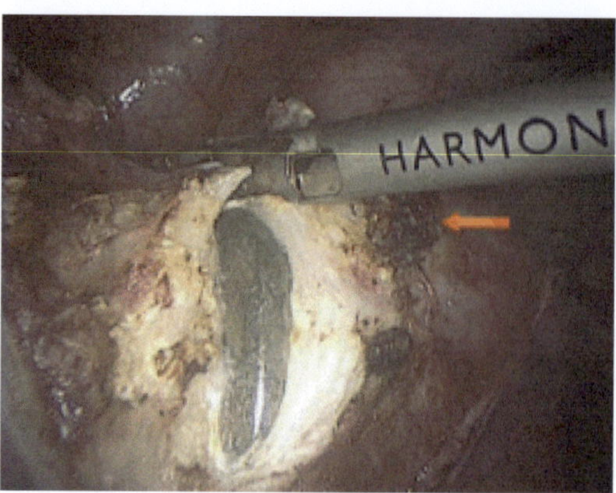

Fig. 9.6 Incision on the vaginal cup

below the level of the cervix (Fig. 9.5) and care is taken to ensure the bladder has been mobilized below the level of intended colpotomy incision. Cephalad deflection of the uterus aids with identification of the vaginal fornices, and the colpotomy is made in a circumferential fashion with monopolar or harmonic device of choice (Fig. 9.6). In cases of a narrow introitus where it is not feasible to employ a uterine manipulator, laparoscopic upward traction is essential in order to distance the ascending uterine vessels from the ureters and allow for safe colpotomy performance. The specimen is then removed through the vagina or morcellated as necessary, either laparoscopically or vaginally. Following specimen retrieval, pneumoperitoneum is maintained by occlusion of the vaginal canal; one useful option for this purpose is a sponge-filled surgical glove. Vaginal cuff closure is performed with laparoscopic suturing techniques, with care to take bites of sufficient distance from the thermal margin and incorporate both the vaginal mucosa as well as rectovaginal and pubocervical fascia.

9.4 Special Considerations

Of particular concern during advanced laparoscopic surgery, and specifically hysterectomy, is the avoidance of injury to ureter or bladder. It is imperative that the surgeon keeps the anatomic course of the ureter in consideration throughout the procedure, with retroperitoneal dissection and ureterolysis as necessary. The transection of the infundibulopelvic ligament and creation of uterine vascular pedicles are steps where the ureter is under particular risk of damage; suggestions for limiting potential ureteral injury are provided in the Operative Technique section earlier (Janssen et al. 2011). Cystoscopy should be employed liberally if there are any concerns about injury to bladder or ureter. However, a normal cystoscopy does not guarantee lack of injury, particularly in cases of thermal damage or partial transection (Dandolu et al. 2003).

In cases of large uteri extending to or above the level of the umbilicus, it may be helpful to place the accessory trocars at a more cephalad position and/or utilize left upper quadrant entry at Palmer's point. The technique of "port hopping" (whereby the laparoscope is moved between umbilical and lateral ports) can also be useful in cases where visualization is limited by a bulky uterus. Another consideration with larger uteri is the limited mobility provided by traditional uterine manipulators. In these cases, injection of dilute vasopressin solution subserosally into the uterus, followed by application of a laparoscopic tenaculum, may provide additional visualization. If there is an obstructed view caused by one or more dominant myomas, it may be beneficial to perform myomectomy first in order to generate more space in the pelvis. Similarly, in cases of planned total hysterectomy of a large uterus, it may be necessary to perform a supracervical transection first, mobilize the uterine specimen out of the pelvis, and then complete the procedure with a trachelectomy.

9.5 Postoperative Care

Laparoscopic hysterectomy patients may be offered the option of same-day discharge after an uncomplicated procedure if appropriate based on patient preferences, comorbid medical conditions, and home support system (Taylor 1994; Thiel and Gamelin 2003; Morrison and Jacobs 2004; Lieng et al. 2005). A randomized trial of day-case versus inpatient laparoscopic supracervical hysterectomy found similar satisfaction rates with lower self-reported short-term quality of life in the day surgery group (Kisic-Trope et al. 2011). Recommendations for patient activity following hysterectomy include 4–6 weeks of pelvic rest (longer for total hysterectomies) and avoidance of heavy lifting or vigorous activity in the immediate recovery period. Patients may be counseled that the majority of activities can be resumed by 2–4 weeks postoperatively (Claerhout and Deprest 2005).

Conclusions

Laparoscopic hysterectomy has demonstrated benefits to patients in terms of decreased morbidity and faster return to normal activities. With the techniques described earlier and sufficient surgical experience, laparoscopic hysterectomy can be implemented in a range of clinical scenarios, including complicated cases with distorted pelvic anatomy or large uteri. Continued emphasis on surgical training and awareness of laparoscopic techniques will allow for increased patient access to minimally invasive hysterectomy.

References

Burnham W (1854) Extirpation of the uterus and ovaries for sarcomatous disease. Nelson's Am Lancet 8:147

Brill AI (2008) Bipolar electrosurgery: convention and innovation. Clin Obstet Gynecol 51(1):153–158

Brill AI, Feste JR, Hamilton TL, Tsarouhas AP, Berglund SR, Petelin JB, Perantinides PG et al (1998) Patient safety during laparoscopic monopolar electrosurgery–principles and guidelines. Consortium on Electrosurgical Safety During Laparoscopy. JSLS 2(3):221–225

Claerhout F, Deprest J (2005) Laparoscopic hysterectomy for benign diseases. Best Pract Res Clin Obstet Gynaecol 19(3):357–375

Cohen SL, Einarsson JI (2011) The role of mechanical bowel preparation in gynecologic laparoscopy. Rev Obstet Gynecol 4:28

Dandolu V, Mathai E, Chatwani A et al (2003) Accuracy of cystoscopy in the diagnosis of ureteral injury in benign gynecologic surgery. Int Urogynecol J Pelvic Floor Dysfunct 14(6):427–431

Einarsson JI, Suzuki Y (2009) Total laparoscopic hysterectomy: 10 steps toward a successful procedure. Rev Obstet Gynecol 2(1):57–64

Gendy R, Walsh CA, Walsh SR et al (2011) Vaginal hysterectomy versus total laparoscopic hysterectomy for benign disease: a metaanalysis of randomized controlled trials. Am J Obstet Gynecol 204:388

Jacoby VL, Autry A, Jacobson G et al (2009) Nationwide use of laparoscopic hysterectomy compared with abdominal and vaginal approaches. Obstet Gynecol 114:1041

Janssen PF, Brolmann HA, Huirne JA (2011) Recommendations to prevent urinary tract injuries during laparoscopic hysterectomy: a systematic Delphi procedure among experts. J Minim Invasive Gynecol 18(3):314–321

Kisic-Trope J, Qvigstad E, Ballard K (2011) A randomized trial of day-case vs inpatient laparoscopic supracervical hysterectomy. Am J Obstet Gynecol 204(4): 307.e1-8

Langenbeck CJM (1817) Geschichte einer von mir glucklich verichteten extirpation der ganger gebarmutter. Bibliotheck Chir Ophthalmol Hanover 1:557

Lieng M, Istre O, Langebrekke A et al (2005) Outpatient laparoscopic supracervical hysterectomy with assistance of the lap loop. J Minim Invasive Gynecol 12: 290–294

Morrison JE, Jacobs VE (2004) Outpatient laparoscopic hysterectomy in a rural ambulatory surgery centre. J Am Assoc Gynecol Laparosc 11:359–364

Nieboer TE, Johnson N, Lethaby A et al (2009) Surgical approach to hysterectomy for benign gynaecological disease. Cochranec Database Syst Rev 3:CD003677

Reich H, de Cripo J, McGlynn F (1989) Laparoscopic hysterectomy. J Gynecol Surg 5:213–215

Semm K (1991) Hysterectomy via laparotomy or pelviscopy. A new CASH method without colpotomy. Geburtshilfe Frauenheilkd 51(12):996–1003

Taylor RH (1994) Outpatient laparoscopic hysterectomy with discharge in 4 to 6 hours. J Am Assoc Gynecol Laparosc 1(2):S35

Thiel J, Gamelin A (2003) Outpatient total laparoscopic hysterectomy. J Am Assoc Gynecol Laparosc 10:481–482

Laparoscopic Subtotal Hysterectomy

Stefanos Chandakas and John Erian

Contents

S. Chandakas, MD, MBA, PhD (✉)
Mitera and Hygeia Hospitals, Vas Sofias 121,
Athens 11524, Greece
e-mail: stefhand@hol.gr

J. Erian, FRCOG
Kings College Hospital, Princess Royal University
Hospital Orpington, BR67SE, Kent
e-mail: johnerian@aol.com

10.1   Introduction

Hysterectomy was mentioned in Greek manuscripts 2,000 years ago (Baskett 2005). Soranus of Ephesus described a vaginal hysterectomy for a prolapsed gangrenous uterus in the second century AD. The first abdominal hysterectomy was performed by Charles Clay in Manchester in 1844. During the eighteenth century the postoperative mortality of the procedure was over 70 % (Sutton 1997), mainly from haemorrhage and sepsis. The first abdominal total hysterectomy was performed by Dr E H Richardson in Baltimore in 1929. He also advocated the removal of the cervix for the prevention of cervical cancer of the cervical stump, which at the time had a reported incidence of 0.4 % (Johns 1997). However, subtotal abdominal hysterectomy remained the operation of choice for benign uterine disease until 1940 (Sutton 1995), when antibiotics were introduced, because not opening the vaginal vault reduced the risk of infection and thus death.

Following an intense debate after the introduction of antibiotics and transfusion in the 1950s, total abdominal hysterectomy prevailed as it offered protection against cervical cancer. The incidence of cervical cancer dropped to 0.14–0.16 % in the 1970s, with a further drop to 0.084 % attributed to the uptake of cervical screening (Quinn et al. 1999).

In 1989, the first total laparoscopic hysterectomy (TLH) was described by Harry Reich in

O. Istre (ed.), *Minimally Invasive Gynecological Surgery*,
DOI 10.1007/978-3-662-44059-9_10, © Springer-Verlag Berlin Heidelberg 2015

Pennsylvania (Reich et al. 1989), and 2 years later the first laparoscopic subtotal hysterectomy was described by Kurt Semm (1991). This was performed via 'pelviscopy' (gynaecological laparoscopy); the word 'laparoscopy' was forbidden because it was associated with great intraoperative morbidity. The procedure carrying the unfortunate acronym CASH (classic abdominal serrated-edge macromorcellator hysterectomy) involved complete excision of the endocervix with the aid of a transcervical guide wire and removal of the uterine corpus. The procedure was long, expensive, had a relatively high morbidity, and required advanced laparoscopic surgical skills. Preservation of the ectocervix also contradicted the belief of gynaecologists, built over three decades, that the cervix is 'better removed'.

During recent years, the interest in subtotal hysterectomy through the laparoscopic approach has been revived. Indeed, the USA has seen a fourfold increase in the number of subtotal hysterectomies performed (Merrill 2008). However, grade A evidence is lacking. As different women have different pathology and are treated by surgeons with different skills, any attempt at randomisation is likely to be impossible. We will describe our own experience with laparoscopic subtotal hysterectomy with reference to the literature when available.

10.2 Preoperative Preparation

Laparoscopic subtotal hysterectomy includes morcellation of the myometrium and of the endometrium; therefore it is very important to exclude endometrial hyperplasia and malignancy. Preoperative endometrial assessment with transvaginal ultrasound scanning and, where appropriate, outpatient hysteroscopy and endometrial sampling is of paramount importance for all women undergoing the procedure.

Women are advised that there is a small chance of developing cyclical bleeding despite diathermy of the endocervix and it is impossible to predict which women will develop this symptom. This cyclical bleeding invariably lasts for 1 day only in a periodical pattern and will never evolve into a heavy period. We believe that women who are informed of the possibility of cyclical bleeding are much less likely to be disturbed by its occurrence and much less likely to request a trachelectomy following a laparoscopic subtotal hysterectomy. The importance of continued cervical screening is also reinforced.

Contraindications to laparoscopic subtotal hysterectomy include the following:

- uterus more than 20 weeks size
- stoma
- adhesions
- unfitness for anaesthesia
- poor compliance with cervical screening
- diskaryosis/cervical intraepithelial neoplasia
- suspected malignancy.

We consider it good practice to offer the results of our own continuous audit to the women attending the clinic.

10.3 Surgical Technique

This is a comprehensive account of our standardised technique. In other units, alternative forms of thermal energy, different types of morcellating devices and uterine manipulators are used with equally good results.

The procedure is performed under general anaesthesia by two surgeons, with the women in the Lloyd–Davies position. Preparation of the woman includes indwelling bladder catheterisation and placement of a Pelosi uterine manipulator (Apple Medical Corporation, Bolton, MA, USA Apple Medical Corporation, Marlboro, MA, USA) in the cervix. This is an articulated manipulator that allows extreme anteversion and retroversion as well as lateral manipulation of the uterus even in the absence of an assistant. The use of an indwelling catheter is essential as it will keep the bladder empty as the suprapubic port is placed later during the procedure and the collecting bag will immediately fill with carbon dioxide if the bladder is injured. If Palmer's point entry is indicated, a nasogastric tube is inserted to decompress the upper gastrointestinal tract after the introduction of anaesthesia.

The procedure is performed through a 4-port operative laparoscopy: a 10 mm infraumbilical port for the laparoscope, two 5 mm lateral ports and a suprapubic 12 mm port for morcellation. The lateral ports are placed high in the abdomen, at the same level as the umbilicus. This allows more space for handling pedicles in large uteruses and also facilitates the angle of coagulation as the line of the instrument is parallel to the lateral margin of the uterus and away from the pelvic sidewall.

Laparoscopic subtotal hysterectomy is a two-surgeon procedure, with both surgeons predominantly operating with their right hand. The surgeon on the left uses the right hand to handle instruments through the left port and the left hand to manipulate the Pelosi uterine manipulator and maximise exposure of the operating field. The surgeon on the right of the woman under surgery uses the right hand to handle instruments through the right port and the left hand to handle the laparoscope.

The laparoscopic steps include coagulation and transection of the infundibulopelvic ligament in the case of bilateral salpingo-oophorectomy or the ovarian ligament in the case of conservation of the ovaries. The round ligament is coagulated and transected. The broad ligament is incised and the uterovesical fold is deflected to allow more space for the Lap Loop (Roberts Surgical Healthcare, Kidderminster, UK) monopolar diathermy device at the level of the cervical isthmus. The broad ligament is incised lateral to the uterus so that the uterine plexus is not inadvertently injured.

Transection of the uterine vessels is performed at the same time as the detachment of the uterine corpus using the Lap Loop monopolar wire after removal of the uterine manipulator. The Lap Loop device is inserted through the suprapubic port to the left of the uterus and the wire is grasped by the surgeon on the right, advanced behind the cervix and attached to the Lap Loop applicator. The pouch of Douglas is checked with the wire under tension to avoid bowel entrapment inside the monopolar wire. The diathermy is set at 100 W coagulation and the surgeon on the left keeps the uterus retroflexed. With this technique, the angle of cutting is vertical and the Lap Loop device provides a conisation effect removing a wedge off the endocervix.

When the uterine vessels are cut with the wire, they remain attached on the sides of the cervical stump instead of retracting to the pelvic sidewall. All pedicles are cross-coagulated, i.e. coagulated from the left and the right side trocars at right angles, by the surgeon and the assistant. Any complementary coagulation to the uterine vessels is easy, does not require any additional dissection and most importantly does not jeopardise the integrity of the ureters and the major vessels of the pelvic sidewall.

The uterus is then morcellated by drawing the specimen into the morcellator using a single-tooth or a gallbladder forceps while the uterus is lifted and stabilised by the surgeon on the right. The tip of the rotating electromechanical morcellator is always kept within 2 cm of the lower abdominal wall (Erian et al. 2007), and the single-tooth forceps is only advanced 3–4 cm beyond the edge of the trocar to avoid inadvertent grasping of bowel or omentum during the morcellation. We routinely use the suprapubic port for the morcellator as we feel this provides more space inferiorly and laterally from the blade of the morcellator to the abdominal viscera and the pelvic sidewall, therefore minimising the risk of accidental damage to vital structures.

After morcellation is completed, the peritoneal cavity is cleared of any collected blood and fragments of myometrium by collection and irrigation with normal saline solution followed by suction. The bowel is not displaced before all the visible fragments are removed to minimise missing uterine corpus fragments in between bowel loops. The clearance of the pelvis, paracolic gutters and upper abdomen (as the woman is in deep head-down position) is of paramount importance as there have been reports of pelvic seeding of morcellated uterine tissue and subsequent development of adenomyotic masses (morcelloma) (Donnez et al. 2007; Hilger and Magrina 2006) in the peritoneal cavity or the cervical stump. Meticulous clearance of the peritoneal cavity has been advocated (Sutton 1995; Johns 1997) because several complications may be attributed to incomplete collection of uterine fragments. The endocervix is cauterised with bipolar diathermy.

Haemostasis is checked after decompressing the peritoneal cavity. Then the abdominal cavity is re-inflated and a 16 gauge drain is passed through the lateral port to the pouch of Douglas. The drain is connected with a decompressed collection container as suction drainage may draw small or large bowel into the drain and cause ischaemia and subsequent perforation (Reed et al. 1992). Finally, the laparoscopic instruments and trocars are removed under direct vision and the port sites are closed with a J-shaped needle and number 1 Vicryl® (polyglactin 910; Ethicon Endo-Surgery, Cincinnati, OH, USA) under laparoscopic control before decompression of the pneumoperitoneum.

10.4 Learning Curve

As with all new procedures, mentoring and preceptorship are essential to minimise the risk of complications (Cutner and Erian 1995). Once introduced as routine practice, the complication rate of minimal access hysterectomy seems to fall by 11–13 % per year reaching a plateau after about 5–7 years of practice (Brummer et al. 2008; Wattiez et al. 2002). The fall in complication rates may be associated with the early identification of potential visceral injury and laparoscopic repair of the injured viscera.

The operating time seems to be longer in the first operations but stabilises after the first 30 procedures (Ghomi et al. 2007). The effect of surgical volume was seen in a double-parallel randomised trial in the UK (Garry et al. 2004), where laparoscopic hysterectomy was performed in a limited number of centres, with participating surgeons performing on average only 13 procedures over 4 years. In this study, the complication rate (including preoperative conversion to laparotomy) for the laparoscopic hysterectomy group remained as high as 11 % (Ghomi et al. 2007). Similarly, cyclical bleeding after the procedure has been demonstrated to be more common with the most inexperienced surgeons (Lieng et al. 2008). This

may be related to the correct level of detachment of the uterine corpus or smoothness of the incision line in the cervical stump. In our experience, the Lap Loop system offers a fairly standard level of a smooth uterine incision even in the hands of less experienced surgeons, which may offer an advantage over the monopolar hook or spatula, ultrasonic hook or Plasma Kinetic (Gyrus Olympus Medical Systems Hamburg Germany) hook technique. However, this advantage has not been assessed by comparative studies.

In our series, the major complication rate was 1.2 % (Erian et al. 2008a), which is in agreement with results found by Wattiez et al. at Clermond Ferrand (Wattiez et al. 2002). All complications associated with haemostasis (haematoma, pelvic collection and transfusion) occurred during the first 81 operations (Erian et al. 2008a) and this reflects the duration of the learning curve. However, visceral injuries occurred later, after the first 100 operations (Erian et al. 2005) or 2 years of practice, probably reflecting the confidence to undertake more difficult procedures in women with a complex previous surgical history. These findings are in accordance with those from previous studies (Wattiez et al. 2002). It is notable that none of the visceral injuries that occurred in our series were related to thermal energy or morcellation.

In our technique, reflection of the bladder is essential prior to the placement of the Lap Loop wire, but we understand that in other units this step is not considered to be essential, with equally good but unpublished results. We have changed the technique of bladder dissection and now each surgeon dissects their side of the bladder. Following this change, we have not had any bladder damage. All bladder injuries in our series (0.75 %) occurred in women with three or four previous caesarean sections (Erian et al. 2008a).

10.5 Laparoscopic Subtotal Hysterectomy as Same-Day Surgery

The Foley indwelling catheter and the drain are removed 4 h after the procedure. Women are reviewed by the medical team 6 h postoperatively and discharged. They are advised to call the 24-h helpline service if they are experiencing any symptoms. If there has been bladder damage during surgery, the home care team will allocate a nurse who will remove the catheter at the appropriate time (5 days postoperatively) and ensure there is an acceptable postvoiding residual of urine. In our series of over 400 women, we have not had to intervene surgically or transfuse any women intra- or postoperatively. The readmission rates seem very low (Erian et al. 2008b) and the duration of surgery is short, even with large uteruses approaching 1 kg in weight. The postoperative management protocol is simple but requires a team effort and multiprofessional education to organise a setting where LSH can be performed safely as a 6-h discharge procedure.

10.6 Urinary Tract Injuries: Diagnosis, Surgical and Postoperative Management

In our series, there was no ureteric injury (0 %) in the first 500 women. This was probably the case because there is no need to dissect the paracervical tissues. The distance between the cervix and the ureter is less than 5 mm in over 10 % of women (Simon et al. 1999); the lateral thermal spread of coagulating devices varies from 2 to 4 mm (Carbonell et al. 2003) and they are usually 2–5 mm wide. It is easy to understand how ureteric thermal injury occurs in these conditions. The possibility of avoiding this area altogether gives laparoscopic subtotal hysterectomy a distinct advantage over total laparoscopic hysterectomy.

In a recent series (Jung and Huh 2008), the incidence of ureteric injury was 0.34 %. It is noteworthy, however, that all ureteric injuries in this series occurred when a colpotomy was used to remove the uterus from the peritoneal cavity. When colpotomy was replaced by morcellation, there was no ureteric injury for over 10 years. We can safely say that ureteric injury during LSH is very rare when morcellation is used to remove the uterine corpus.

Bladder injury is not so uncommon. If a suprapubic trocar is used, catheterisation is absolutely essential. In our experience, bladder injury only occurred in the presence of multiple (more than 2) previous caesarean sections and this is a counselling point that needs to be stressed. The results by Donnez et al. (2009) are in agreement with this point as all their bladder injuries happened in women with previous caesarean sections as well. The incidence reported was 0.25 %, which is lower than that in our series (0.75 %). Bladder injuries are easy to detect intraoperatively as the catheter bag is inflated with carbon dioxide that escapes through the bladder incision. Bladder injury is repaired by laparoscopic suturing using a single-layer closure (Thakar et al. 2002). Antibiotic prophylaxis is administered and the bladder is catheterised for 5 days on free flow (the catheter is draining freely in a urine collector and no tap is used ensuring continuous decompression of the bladder) on an outpatient basis. The catheter is then removed at home and the postvoiding residual urine is measured.

10.7 Satisfaction with the Procedure

In our series, 98 % of the women were satisfied with the operation and the same number would recommend the procedure to a friend. In previous studies (Ghomi et al. 2007), there was clear evidence that the laparoscopic approach resulted in a shorter convalescence time, less postoperative pain and rapid improvement in quality-of-life indicators (Simon et al. 1999). This percentage is higher than that in a recent report (Lieng et al. 2008), which presented a satisfaction rate of 90 %. However, in that study about half the women did not expect to have any bleeding postoperatively. In our opinion, the procedure is offered to treat menorrhagia and not to induce complete amenorrhea. When this is clearly conveyed to the women preoperatively, they are less likely to be disappointed because of cyclical bleeding. The incidence of cyclical bleeding in our series was 2 % and some surgeons would argue that this is the reason why our satisfaction rate is 98 % (Erian et al. 2008a). This is incorrect as there are women who are dissatisfied because of other problems such as residual pain, postoperative infection, communication with medical and nursing staff and waiting time.

10.8 Laparoscopic Subtotal Hysterectomy and Cervical Cancer

One of the main arguments of those supporting total hysterectomy is the potential for the cervical stump to develop cervical intraepithelial neoplasia (CIN) or cancer. We do not offer a laparoscopic subtotal hysterectomy to women with smear abnormalities. A study of 1.87 million has shown that the risk of cervical cancer after a normal smear history is 1:5546 (0.018 %) (Morrell et al. 2005). The incidence of cervical cancer in women who have undergone subtotal hysterectomy is 0.1–0.2 % (Brummer et al. 2008). To put this into context, the risk of cervical cancer in women who undergo laparoscopic subtotal hysterectomy is smaller than the risk of uterine rupture in labour in women with a previous caesarean section (0.3 %)—and vaginal birth after a caesarean section is considered routine practice.

In the rare case when cervical cancer does occur in the cervical stump, the prognosis is no different to that in women who have not had a hysterectomy (Hellström et al. 2001). However, the treatment of CIN with large loop excision of the transformation zone (LLETZ) is more hazardous as the uncontrolled spread of thermal energy toward the bladder in the absence of a uterine corpus may result in fistulae. In these circumstances, laparoscopic dissection of the anterior peritoneum with a relatively full bladder, acting as a heat sink, should be considered.

10.9 Cervical Stump Symptoms

The rate of persistent vaginal bleeding in other series can be as high as 24 % (Lieng et al. 2006; Lieng et al. 2008), but 90 % of the women are satisfied with the procedure and this reinforces the need for appropriate preoperative counselling regarding this potential symptom. In our series, 2 % of the women complained of chronic vaginal bleeding and this low rate may be attributed to the low amputation of the cervical stump with the Lap Loop device and the meticulous destruction of the cervical canal with high-frequency pulsatile bipolar diathermy.

Disturbing symptoms, namely pain and bleeding from the cervical stump, have been reported to be more common in women who have endometriosis (Okaro et al. 2001). However, later studies have contradicted this notion (Ghomi et al. 2005). The degree of treatment of peritoneal disease, the presence of ovaries and the pre- and postoperative medical treatment of the disease would affect these results. There has not been a study assessing the resolution of symptoms, which is thought to result from the retained cervix after a trachelectomy.

In a large retrospective Scandinavian study (Brandsborg et al. 2007), at least a third of the women undergoing hysterectomy had chronic pain 1 year later and the main risk factors appeared to be pelvic pain, pain in another part of their body and of course endometriosis. In women who have persistent pain, therefore, other causes of pain must also be considered, in addition to the retained cervical stump (Garry 2008).

Conclusion

Laparoscopic subtotal hysterectomy is an effective procedure that can be performed safely in a day care setting. It is not proven to be superior or inferior to total laparoscopic hysterectomy, but it seems to carry less febrile morbidity and a lower risk of hospital admission, making it more suitable for same-day surgery. The procedure offers an early return to normal activities and an early resumption of sexual function.

Advances in coagulation and morcellation technology have reduced the operating time and have dramatically changed the safety profile of the procedure compared with the 1990s. The long-term risks are small and mostly theoretical, whereas the benefits in the immediate and late postoperative period are documented and substantial.

References

Baskett TF (2005) Hysterectomy: evolution and trends. Best Pract Res Clin Obstet Gynaecol 19(3):295–305

Brandsborg B, Nikolajsen L, Hansen CT, Kehlet H, Jensen TS (2007) Risk factors for chronic pain after hysterectomy: a nationwide questionnaire and database study. Anesthesiology 106(5):1003–1012

Brummer TH, Seppälä TT, Härkki PS (2008) National learning curve for laparoscopic hysterectomy and trends in hysterectomy in Finland 2000–2005. Hum Reprod 23:840–845

Carbonell AM, Joels CS, Kercher KW, Matthews BD, Sing RF, Heniford BT (2003) A comparison of laparoscopic bipolar vessel sealing devices in the hemostasis of small-, medium-, and large-sized arteries. J Laparoendosc Adv Surg Tech A 13:377–380

Cutner A, Erian J (1995) Training in minimal access surgery. Br J Hosp Med 53(5):226–228

Donnez O, Squifflet J, Leconte I, Jadoul P, Donnez J (2007) Posthysterectomy pelvic adenomyotic masses observed in 8 cases out of a series of 1405 laparoscopic subtotal hysterectomies. J Minim Invasive Gynecol 14(2):156–160

Donnez O, Jadoul P, Squifflet J, Donnez J (2009) A series of 3190 laparoscopic hysterectomies for benign disease from 1990 to 2006: evaluation of complications compared with vaginal and abdominal procedures. BJOG 116:492–500

Erian J, El-Toukhy T, Chandakas S, Theodoridis T, Hill N (2005) One hundred cases of laparoscopic subtotal hysterectomy using the PK and Lap Loop systems. J Minim Invasive Gynecol 12(4):365–369

Erian J, Hassan M, Hill N (2007) Electromechanical morcellation in laparoscopic subtotal hysterectomy. Int J Gynaecol Obstet 99(1):67–68

Erian J, Hassan M, Pachydakis A, Chandakas S, Wissa I, Hill N (2008a) Efficacy of laparoscopic subtotal hysterectomy in the management of menorrhagia: 400 consecutive cases. BJOG 115(6):742–748

Erian J, Lee C, Chandakas S, Watkinson S, Hill N (2008b) Feasibility of 6 hour discharge following laparoscopic subtotal hysterectomy; analysis of 492 consecutive cases. J Minim Invasive Gynecol 15:5S

Garry R (2008) The place of subtotal/supracervical hysterectomy in current practice. BJOG 115:1597–1600

Garry R, Fountain J, Mason S, Napp V, Brown J, Hawe J et al (2004) The eVALuate study: two parallel randomised trials, one comparing laparoscopic with abdominal hysterectomy, the other comparing laparoscopic with vaginal hysterectomy. Br Med J 328:129–136

Ghomi A, Hantes J, Lotze EC (2005) Incidence of cyclical bleeding after laparoscopic supracervical hysterectomy. J Minim Invasive Gynecol 12(3):201–205

Ghomi A, Littman P, Prasad A, Einarsson JI (2007) Assessing the learning curve for laparoscopic supracervical hysterectomy. JSLS 11(2):190–194

Hellström AC, Sigurjonson T, Pettersson F (2001) Carcinoma of the cervical stump. The radiumhemmet series 1959–1987. Treatment and prognosis. Acta Obstet Gynecol Scand 80(2):152–157

Hilger WS, Magrina JF (2006) Removal of pelvic leiomyomata and endometriosis five years after supracervical hysterectomy. Obstet Gynecol 108(3 Pt 2):772–774

Johns A (1997) Supracervical versus total hysterectomy. Clin Obstet Gynecol 40(4):903–913

Jung SK, Huh CY (2008) Ureteral injuries during classic intrafascial supracervical hysterectomy: an 11-year experience in 1163 patients. J Minim Invasive Gynecol 15(4):440–445

Lieng M, Istre O, Busund B, Qvigstad E (2006) Severe complications caused by retained tissue in laparoscopic supracervical hysterectomy. J Minim Invasive Gynecol 13(3):231–233

Lieng M, Qvigstad E, Istre O, Langebrekke A, Ballard K (2008) Long-term outcomes following laparoscopic supracervical hysterectomy. BJOG 115(13):1605–1610

Merrill RM (2008) Hysterectomy surveillance in the United States, 1997 through 2005. Med Sci Monit 14(1):CR24–CR31

Morrell S, Taylor R, Wain G (2005) A study of Pap test history and histologically determined cervical cancer in NSW women, 1997–2003. J Med Screen 12(4): 190–196

Okaro EO, Jones KD, Sutton C (2001) Long term outcome following laparoscopic supracervical hysterectomy. BJOG 108(10):1017–1020

Quinn M, Babb P, Jones J, Allen E (1999) Effect of screening on incidence of and mortality from cancer of cervix in England: evaluation based on routinely collected statistics. BMJ 318:904–908

Reed MWR, Wyman A, Thomas WE, Zeiderman MR (1992) Perforation of the bowel by suction drains. Br J Surg 79:679

Reich H, DeCaprio J, McGlynn E (1989) Laparoscopic hysterectomy. J Gynecol Surg 5:213–216

Semm K (1991) Hysterectomy via laparotomy or pelviscopy. A new CASH method without colpotomy [article in German]. Geburtshilfe Frauenheilkd 51:996–1003

Simon NV, Laveran RL, Cavanaugh S, Gerlach DH, Jackson JR (1999) Laparoscopic supracervical hysterectomy vs. abdominal hysterectomy in a community hospital. A cost comparison. J Reprod Med 44(4):339–345

Sutton C (1995) Subtotal hysterectomy revisited. Endosc Surg Allied Technol 3(2–3):105–108

Sutton C (1997) Hysterectomy: a historical perspective. Baillières Clin Obstet Gynaecol 11(1):1–22, Hysterectomy

Thakar R, Ayers S, Clarkson P, Stanton S, Manyonda I (2002) Outcomes after total versus subtotal abdominal hysterectomy. N Engl J Med 347:1318–1325

Wattiez A, Soriano D, Cohen SB, Nervo P, Canis M, Botchorishvili R et al (2002) The learning curve of total laparoscopic hysterectomy: comparative analysis of 1647 cases. J Am Assoc Gynecol Laparosc 9:339–345

How to Avoid Laparotomy Doing Laparoscopic Hysterectomy

11

Olav Istre

Contents

O. Istre, MD, PhD, DMSc,
Minimal Invasive Gynecology,
University of Southern Denmark,
Odense, Denmark

Department of Gynecology,
Aleris-Hamlet Hospital, Scandinavia
e-mail: oistre@gmail.com

Uterine fibroids are benign smooth muscle tumors of the uterus. They are seen in approximately one in three women and cause significant symptoms in at least half of them (Gentry et al. 2001). Hysterectomy is the ultimate treatment for women suffering from symptomatic myomas, menstrual disorders, endometriosis, and malignancy in the uterus. In Scandinavia, the prevalence of hysterectomy is mostly the same in Denmark, Norway, and Sweden, while the prevalence is almost threefold in Finland (Scott and Scott 1995). About 15 % of Norwegian women will have had a hysterectomy at the age of 60, while the figure will be approximately 40 % among American women (Backe and Lilleeng 1993; Lepine et al. 1997). The difference from one country to another may reflect to what degree women accept symptoms and the impact of doctors' advice in the current situation. This difference also reflects the treatment modalities chosen by the doctor, in particular with bleeding disorders (i.e., hysterectomy vs. transcervical resection [TCRE] or insertion of levonorgestrel intrauterine device). Since Harry Reich first described total laparoscopic hysterectomy (LH) in 1988 (Reich 1992), endoscopic hysterectomies have become a routine procedure in many gynecologic departments, even though open abdominal hysterectomy is still the dominant surgical technique worldwide. Many advocate the vaginal approach for hysterectomy as an excellent alternative to both abdominal and laparoscopic

O. Istre (ed.), *Minimally Invasive Gynecological Surgery*,
DOI 10.1007/978-3-662-44059-9_11, © Springer-Verlag Berlin Heidelberg 2015

hysterectomy techniques (Garry et al. 2004). To perform hysterectomy in uterus myomatosus, there are several surgical techniques. For a uterine weight of >1,000 g, after a caesarean section and in nullipara per vaginam, the most common surgical technique for hysterectomy in patients is hysterectomy per laparotomy. There are several surgical techniques: vaginal hysterectomy, abdominal hysterectomy, laparoscopic assisted vaginal hysterectomy, laparoscopic supracervical hysterectomy, and total laparoscopic hysterectomy, according to the wishes of the patient, her parity, and the clinical findings, e.g., adhesions. With a uterine weight of >1,000 g, after a caesarean section and as a nullipara per vaginam, the patient was classified as a difficult minimal-invasive case regarding surgical intervention.

11.1 Methods

In the present study, we investigated 406 consecutive patient operated for benign reason at a private hospital in Copenhagen Denmark. No rejection of referred patient and the patients were recruited from the primary health care sector by specialists in gynecology and were referred to the Minimal Invasive Gynecological Surgery (MIGS) unit at Aleris-Hamlet Hospital in Copenhagen, Denmark. The data were obtained from the patients records in the hospital and all patients were informed about the investigation.

All patients underwent pelvic examination and transvaginal ultrasound in the outpatient department. Patients were then scheduled for surgery within 3 weeks. We were able to perform 100 % laparoscopic approach apart from vaginal hysterectomy. The technique was a 4 port laparoscopic approach; in the smaller uterus the port placement was the camera in the umbilicus and 2 lateral ports and one in the middle 6 cm from the umbilicus. In the bigger uterus more than 400 g, the mid port and the camera was changed to be 6 cm from umbilicus upward (Fig. 11.1).

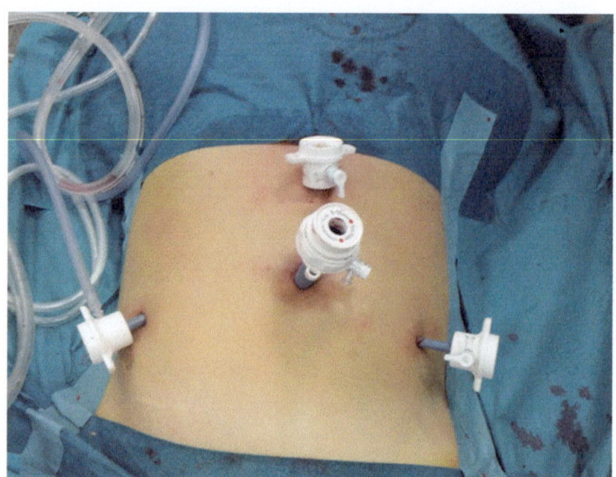

Fig. 11.1 Port placement in large fibroids

11.2 Results

In the present series only one laparotomy was performed in a 2.2 kg uterus where heavy bleeding encountered when the laparoscopic dissection of the uterus was performed, otherwise laparoscopic approach was utilized. Both in the TLH group and the LSH group the time was 75 min, however in larger uterus and fibroids very often LSH was the preferred technique, no malignancies was seen. Power morcellation was performed in the LSH group without any problems.

11.3 Complications

In the 445 patients so far the complications rate is low 6 % compared to the 16 % in the database for hysterectomy database Denmark. The most serious we had were 2 vesicoc-vaginal fistula and one urether lesion, one bladder perforation during the surgery.

Hematoma and postoperative infection encountered in 5 % of the patient (Table 11.1).

In 44 cases the uterine size exceeded 700 g and from Table 11.2 you can see that the operating time amount of bleeding increased significantly.

Lately, there has been discussions and concern of remnants of fibroid tissue left behind in the

Table 11.1 Laparoscopic hysterectomy ($N=404$, year 2014)

	LSH	TLH	Vag Hyst	Tot
	$N=206$, BMI=24	$N=156$, BMI=25	$N=41$, BMI=25	
	Age 47	Age 48	Age 61	$N=406$
OR time	75 (35–175)	75 (35–150)	85 (50–120)	78
Uterine weight (g)	394 (60–1,750)	263 (56–1,035)	75 (42–79)	315
Bleeding (ml)	77 (5–800)	57 (10–300)	63 (20–200)	81
Normal activity (days)	5 (1–14)	6 (1–14)	6 (1–14)	5.5
Back to work (days)	14 (1–42)	17 (7–35)	24 (14–49)	16
Postop complication $N=100$	4 (3 %)	7 (6.8%)	2 (4 %)	12 (4.5 %)

Table 11.2 Operation details in pat with weight >700 g

	Or time (min)	Weight (g)	Bleeding (ml)
Mean	108	1,006	201
Max	200	1,552	703
Range	130	1,950	600

abdominal cavity after power morcellation (FDA Issues Safety Communication on Laparoscopic Uterine Power Morcellation in Hysterectomy and Myomectomy 2014). It is feared to cause spread of malignancies. This could be reduced using a bag, as this technique facilitates safely morcellation of uterus and fibroids (Fig. 11.2).

11.4 Discussion

In the present study we were able to perform all the hysterectomies with the laparoscopic technique and with the use of morcellating in the larger uteri and fibroids, this is also in line with other studies in the literature. A retrospective cohort study of 957 patients who underwent laparoscopic supracervical (LSH), total (TLH), and assisted vaginal (LAVH) hysterectomies between January 2003 and December 2009. Among 957 hysterectomies LH, 799 (83.5 %) were LSH, 62 (6.4 %) TLH, and 96 (10.1 %) LAVH. Estimated blood loss, operating time, and length of hospital stay were significantly reduced with LSH. Meaning that the morcellation technique is beneficial and that the larger fibroid can come out this way avoiding big laparotomies.

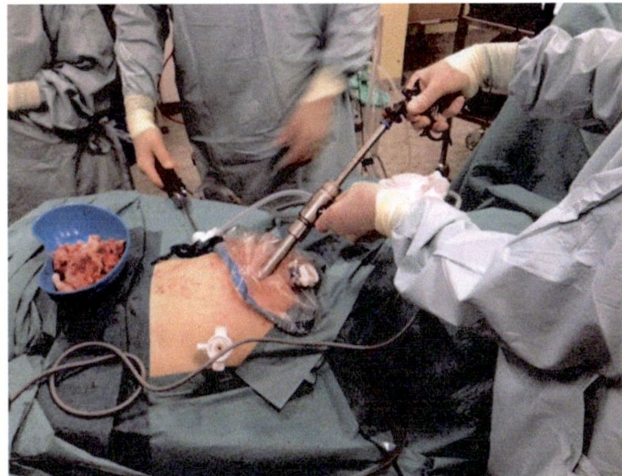

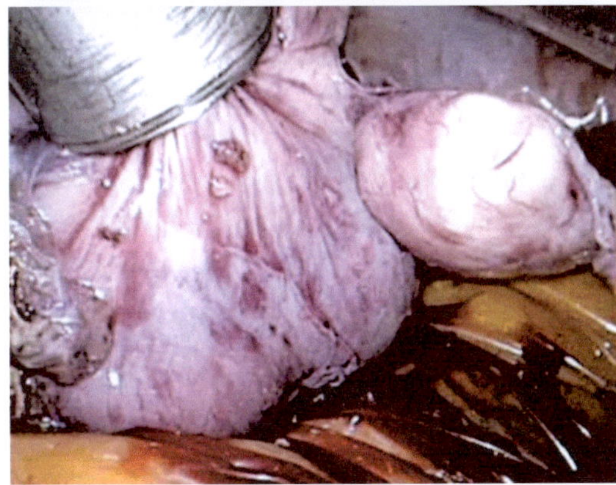

Fig. 11.2 Safe morcelation in a bag. Peritoneum completely cover in a articificiel space

Abdominal hysterectomy in Denmark is the main treatment for enlarged uterus in Denmark 53 % (The Danish hysterectomy database 2011) 8. Laparoscopic hysterectomy is performed in 12 % and vaginal route is utilized in 35 % in the smaller uterus. Complication rate was 18 %, readmission rate 5.4 %, and repeat surgery 4 % (The Danish Hysterectomy database 2010). In our intuition we have specialized in doing the hysterectomies even with large fibroid with the laparoscopic route. The benefits of minimally invasive surgery (MIS) for treating a variety of gynecologic conditions are well documented (Wright et al. 2012; Warren et al. 2009; Kongwattanakul and Khampitak 2012; Lenihan et al. 2004; Nieboer et al. 2012; Wiser et al. 2013). Nearly half of the estimated 400,000 inpatient-based hysterectomies performed annually in the United States for benign indications employ these innovative techniques. Thousands more women benefit from MIS in uterus-sparing procedures such as myomectomy. The ability to offer less invasive surgery to women often requires the removal of large tissue specimens through small incisions, which may be facilitated by morcellation. The term morcellation encompasses a variety of surgical techniques, some used in concert with specific devices, used to enable removal of large specimens from the peritoneal cavity, avoiding the need for laparotomy. In order to overcome the problem with spread of remnants from morcellation we have introduced the use of bags. In many ways this technique represents major benefits, the tissue and blood will stay within the bag so less cleaning at the end is needed however, more studies of this issue will be needed.

References

Backe B, Lilleeng S (1993) Hysterectomy in Norway. Quality of data and clinical practice. Tidsskr Nor Laegeforen 113:971–974

Garry R, Fountain J, Mason S et al (2004) The eVALuate study: two parallel randomised trials, one comparing laparoscopic with abdominal hysterectomy, the other comparing laparoscopic with vaginal hysterectomy. BMJ 328:129

Gentry CC, Okolo SO, Fong LF, Crow JC, Maclean AB, Perrett CW (2001) Quantification of vascular endothelial growth factor-A in leiomyomas and adjacent myometrium. Clin Sci (Lond) 101(6):691–695

Kongwattanakul K, Khampitak K (2012) Comparison of laparoscopically assisted vaginal hysterectomy and abdominal hysterectomy: a randomized controlled trial. J Minim Invasive Gynecol 19(1):89–94

Le Huu Nho R, Mege D, Ouaissi M, Sielezneff I, Sastre B (2012) Incidence and prevention of ventral incisional hernia. J Visc Surg 149(5 Suppl):3–14

Lenihan JP Jr, Kovanda C, Cammarano C (2004) Comparison of laparoscopic- assisted vaginal hysterectomy with traditional hysterectomy for cost-effectiveness to employers. Am J Obstet Gynecol 190(6):1714–1720; discussion 1720–1722

Lepine LA, Hillis SD, Marchbanks PA et al (1997) Hysterectomy surveillance: United States, 1980–1993. MMWR CDC Surveill Summ 46:1–15

Nieboer TE, Johnson N, Lethaby A, Tavender E, Curr E, Garry R et al (2009) Surgical approach to hysterectomy for benign gynaecological disease. Cochrane Database Syst Rev 8(3):CD003677

Nieboer TE, Hendriks JC, Bongers MY, Vierhout ME, Kluivers KB (2012) Quality of life after laparoscopic and abdominal hysterectomy: a randomized controlled trial. Obstet Gynecol 119(1):85–91

Reich H (1992) Laparoscopic hysterectomy. Surg Laparosc Endosc 2:85–88

Scott HM, Scott WG (1995) Hysterectomy for nonmalignant conditions: cost to New Zealand society. N Z Med J 108:423–426

The Danish Hysterectomy database 2010. https://www.sunhed.dk /../1869 hystektomi 2011

Warren L, Ladapo JA, Borah BJ, Gunnarsson CL (2009) Open abdominal versus laparoscopic and vaginal hysterectomy: analysis of a large United States payer measuring quality and cost of care. J Minim Invasive Gynecol 16(5):581–588

Wiser A, Holcroft CA, Tolandi T, Abenhaim HA (2013) Abdominal versus laparoscopic hysterectomies for benign diseases: evaluation of morbidity and mortality among 465,798 cases. Gynecol Surg 10:117–122

Wright KN, Jonsdottir GM, Jorgensen S, Shah N, Einarsson JI (2012) Costs and outcomes of abdominal, vaginal, laparoscopic and robotic hysterectomies. JSLS 16(4):519–524

Robotic Approach to Management of Fibroids

Olga A. Tusheva, Sarah L. Cohen, and Karen C. Wang

Contents

12.1   Introduction

The integration of robotics into the field of gynecologic surgery initially involved a voice-recognition system and robotic control of laparoscopic camera movement (AESOP® Endoscope Positioner (Computer Motion Inc., Goleta, CA)). This technology further evolved with the ZEUS® Surgical System (Computer Motion Inc., Goleta, CA) to include two robotic arms, thereby allowing the surgeon to operate from a console away from the operative table. The da Vinci Surgical System® (Intuitive Surgical, Sunnyvale, CA, USA), which was approved for gynecologic surgery in 2005 by the United States Food and Drug Administration, incorporates three or four robotic arms to allow surgeon control of the visual field and up to three laparoscopic instruments.

Advantages of the robotic platform for laparoscopic surgery include: three-dimensional stereoscopic vision, wristed instrumentation with seven degrees of freedom, diminished tremor effect, and enhanced ergonomics for the operator. In addition, the surgeon is able to control virtually all aspects of the operation from the surgeon console (aside from uterine manipulation) with the use of foot pedals and clutches. Disadvantages compared to traditional laparoscopy include lack of haptic feedback, which may result in inadvertent administration of excessive tension on tissues or suture materials.

Robotic tubal reanastomosis was the first surgery in gynecology performed with robotic

O.A. Tusheva • S.L. Cohen, MD, MPH
K.C. Wang, MD (✉)
Division of Minimally Invasive Gynecologic Surgery,
Department of Obstetrics and Gynecology,
Brigham and Women's Hospital, Boston, MA, USA
e-mail: kc.wang@partners.com

O. Istre (ed.), *Minimally Invasive Gynecological Surgery*,
DOI 10.1007/978-3-662-44059-9_12, © Springer-Verlag Berlin Heidelberg 2015

assistance in 1999 (Falcone et al. 1999). An early application of robotics in reproductive surgery and in particular to tubal reanastomosis is not surprising considering enhanced microsurgical capability of robotic approach. Hysterectomy was the next gynecologic procedure to adapt the robotic approach in 2002 (Diaz-Arrastia et al. 2002), followed by several studies supporting the feasibility of this method (Marchal et al. 2005; Fiorentino et al. 2006; Advincula 2006). Reports of robotic approach to multiple procedures in benign and reproductive gynecology, gynecologic oncology, and urogynecology eventually emerged, including surgical management of endometriosis (Nezhat et al. 2010), leiomyomas (Nezhat et al. 2009b), adnexectomy (Nezhat et al. 2009a; Magrina et al. 2009), ovarian (Magrina et al. 2011), uterine (Paley et al. 2011), and endometrial (Hong et al. 2011) cancer staging and resection, as well as sacrocolpopexy (Geller et al. 2008; Germain et al. 2013).

Surgical management of uterine fibroids includes hysterectomy or myomectomy, depending on the number and location of fibroids, as well as child-bearing potential of a woman. Myomectomy is a common indication for women desiring fertility preservation.

12.2 Robotic Myomectomy

Laparoscopic management of uterine fibroids has been established as a safe, feasible, and potentially advantageous method compared to laparotomy (Advincula et al. 2004; Pitter et al. 2008; Nezhat et al. 2009b). When appropriate, robotic approach to the management of uterine fibroids can be indicated. One of the purported advantages of using a robotic platform for laparoscopic removal of fibroids is the ease of suturing utilizing the wristed instrumentation when compared to conventional laparoscopy.

12.2.1 Surgical Outcomes

12.2.1.1 Robotic Versus Open Approach

Several studies compared the outcomes of robotic vs open approach to myomectomy, as well as laparoscopic vs robotic myomectomy outcomes. A retrospective cohort study by Advincula et al. reported reduced blood loss and shortened hospital stay in patients who underwent robotic myomectomy compared to the open abdominal approach group. Robotic approach was also associated with prolonged operative times and increased cost (Advincula et al. 2007). These outcomes of increased operative times and increased cost are supported by two retrospective studies of 38 Canadian and 27 US-based patients undergoing robotic myomectomy and compared to 21 and 106 historical controls, respectively, treated by open approach (Mansour et al. 2012; Nash et al. 2012). Robotic approach was also associated with decreased post-operative pain and shortened hospital stay but not blood loss or complication rate (Nash et al. 2012).

Since increased cost appears to be a major drawback associated with robotic surgery, a decision model was developed for cost analysis of different approaches to myomectomy (Behera et al. 2012). Based on the cost-minimization analysis, abdominal myomectomy was least expensive if length of stay was less than 4.6 days and cost was less than $2410. Otherwise, laparoscopic myomectomy was found to be the least expensive method. Robotic approach was associated with a significantly increased cost unless robotic disposable equipment costs were less than $1400.

12.2.1.2 Robotic Versus Laparoscopic Approach

Several studies compared robotic and laparoscopic approaches to myomectomy and reported the following outcomes. Bedient et al. conducted a retrospective case control analysis of 40 robotic and 41 laparoscopic myomectomy cases (Bedient et al. 2009). No statistically significant differences in surgical outcomes, including blood loss, mean operating time, hospital stay <2 days, or complications were reported after adjusting for uterine and fibroid size and number. A retrospective case–control analysis of 15 robotic cases by Nezhat concluded that robotic myomectomy is associated with a significantly longer operating time with no difference in other surgical outcomes and overall lacked any major advantage in the hands of a skilled laparoscopic surgeon

(Nezhat et al. 2009c). Two other retrospective studies of 75 and 89 robotic cases reported prolonged operating times but improved surgical parameters with the robotic approach, including reduced blood loss, hospital stay, improved febrile morbidity, and faster return of a bowel function (Ascher-Walsh and Capes 2010; Barakat et al. 2011). Finally, a retrospective cohort study of 115 laparoscopic and 174 robotic myomectomies reported significantly longer operating times associated with robotic approach, although this can be partially attributed to the choice of suture for defect repair (Gargiulo et al. 2012a). In particular, all robotic cases were performed with conventional suture, while laparoscopic myomectomy team utilized barbed suture known to decrease operative times and perioperative blood loss (Alessandri et al. 2010; Einarsson et al. 2011a). This difference in closure technique and material may have contributed to increased blood loss associated with robotic myomectomy (110 mL vs 85.9 mL), although the estimate-based scale used to report the blood loss could be another factor responsible for the difference observed. Other short-term outcomes and complication rates were comparable between the two approaches.

The evidence outlined earlier suggests that when indicated, robotic myomectomy compares favorably with an open approach in terms of blood loss and postoperative stay, yet is associated with increased operative times and increased cost. The difference in outcomes between the standard laparoscopy and robotic approach to myomectomy appears less defined, with most studies, agreeing on prolonged surgical times associated with robotic myomectomy. This is likely a result of several contributing factors, including time spent on set-up and undocking of robotic system, difference in surgeon's skill, and variation in procedural techniques and approaches, such as use of conventional versus barbed suture. Other outcomes, including blood loss and hospital stay, appear to be similar between the two approaches.

12.2.2 Reproductive Outcomes

Since the majority of patients undergoing myomectomy are interested in preserving or restoring their fertility, ensuring satisfactory reproductive outcomes following robotic myomectomy is a task of an utmost importance. While safety and reproductive benefits of laparoscopic myomectomy compared to the open abdominal approach have been established in literature (Mais et al. 1996; Seracchioli et al. 2000; Palomba et al. 2007), limited data is available about the robotic myomectomy. One prospective observational study reported the pregnancy rate of 68 % in 22 women interested in conception following robotic myomectomy for symptomatic deep intramural myomas (Lönnerfors and Persson 2011). The authors reported 18 pregnancies resulting in 3 miscarriages, 2 terminated pregnancies, 10 successful term deliveries, and 3 ongoing pregnancies. The rate of natural conception was 55 %. Five women (50 %) delivered vaginally, while five underwent a c-section. Another retrospective cohort study reported the pregnancy rate of 75 % among 16 patients attempting conception following robotic myomectomy procedure with no reported complications, including entry to the uterine cavity (Tusheva et al. 2013). The rate of natural conception was 67 %, while 33 % of patients conceived with the help of ART. Of those who conceived, one patient (8 %) underwent three consecutive miscarriages, and two patients (17 %) delivered prematurely at 28 and 32 weeks, respectively. All 11 deliveries were done via c-section. No incidents of uterine rupture were reported in either study.

12.2.3 Patient Selection

Appropriate patient selection is vital to ensure successful outcomes following robotic myomectomy. From the surgical standpoint, robotic myomectomy may be contraindicated in patients with one of the following (Seracchioli et al. 2000; Prentice et al. 2004; Quaas et al. 2010):

- a uterus larger than 16-week size or palpable above the umbilicus
- more than 15 total fibroids
- a single fibroid larger than 15 cm
- myomas close or originating from the cervix, broad ligament, uterine arteries, uterine cornua

- diffuse adenomyosis diagnosed by magnetic resonance imaging (MRI)
- women whose uterine cavity cannot be clearly visualized by MRI

A recent study by Nash et al. supports these findings from the efficiency standpoint by demonstrating a significant positive correlation between the specimen size and operating time during robotic myomectomy as compared to the open approach (Nash et al. 2012). Decreasing operating efficiency with the increasing specimen size is likely due to prolonged time spent on morcellation and would be expected to significantly improve with the development of newer more efficient methods of specimen retrieval.

Another consideration with robotic approach to myomectomy is the patient's BMI. Several studies demonstrated improved surgical outcomes compared to laparoscopy in patients with BMI>30 undergoing robotic adnexectomy for adnexal mass and robotic hysterectomy with pelvic–aortic lymphadenectomy for endometrial cancer, as well as robotic surgery for uterine cancer staging (Magrina et al. 2009; Paley et al. 2011; Seamon et al. 2008). With respect to robotic myomectomy, one study reported no association between increased BMI in the morbid range and poor surgical outcomes. Although additional data is needed to investigate the possibility of improved outcomes, it is reasonable to conclude that robotic myomectomy can be safely performed in patients with BMI>30.

12.2.4 Tips and Techniques

In this chapter, we briefly describe the technique of robotic myomectomy as performed at our institution along with useful tips and advice on how to achieve best outcomes and avoid complications.

Preoperative preparation is important when planning a robotic myomectomy. High quality MRI imaging is important in the work up as it partially compensates for the loss of tactile feedback by mapping all existing uterine masses, in order to develop an effective strategy of their surgical management. The goals of preoperative imaging include identifying the number, size, and locations of all fibroids; assessing for the presence of adenomyosis; and evaluating the malignant potential of uterine masses (Gargiulo and Nezhat 2011). Smaller fibroids may be better assessed with transvaginal ultrasound (Gargiulo and Nezhat 2011), while large masses commonly require MRI with gadolinium enhancement in order to identify the uterine cavity (Gargiulo and Nezhat 2011). As previously noted, evidence of diffuse adenomyosis on MRI is a relative contraindication for the robotic approach, while isolated adenomyomas can still be successfully tackled with robotic surgery (Gargiulo and Nezhat 2011). It is also important to rule out the possibility of malignancy as morcellation is contraindicated in such patients.

Once in the operating room, the patient should be placed in a dorsal lithotomy position lying on top of antiskid material (egg crate foam, bean bag, gel pad) to avoid movement during steep Trendelenburg position with arms padded and fully adducted, and knees placed in Allen or Yellofin stirrups in the same plane as pelvic girdle. The uterine positioning system may be used to assist with uterine manipulation and to check for endometrial perforation if suspected following myoma enucleation.

Several approaches to trocar placement during robotic myomectomy have been employed at our institution. A three-arm minimally invasive approach (Fig. 12.1) allows for superior cosmetic result at the cost of a limited robotic assistance (Gargiulo 2011). This approach may be utilized in younger patients with small fibroid(s) and non-significantly distended uterus. A preferred approach includes the use of four robotic arms and a 12 mm assistant port in the right lower quadrant for suction, irrigation, passage of needles, tissue retraction, and morcellation (Quaas et al. 2010) (Fig. 12.2). One advantage of placing an assistant trocar in this location is the ability to pass needles and other instruments in the field of direct view, thus minimizing the chance of needle loss or bowel injury (Quaas et al. 2010) as well as limiting inadvertent collision of the surgical assistant instruments with the robotic instrument on the same side. Additionally, should there be a need to convert to laparoscopy, the assistant port can be successfully converted to the "ultra lateral" port described by Koh et al. (Gargiulo and Nezhat 2011; Koh and Janik 2003). It is also critical to place trocars at an adequate distance from enlarged pathology to avoid limited visualization with the endoscope as well as limited access with the robotic instruments. A good guideline is to ensure that the endoscope is placed at least 8–10 cm above to the top most portion of the uterine fundus when pushing the uterus cephalad on bimanual examination. Robotic trocars and

the assistant port would similarly be placed higher in order to adequately access the leiomyomas and allow for optimal movement of the robotic instruments.

Patients with large intramural myomas >10 cm in diameter may be best treated with hybrid robotic myomectomy technique (Quaas et al. 2010). With this approach, enucleation of myoma is performed by laparoscopy, while suturing is done robotically. Major benefits of the hybrid approach in management of large fibroids include preservation of tactile feedback during separation of large mass from the delicate surrounding tissues; the ability to use a rigid tenaculum needed to exert significant pull force during enucleation; and easy access and navigation through all four pelvic quadrants, which may be limited during the robotic procedure.

Regardless of timing, docking of robotic system can be done in various ways. One traditional approach involves positioning of the robot between the patient legs (Fig. 12.3). Vaginal access in this midline approach is limited which makes uterine manipulation difficult. More recently, side docking was developed and successfully adopted for the majority of robotic procedures (Einarsson et al. 2011b). With side docking, the robot is positioned at the left or right patient's knee at a 45° angle from the lower torso (Fig. 12.4). Parallel docking simi-

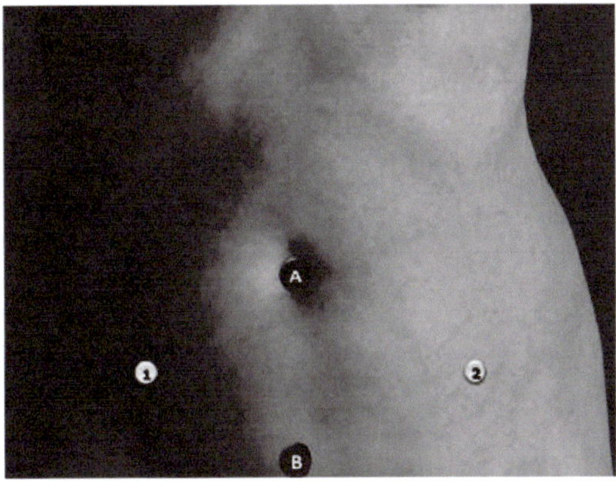

Fig. 12.1 A three-arm approach to port placement for improved cosmesis (From Gargiulo 2011)

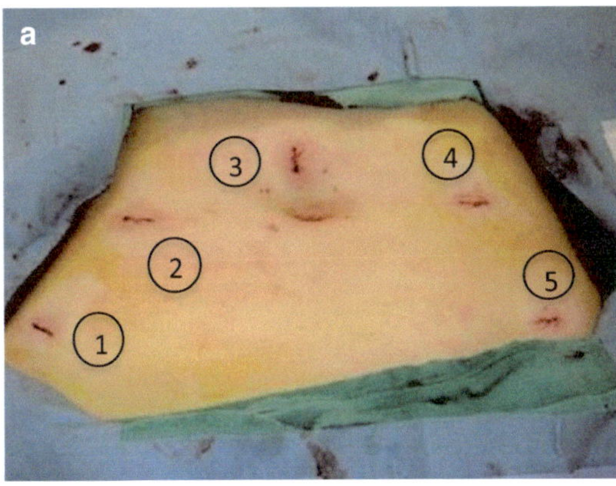
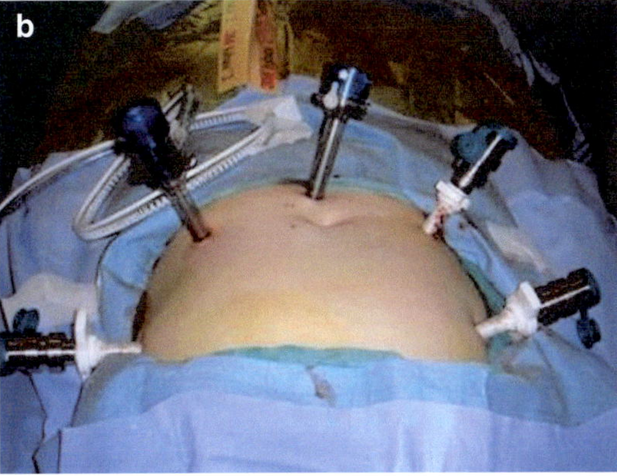
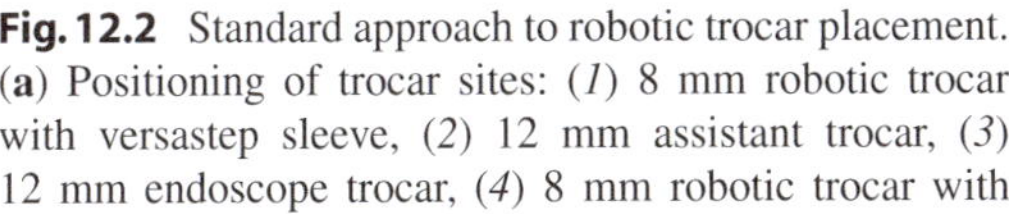

Fig. 12.2 Standard approach to robotic trocar placement. (**a**) Positioning of trocar sites: (*1*) 8 mm robotic trocar with versastep sleeve, (*2*) 12 mm assistant trocar, (*3*) 12 mm endoscope trocar, (*4*) 8 mm robotic trocar with versastep sleeve, (*5*) 8 mm robotic trocar with versastep sleeve. (**b**) Insufflated abdomen with robotic trocars in place (Courtesy of Karen Wang, MD)

Fig. 12.3 Traditional docking of the robot between the patient's legs

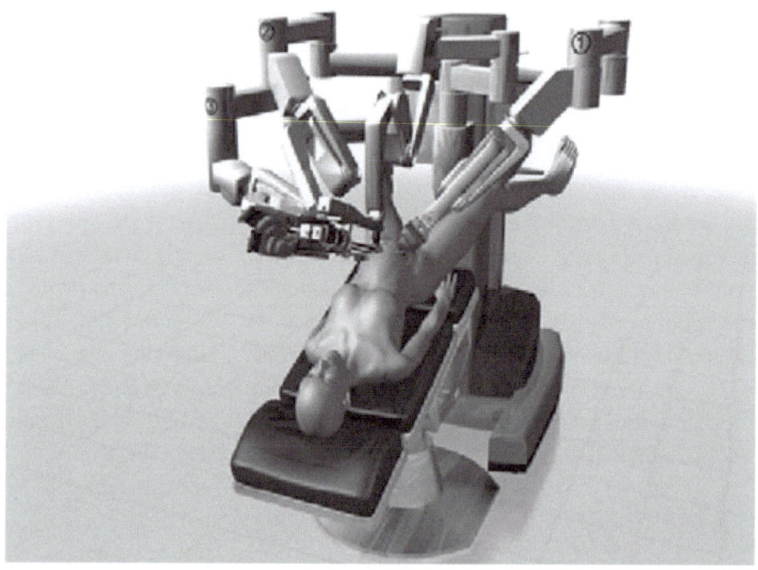

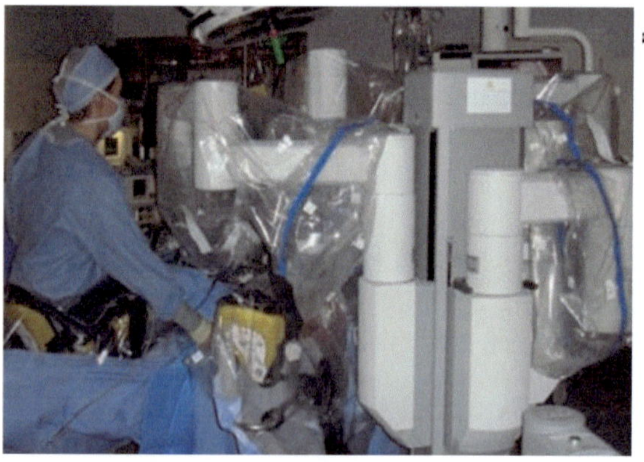

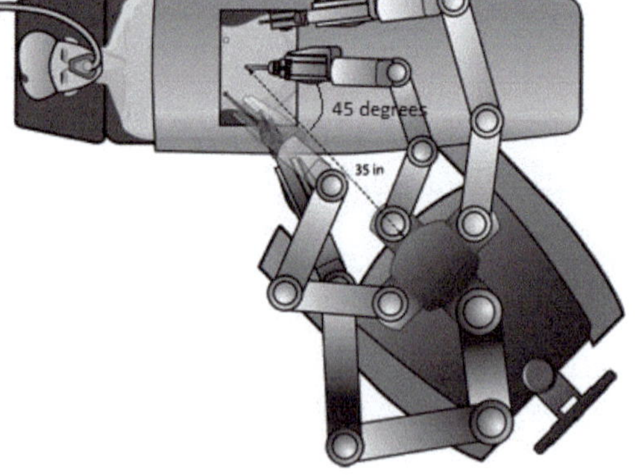

Fig. 12.4 Robotic side docking (From Einarsson et al. 2011b)

larly positions the robot at the patient's side with the robot parallel to the operative table (Silverman et al. 2012) (Fig. 12.5). Such side-access set ups allow for significantly improved vaginal access and ability to use and adjust uterine manipulator intraoperatively.

Several approaches to blood loss control during myomectomy have been described, including tourniquet application, uterine vessel clipping, vasopressin injection, and others. While approved by the US Food and Drug Administration, vasopressin use is not permitted in several European countries. Vasopressin, as well as misoprostol,

bupivacaine plus epinephrine, tranexamic acid, gelatin–thrombin matrix, pericervical tourniquet, and mesna, but not oxytocin or morcellation, were found to significantly reduce bleeding during myomectomy (Kongnyuy and Wiysonge 2011). Clipping of uterine vessels is another method shown to effectively reduce blood loss during the procedure (Sinha et al. 2004; Vercellino et al. 2012; Rosen et al. 2009).

Following the appropriate measures to ensure intraoperative hemostasis, the uterine incision is made in a longitudinal or transverse manner (Quaas et al. 2010). The approach to myoma enu-

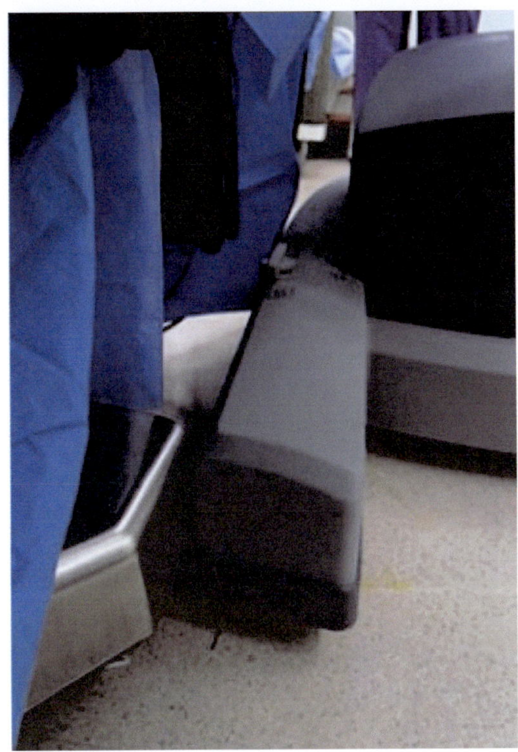

Fig. 12.5 Robotic parallel docking (From Silverman et al. 2012)

cleation is similar to one employed during an open procedure, with robotic tenaculum, robotic bipolar coagulator, and ultrasonic or monopolar energy employed to assist in this process (Fig. 12.6a–h). The bedside assistant can place additional traction on myoma(s).

Following removal, the myoma is placed in the posterior cul-de-sac or upper quadrant(s) to allow unobstructed access to the uterus; it is later morcellated. Whether morcellating with a power morcellotor device or via minilaparotomy, efforts should be made to contain all tissue fragments and avoid tissue dissemination during this process. It is also important to keep track of the number of fibroids extracted to ensure that all are removed at the end of the procedure.

The closure of the myometrial defect is best performed in a multilayer fashion in order to minimize the risk of uterine rupture (Parker et al. 2010). Other factors to consider include

the judicious use of electrosurgery, CO_2 pneumoperitoneum effect on wound healing, and individual wound healing characteristics, including thinning myometrium (Parker et al. 2010). Successful application of the bidirectional barbed suture in laparoscopic myomectomy was previously tested and described (Greenberg and Einarsson 2008). In our practice, Quill™ (Angiotech Pharmaceuticals, Inc., Vancouver, BC, Canada), V-lock™ (Covidien, Mansfield, MA) or STRATAFIX™ (Ethicon, Somerville NJ) have been successfully utilized, and their choice depends on surgeon's preference. The use of bidirectional suture decreases operative time and could be one of the key reasons behind the longer operating times associated with robotic myomectomy in a recent comparison of the two minimally invasive techniques at our institution (Gargiulo et al. 2012a).

With the advancements in the field of minimally invasive surgery, additional approaches to laparoscopic myomectomy are now available. A single port laparoscopic myomectomy technique has been successfully attempted in the past (Einarsson 2010), and more recently, applied to robotics (Gargiulo et al. 2012b) (Fig. 12.7). Although safe and reproducible with outcomes comparable to conventional robotic myomectomy, robot-assisted single-incision laparoscopic approach was found to be associated with additional technical challenges typical for single incision surgery, such as crowding of instruments, loss of optimum instrument triangulation, and inability to use all three robotic arms. In particular, partial loss of dexterity was noted by authors due to crowding of 8 mm instruments.

Although robot-assisted single-incision laparoscopic myomectomy may be beneficial in patients with higher BMIs due to excellent cosmetic outcomes achieved with 4 cm skin incision (Gargiulo et al. 2012b), further studies are needed in order to definitively investigate the risk of umbilical hernia formation in this subset of patients based on its recently reported association with laparoscopic single-site approach (Gunderson et al. 2012).

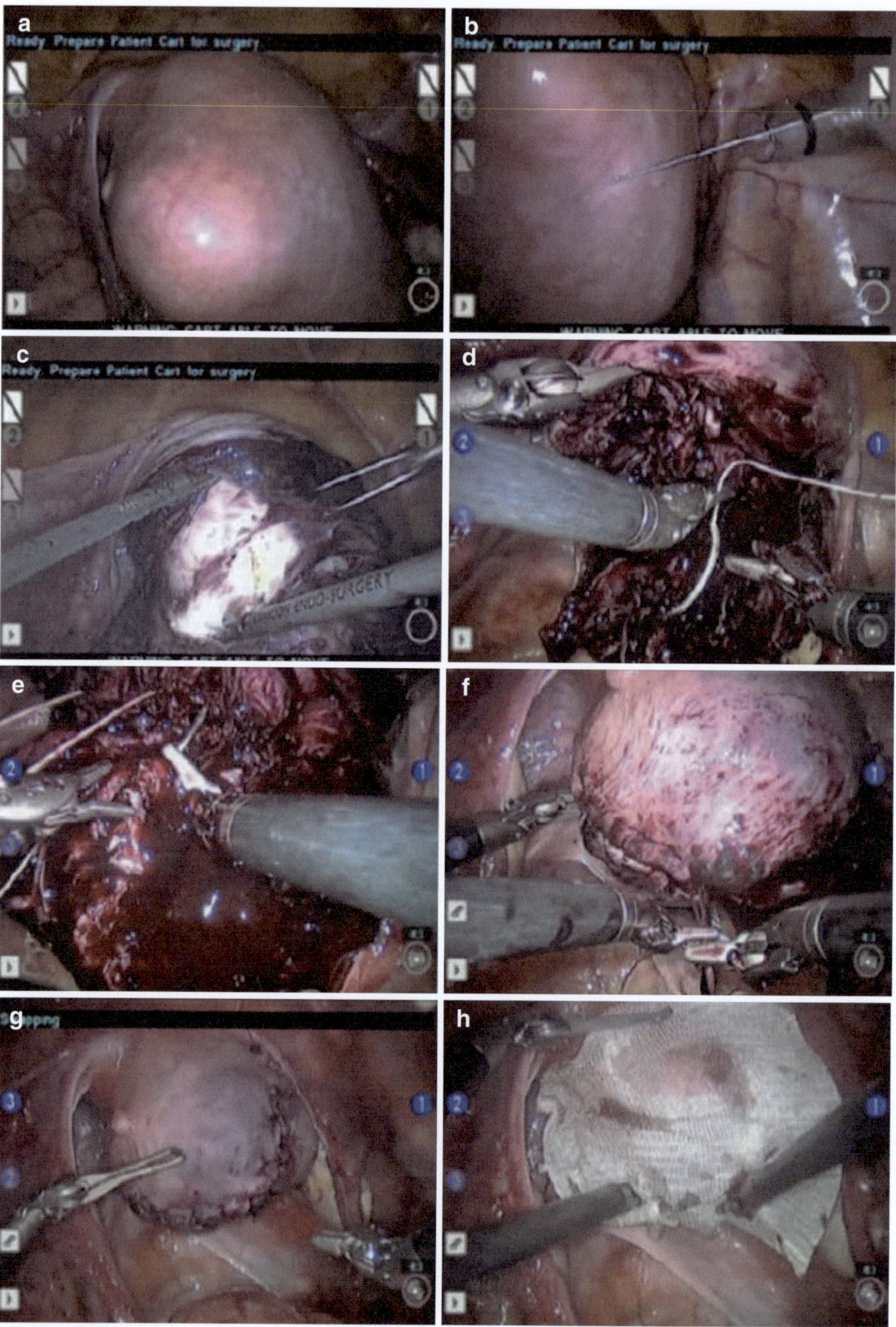

Fig. 12.6 Technique of robotic myomectomy. (**a**, **b**) After the fibroid location has been exactly determined, a dilute concentration of vasopressin is injected into the myometrium surrounding the myoma. (**c**) Using the robotic harmonic shears, a hysterotomy is made over the myoma. (**d–g**) A multilayer closure is performed employing sutures and suturing techniques that are identical to those of an open myomectomy. (**h**) An adhesion barrier may be placed onto the closed hysterotomy to prevent future scar tissue formation (From Quaas et al. 2010)

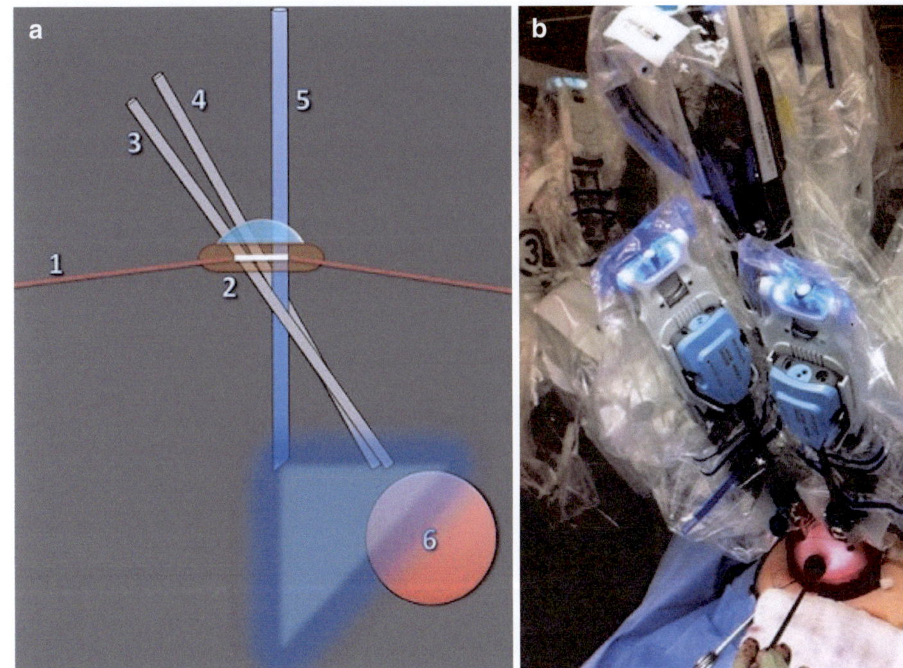

Fig. 12.7 Single port robotic myomectomy: schematic (**a**) and live (**b**) set up. (*1*) Anterior abdominal wall; (*2*) GelPOINT device; (*3*) robotic arm one; (*4*) robotic arm three; (*5*) 30° "up" laparoscope; (*6*) uterine mass (From Gargiulo et al. 2012b)

Another useful adjunct to robotic myomectomy successfully implemented at our institution is flexible CO_2 laser (Barton and Gargiulo 2012) (Fig. 12.8). The low thermal spread of laser energy, preserved seven degrees of freedom, sturdy design suitable for blunt dissection, as well as reliable hemostatic effect due to helium gas flow, make flexible CO_2 laser a useful and practical tool in a variety of gynecologic applications, including robotic myomectomy. In particular, use of CO_2 laser is expected to minimize the thermal damage of the myometrium, and therefore facilitate the healing process. Potential disadvantages of this approach include cost and fiber failure during extensive angling. At our institution, CO_2 laser is considered based on surgeon preference in cases with leading tumor size <8 cm in diameter. In cases when the leading tumor diameter is >8 cm, the preference goes to the ultrasonic scalpel due to its better ability to control bleeding.

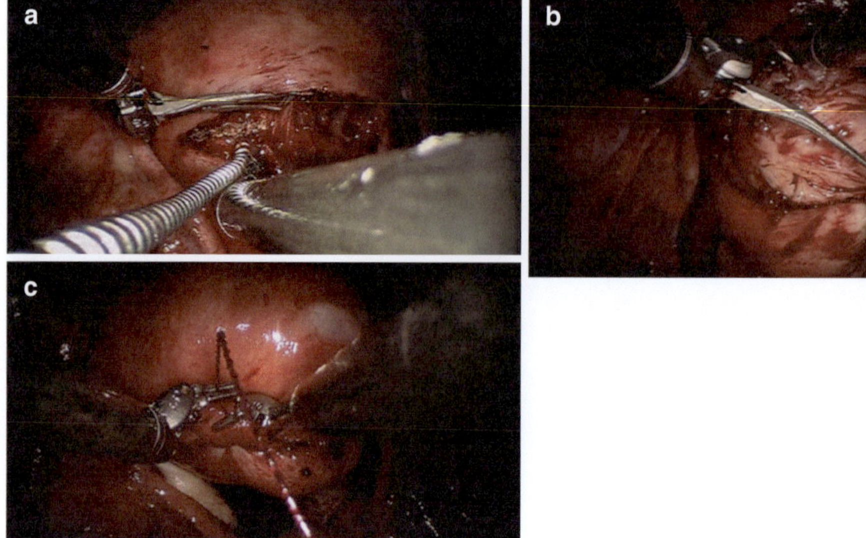

Fig. 12.8 CO_2 Laser application during single incision robotic myomectomy. (**a**) Flexible laser fiber introduced through the assistant port is used for hysterotomy. (**b**) Tenaculum is used in conjunction with robotic shears and the assistant countertraction with Allis forceps. (**c**) After enucleation, the hysterotomy is closed in layers with large needle drivers (From Gargiulo et al. 2012b)

Conclusion

Despite evidence supporting the safety, feasibility, and improved outcomes following the minimally invasive approach to myomectomy, the majority of cases in the United States are performed by laparotomy (Liu et al. 2010). This may be due to the fact that majority of benign procedures are performed by community surgeons presented with unique challenges of mastering the minimally invasive techniques, including inconsistent training across generations and programs, dependency on various nonstandardized review courses to initiate learning, "on the job" training to attain competency, and perceived long learning curves needed to become proficient (Payne and Pitter 2011; Lenihan et al. 2008). Some of the challenges associated with adopting the laparoscopic technique include increased need for dexterity and hand–eye coordination in a two-dimensional field of view, long rigid instruments, tremor amplification, and nonergonomic body positioning of the surgeon (Stylopoulos and Rattner 2003). In addition to providing the benefits of three-dimensional view, tremor reduction and increased dexterity with seven degrees of freedom, the robotic approach acts as an enabling technology by facilitating successful completion of minimally invasive laparoscopic procedures with the same outcomes as more advanced surgeons (Lenihan et al. 2008). Lim et al. estimated the learning curve for robotic surgeries to be half the number of cases required to attain the same level of proficiency in laparoscopy (Lim et al. 2011). Other studies did not find significant difference in learning curve between the robotic and laparoscopic approach (Lenihan et al. 2008; Yacoub et al. 2010). Such variation in findings could be due to the differences in prior level of proficiency in laparoscopic and robotic surgery among the surgeons participating in the study. On average, 20–75 procedures are required to transcend the early learning curves associated with robot-assisted surgery (Geller et al. 2011).

Recent introduction of a dual console robotic system and greater recognition of the importance of minimally invasive training among residents and fellows at many programs across the country has led to interest in evaluating the outcomes of these approaches. Due to limitations in residency work duty hours, the amount of time spent on surgical training has also decreased and poses additional challenges to incorporating the novel minimally invasive approach into residency and fellowship training curriculum (Advincula and Wang 2009). In this context, the benefits provided by the dual console training are especially important since they provide an opportunity for the trainee to operate under direct supervision and at the same time as an attending physician (Smith et al. 2012). Potential obstacles for dual console training implementation include the possibility of litigation issues for the instructors and the need for designing protective measures (Lee et al. 2012).

With accessibility of the robotic approach in mind, it is important to remember that it is not intended to replace laparoscopy. Although safe and efficient, with outcomes at least on par with laparoscopy, robotic surgery is associated with significantly increased cost of procedure and prolonged operative times (Weinberg et al. 2011). The lack of tactile feedback is another sensible disadvantage in robotic myomectomy and other procedures depending on haptic feedback (Weinberg et al. 2011). Continued advancements and innovations in robotic sector are likely to eventually overcome the limitations currently posed by robotic approach and may lead to a paradigm shift in the field of gynecologic minimally invasive surgery.

References

Advincula AP (2006) Surgical techniques: robot-assisted laparoscopic hysterectomy with the da Vinci surgical system. Int J Med Robot 2(4):305–311

Advincula AP, Wang K (2009) Evolving role and current state of robotics in minimally invasive gynecologic surgery. J Minim Invasive Gynecol 16(3):291–301

Advincula AP, Song A, Burke W, Reynolds RK (2004) Preliminary experience with robot-assisted laparoscopic myomectomy. J Am Assoc Gynecol Laparosc 11(4):511e8

Advincula AP, Xu X, Goudeau S 4th, Ransom SB (2007) Robot-assisted laparoscopic myomectomy versus abdominal myomectomy: a comparison of short-termsurgical outcomes and immediate costs. J Minim Invasive Gynecol 14(6):698e705

Alessandri F, Remorgida V, Venturini PL, Ferrero S (2010) Unidirectional barbed suture versus continuous suture with intracorporeal knots in laparoscopic myomectomy: a randomized study. J Minim Invasive Gynecol 17(6):725–729

Ascher-Walsh CJ, Capes TL (2010) Robot-assisted laparoscopic myomectomy is an improvement over laparotomy in women with a limited number of myomas. J Minim Invasive Gynecol 17(3):306e10

Barakat EE, Bedaiwy MA, Zimberg S, Nutter B, Nosseir M, Falcone T (2011) Robotic assisted, laparoscopic, and abdominal myomectomy: a comparison of surgical outcomes. Obstet Gynecol 117:256e65

Barton SE, Gargiulo AR (2012) Robot-assisted laparoscopic myomectomy and adenomyomectomy with a flexible CO2 laser device. J Robotic Surg 1–6. doi:10.1007/s11701-012-0360-5

Bedient CE, Magrina JF, Noble BN, Kho RM (2009) Comparison of robotic and laparoscopic myomectomy. Am J Obstet Gynecol 201(6):566.e1e5

Behera MA, Likes CE 3rd, Judd JP, Barnett JC, Havrilesky LJ, Wu JM (2012) Cost analysis of abdominal, laparoscopic, and robotic-assisted myomectomies. J Minim Invasive Gynecol 19(1):52–57

Diaz-Arrastia C, Jurnalov C, Gomez G, Townsend C Jr (2002) Laparoscopic hysterectomy using a computer-enhanced surgical robot. Surg Endosc 16(9):1271–1273

Doyle PJ, Kilic GS, Breitkopf D, Xu Y, King B (2011) Initial experience of residents with robotic assisted hysterectomies. Abstract. J Minim Invasive Gynecol 18:S91–S113

Einarsson JI (2010) Single-incision laparoscopic myomectomy. J Minim Invasive Gynecol 17(3):371–373

Einarsson JI, Chavan NR, Suzuki Y, Jonsdottir G, Vellinga TT, Greenberg JA (2011a) Use of bidirectional barbed suture in laparoscopic myomectomy: evaluation of perioperative outcomes, safety, and efficacy. J Minim Invasive Gynecol 18(1):92–95

Einarsson JI, Hibner M, Advincula AP (2011b) Side docking: an alternative docking method for gynecologic robotic surgery. Rev Obstet Gynecol 4(3–4):123–125

Falcone T, Goldberg J, Garcia-Ruiz A, Margossian H, Stevens L (1999) Full robotic assistance for laparoscopic tubal anastomosis: a case report. J Laparoendosc Adv Surg Tech A 9(1):107–113

Fiorentino RP, Zepeda MA, Goldstein BH, John CR, Rettenmaier MA (2006) Pilot study assessing robotic laparoscopic hysterectomy and patient outcomes. J Minim Invasive Gynecol 13(1):60–63

Gargiulo AR (2011) Fertility preservation and the role of robotics. Clin Obstet Gynecol 54(3):431–448

Gargiulo AR, Nezhat C (2011) Robot-assisted laparoscopy, natural orifice transluminal endoscopy, and single-site laparoscopy in reproductive surgery. Semin Reprod Med 29(2):155–168

Gargiulo AR, Srouji SS, Missmer SA, Correia KF, Vellinga T, Einarsson JI (2012a) Robot-assisted laparoscopic myomectomy compared with standard laparoscopic myomectomy. Obstet Gynecol 120:284–291

Gargiulo AR, Bailey AP, Srouji SS (2012b) Robot-assisted single-incision laparoscopic myomectomy: initial report and technique. J Robot Surg. doi:10.1007/s11701-012-0356-1

Geller EJ, Siddiqui NY, Wu JM, Visco AG (2008) Short-term outcomes of robotic sacrocolpopexy compared with abdominal sacrocolpopexy. Obstet Gynecol 112(6):1201–1206

Geller EJ, Schuler KM, Boggess JF (2011) Robotic surgical training program in gynecology: how to train residents and fellows. J Minim Invasive Gynecol 18:224–229

Germain A, Thibault F, Galifet M, Scherrer ML, Ayav A, Hubert J, Brunaud L, Bresler L (2013) Long-term outcomes after totally robotic sacrocolpopexy for treatment of pelvic organ prolapse. Surg Endosc 27:525–529

Greenberg JA, Einarsson JI (2008) The use of bidirectional barbed suture in laparoscopic myomectomy and total laparoscopic hysterectomy. J Minim Invasive Gynecol 15(5):621–623

Gunderson CC, Knight J, Ybanez-Morano J, Ritter C, Escobar PF, Ibeanu O, Grumbine FC, Bedaiwy MA, Hurd WW, Fader AN (2012) The risk of umbilical hernia and other complications with laparoendoscopic single-site surgery. J Minim Invasive Gynecol 19(1):40–45

Hong DG, Lee YS, Park NY, Chong GO, Park IS, Cho YL (2011) Robotic uterine artery preservation and nerve-sparing radical trachelectomy with bilateral pelvic lymphadenectomy in early-stage cervical cancer. Int J Gynecol Cancer 21(2):391–396

Koh C, Janik G (2003) Laparoscopic myomectomy: the current status. Curr Opin Obstet Gynecol 15(4):295–301

Kongnyuy EJ, Wiysonge CS (2011) Interventions to reduce haemorrhage during myomectomy for fibroids. Cochrane Database Syst Rev (11):CD005355

Lee YL, Kilic G, Phelps JY (2012) Liability exposure for surgical robotics instructors. J Minim Invasive Gynecol 19(3):376–379

Lenihan JP Jr, Kovanda C, Seshadri-Kreaden U (2008) What is the learning curve for robotic assisted gynecologic surgery? J Minim Invasive Gynecol 15:589–594

Lim PC, Kang E, Park do H (2011) A comparative detail analysis of the learning curve and surgical outcome for robotic hysterectomy with lymphadenectomy versus laparoscopic hysterectomy with lymphadenectomy in treatment of endometrial cancer: a case-matched controlled study of the first one hundred twenty two patients. Gynecol Oncol 120:413–418

Liu G, Zolis L, Kung R, Melchior M, Singh S, Cook EF (2010) The laparoscopic myomectomy: a survey of Canadian gynaecologists. J Obstet Gynaecol Can 32(2):139–148

Lönnerfors C, Persson J (2011) Pregnancy following robot-assisted laparoscopic myomectomy in women with deep intramural myomas. Acta Obstet Gynecol Scand 90(9):972–977

Magrina JF, Espada M, Munoz R, Noble BN, Kho RMC (2009) Robotic adnexectomy compared with laparoscopy for adnexal mass. Obstet Gynecol 114(3):581–584

Magrina JF, Zanagnolo V, Noble BN, Kho RM, Magtibay P (2011) Robotic approach for ovarian cancer: perioperative and survival results and comparison with laparoscopy and laparotomy. Gynecol Oncol 121(1):100–105

Mais V, Ajossa S, Guerriero S et al (1996) Laparoscopic versus abdominal myomectomy: a prospective, randomized trial to evaluate benefits in early outcome. Am J Obstet Gynecol 174:654–658

Mansour FW, Kives S, Urbach DR, Lefebvre G (2012) Robotically assisted laparoscopic myomectomy: a Canadian experience. J Obstet Gynaecol Can 34(4):353–358

Marchal F, Rauch P, Vandromme J, Laurent I, Lobontiu A, Ahcel B, Verhaeghe JL, Meistelman C, Degueldre M, Villemot JP, Guillemin F (2005) Telerobotic-assisted laparoscopic hysterectomy for benign and oncologic pathologies: initial clinical experience with 30 patients. Surg Endosc 19(6):826–831

Nash K, Feinglass J, Zei C, Lu G, Mengesha B, Lewicky-Gaupp C, Lin A (2012) Robotic-assisted laparoscopic myomectomy versus abdominal myomectomy: a comparative analysis of surgical outcomes and costs. Arch Gynecol Obstet 285(2):435–440

Nezhat C, Lavie O, Lemyre M, Unal E, Nezhat CH, Nezhat F (2009a) Robot-assisted laparoscopic surgery in gynecology: scientific dream or reality? Fertil Steril 91(6):2620–2622

Nezhat C, Lavie O, Hsu S, Watson J, Barnett O, Lemyre M (2009b) Robotic-assisted laparoscopic myomectomy compared with standard laparoscopic myomectomy–a retrospective matched control study. Fertil Steril 91(2):556–559

Nezhat C, Lavie O, Hsu S, Watson J, Barnett O, Lemyre M (2009c) Robotic-assisted laparoscopic myomectomy compared with standard laparoscopic myomectomy: retrospective matched control study. Fertil Steril 91(2):556e9

Nezhat C, Lewis M, Kotikela S et al (2010) Robotic versus standard laparoscopy for the treatment of endometriosis. Fertil Steril 94(7):2758–2760

Paley PJ, Veljovich DS, Shah CA, Everett EN, Bondurant AE, Drescher CW, Peters WA 3rd (2011) Surgical outcomes in gynecologic oncology in the era of robotics: analysis of first 1000 cases. Am J Obstet Gynecol 204(6):551.e1–9

Palomba S, Zupi E, Falbo A et al (2007) A multicenter randomized, controlled study comparing laparoscopic versus minilaparotomic myomectomy: reproductive outcomes. Fertil Steril 88:933–941

Parker WH, Einarsson J, Istre O, Dubuisson JB (2010) Risk factors for uterine rupture after laparoscopic myomectomy. J Minim Invasive Gynecol 17(5):551–554

Payne TN, Pitter MC (2011) Robotic-assisted surgery for the community gynecologist: can it be adopted? Clin Obstet Gynecol 54(3):391–411

Pitter MC, Anderson P, Blissett A, Pemberton N (2008) Robotic-assisted gynaecological surgery-establishing training criteria; minimizing operative time and blood loss. Int J Med Robot 4(2):114–120

Prentice A, Taylor A, Sharma MA, Magos A (2004) Laparoscopic versus open myomectomy for uterine fibroids. Cochrane Database Syst Rev (1)

Quaas AM, Einarsson JI, Srouji S, Gargiulo AR (2010) Robotic myomectomy: a review of indications and techniques. Rev Obstet Gynecol 3(4):185–191

Rosen DM, Hamani Y, Cario GM, Chou D (2009) Uterine perfusion following laparoscopic clipping of uterine arteries at myomectomy. Aust N Z J Obstet Gynaecol 49(5):559–560

Seamon LG, Cohn DE, Richardson DL, Valmadre S, Carlson MJ, Phillips GS, Fowler JM (2008) Robotic hysterectomy and pelvic-aortic lymphadenectomy for endometrial cancer. Obstet Gynecol 112(6): 1207–1213

Seracchioli R, Rossi S, Govoni F et al (2000) Fertility and obstetric outcome after laparoscopic myomectomy of large myomata: a randomized comparison with abdominal myomectomy. Hum Reprod 15:2663–2668

Silverman S, Orbuch L, Orbuch I (2012) Parallel side-docking technique for gynecologic procedures utilizing the da Vinci robot. J Robot Surg 6:247–249

Sinha RY, Hegde A, Warty N et al (2004) Laparoscopic devascularization of uterine myomata followed by enucleation of the myomas by direct morcellation. J Am Assoc Gynecol Laparosc 11:99–102

Smith AL, Krivak TC, Scott EM, Rauh-Hain JA, Sukumvanich P, Olawaiye AB, Richard SD (2012) Dual-console robotic surgery compared to laparoscopic surgery with respect to surgical outcomes in a gynecologic oncology fellowship program. Gynecol Oncol 126(3):432–436

Stylopoulos N, Rattner D (2003) Robotics and ergonomics. Surg Clin North Am 83:1321–1337

Tusheva OA, Gyang A, Patel SD (2013) Reproductive outcomes following robotic assisted laparoscopic myomectomy (RALM). J Robot Surg 7(1):65–69

Vercellino G, Erdemoglu E, Joe A, Hopfenmueller W, Holthaus B, Köhler C, Schneider A, Hasenbein K, Chiantera V (2012) Laparoscopic temporary clipping of uterine artery during laparoscopic myomectomy. Arch Gynecol Obstet 286(5):1181–1186

Weinberg L, Rao S, Escobar PF (2011) Robotic surgery in gynecology: an updated systematic review. Obstet Gynecol Int 2011:852061. doi: 10.1155

Yacoub A, Ferdynus C, Tixier H, Mourtialon P, Pinard E, Dunand A, Sagot P, Douvier S (2010) Laparoscopic (LSC) Versus Robotic (RASC) Sacrocolcopexy. Comparison of learning curve of a single laparoscopic experimented surgeon in Dijon Teaching Hospital, France. Abstract. J Minim Invasive Gynecol 17:S178–S188

Olav Istre

Contents

O. Istre, MD, PhD, DMSc
Gynecology Aleris-Hamlet Hospital, Scandinavia

Head of Gynecology Aleris-Hamlet Hospital,
Scandinavia Professor in Minimal Invasive
Gynecology, University of Southern Denmark,
Odense, Denmark
e-mail: oistre@gmail.com

13.1 Introduction

Traditional operative treatments for symptomatic fibroids are laparotomy with hysterectomy or myomectomy, involving considerable morbidity (Guarnaccia and Rein 2001; Dicker et al. 1982). Myomectomy involves the shelling out of fibroids from the myometrium, and in the case of submucosal fibroids these can be removed surgically via hysteroscopic procedures (Fernandez et al. 2001). Although morbidity is reduced with endoscopic surgery, this technique is not widely available and has limitations.

13.1.1 New Treatment Options

A number of minimally invasive treatments options are now available for the treatment of symptomatic fibroids. Surgical treatments with endoscopic technique include hysterectomy, myomectomy, and myolysis (Dubuisson et al. 1997). Multiple fibroids pose a significant problem for treatment. When myomectomy or myolysis is performed and all clinically identified fibroids are removed or "killed," in approximately half of the patients fibroids are seen at a later time (Nezhat et al. 1998). Medical therapy like ulipristal acetate was noninferior to once-monthly leuprolide acetate in controlling uterine bleeding and was significantly less likely to cause hot flashes, and treatment with ulipristal acetate for 13 weeks effectively controlled excessive

O. Istre (ed.), *Minimally Invasive Gynecological Surgery*,
DOI 10.1007/978-3-662-44059-9_13, © Springer-Verlag Berlin Heidelberg 2015

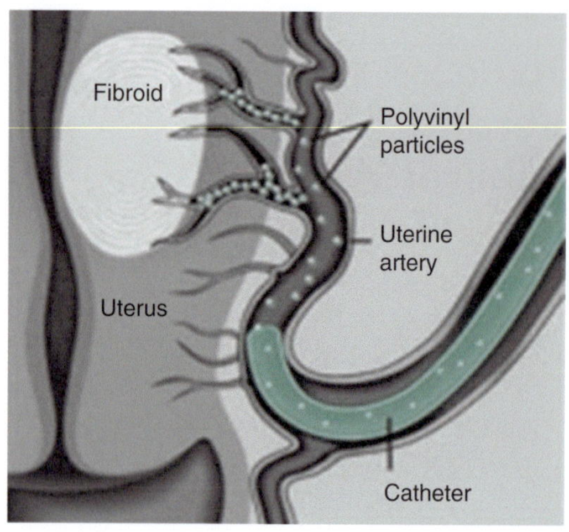

Fig. 13.1 Embolization of the fibroids

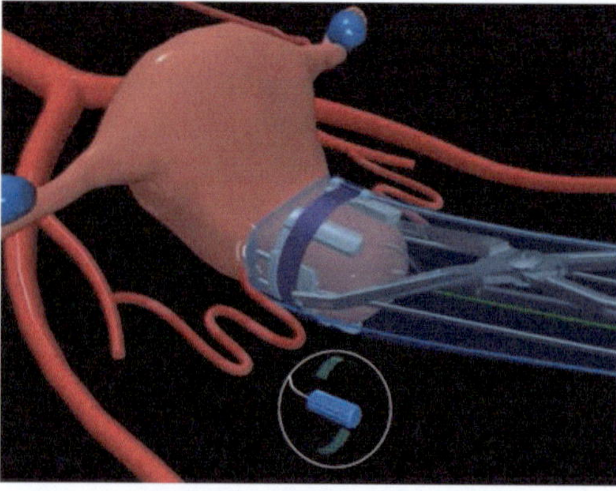

Fig. 13.2 Temporary clamping of the uterus

bleeding due to uterine fibroids and reduced the size of the fibroids before surgery (Donnez et al. 2012). However, medical therapy of fibroids will not be discussed further in this chapter.

Nonsurgical treatments include medical therapy and treatments interfering with the blood supply to the uterus or the fibroids, uterine artery embolization performed by interventional radiologist, or laparoscopic uterine artery occlusion by the gynecologist. Even simpler treatment is the nonincision temporary uterine clamp, placed in the side fornices in the vagina directed with Doppler ultrasound.

The continued therapy goal for symptomatic fibroids must take into consideration the needs and desires of the patients, i.e., length of hospital stay, time to return to work, adverse events, and childbearing plans. Hysterectomy continues to be costly in billions of dollars spent annually, as well as in the more fundamental terms of morbidity and mortality when compared with the less invasive alternatives (Goldfarb 2000) (Figs. 13.1 and 13.2).

13.2 Uterus Circulation

Uterus has a very rich blood supply through two extrinsic arterial systems, the uterine and ovarian arteries. Intrinsic uterine arteries consist of ascending uterine, arcuate, radial, and peripheral arteries implicating free flow through the uterus. Fibroids receive their blood supply from the intrinsic arteries, primary from branches of arcuate arteries, and the vessels are located in the pseudocapsule around the fibroids. The ipsilateral uterine and ovarian arteries are connected by communicating branches. In addition to its primary (uterine artery) and secondary (ovarian artery) extrinsic blood supply, the uterus enjoys a vast network of lesser known arterial collaterals (Burbank and Hutchins 2000). If the blood supply from the right or left uterine artery is occluded, blood from the left or right artery will supply the myometrium by communications through arcuate arteries. Finally, if both uterine arteries are occluded, blood flow to the myometrium will develop from the ovarian arteries through communicating arteries. In addition to the primary and secondary blood flow, the uterus has a vast network of collateral arterial communication from the aorta external iliac and femoral artery branch (Chait et al. 1968) (Fig. 13.3).

Diagram showing the extrinsic arteries of the left side of the uterus, including the aorta and the renal and ovarian arteries arising from the abdominal aorta, the uterine artery arising from the internal iliac artery, and the utero-ovarian communicating artery. Symmetrical arteries are present on the right but are not shown.

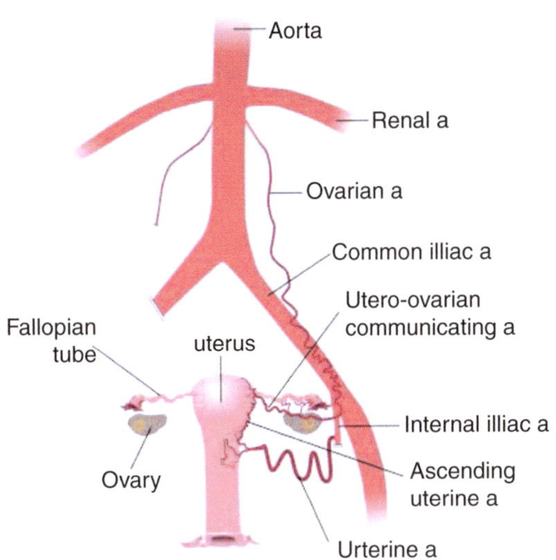

Fig. 13.3 Blood supply to uterus

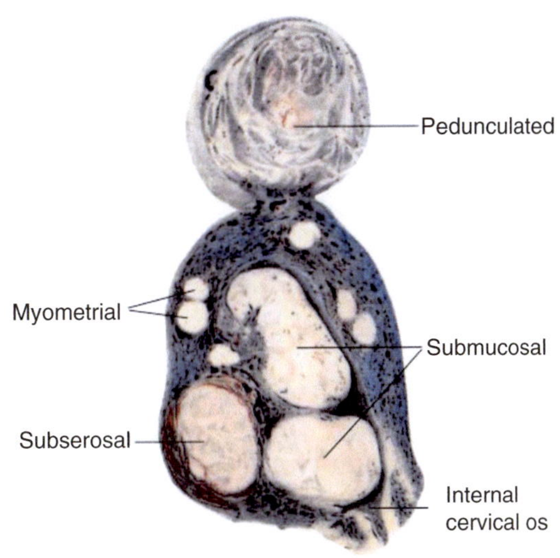

Fig. 13.4 Different types of fibroids and degeneration

13.3 Fibroid Life Cycle

Fibroid degeneration is the physiological way of terminating further growth of fibroids. Fibroids are particularly susceptible to degeneration because their rapid growths need increased blood supply. Fibroids have unsubstantiated connection to the uterine blood supply and as a consequence they frequently outgrow their blood supply, and consequently two thirds of the fibroids show degeneration (Huang et al. 1996). Larger fibroids are more frequently associated with degenerative changes compared to the smaller ones (Cramer et al. 1996). The different types of degenerative changes are hyaline or myxoid degeneration (75 %), calcification (10 %), cystic degeneration (10 %), fatty degeneration, and red degeneration during pregnancy (Fig. 13.4).

the breakdown of glycogen through the glycolytic pathway (Laudanski 1985). After the uterine arteries are occluded, most blood stops flowing in myometrial arteries and veins, and the uterus becomes ischemic. It is postulated that myomas are killed by the same process that kills trophoblasts – transient uterine ischemia (Burbank 2004).

Over time, stagnant blood in these arteries and veins clots. Then, tiny collateral arteries in the broad ligament including communicating arteries from the ovarian arteries open and cause clots within myometrium to lyse and the uterus to reperfuse. Fibroids, however, do not survive this period of ischemia (Lichtinger et al. 2003). This is a unique organ response to clot formation and ischemia. After the uterine arteries are bilaterally occluded, either by uterine artery embolization or by laparoscopic obstruction, women with fibroids experience symptomatic relief after some time.

13.4 Implication of Uterine Ischemia

When the uterine circulation is interrupted, unperfused myometrium quickly becomes hypoxic which will create pain. During ischemia, myometrial energy is derived anaerobically from

13.5 Practical Aspects of Procedure: Uterine Artery Occlusion

In 1964, Bateman reported the successful treatment of menorrhagia in four patients with fibroids and three with functional uterine bleeding

(Bateman 1964). This was the first published article that demonstrates that uterine artery occlusion by ligation, division, or excision is an effective treatment for menorrhagia associated with fibroids and in patients without pathology.

Laparoscopic bipolar coagulation of uterine arteries and anastomotic sites of uterine arteries with ovarian arteries represents another modality of avoiding hysterectomy in some women (Liu 2000; Liu et al. 2001). This procedure was first described in 2000 in three women with symptomatic fibroids who required conventional surgical treatment. Uterine size and dominant fibroid size were assessed by ultrasonography before and after surgery. Both uterine arteries, as well as anastomosis zone of uterine arteries with ovarian arteries, were occluded in all three women. Surgery was uneventful, and patients were hospitalized for only 2 days. All women experienced improvement in symptoms with no complications. Postoperative ultrasound showed progressive reduction in size of the dominant fibroid (Liu 2000).

In another study 46 premenopausal women, age 43 (34–51) years with symptomatic uterine fibroids, undergoing radiologic embolization ($n=24$) or laparoscopic closure of the uterine arteries ($n=22$) (Hald et al. 2004, 2007; Istre et al. 2004). The laparoscopic technique reduced picture blood assessment score after 6 months by 50 % in both groups. Uterus volume was also reduced by 35–40 % in both groups. Postoperative pain and use of pain relief differed significantly, as patients required more pain medication after embolization: ketobemidon 38 mg compared with 16 mg in the laparoscopic group (P=0.008). In conclusion, we found that laparoscopic occlusion of uterine vessels is a promising new method for treating fibroid-related symptoms, with less postoperative pain than embolization and comparable effects on symptoms.

Women with fibroid(s) unsuitable for laparoscopic myomectomy (LM) were treated with uterine artery embolization (UAE) or laparoscopic uterine artery occlusion (LUAO). Before the procedure, patients treated with UAE ($n=100$) had a dominant fibroid greater in size (68 vs. 48 mm) and a mean age lower (33.1 vs. 34.9 years) than surgically treated patients ($n=100$). After 6 months, mean shrinkage of fibroid volume was 53 % after UAE and 39 % after LUAO ($p=0.063$); 82 % of women after UAE, but only 23 % after LUAO, had complete myoma infarction ($p=0.001$). Women treated with UAE had more complications (31 vs. 11 cases, $p=0.006$) and greater incidence of hysteroscopically verified intrauterine necrosis (31 vs. 3 %, $p=0.001$). Both groups were comparable in markers of ovarian functions and number of nonelective reinterventions. The groups did not differ in pregnancy (69 % after UAE vs. 67 % after LUAO), delivery (50 vs. 46 %), or abortion (34 vs. 33 %) rates. The mean birth weight of neonates was greater (3,270 vs. 2,768 g, $p=0.013$) and the incidence of intrauterine growth restriction lower (13 vs. 38 %, $p=0.046$) in post-UAE patients.

Both methods are effective in the treatment of women with future reproductive plans and fibroids not suitable for LM. UAE is more effective in causing complete ischemia of fibroids, but it is associated with greater risk of intrauterine necrosis. Both methods are an effective treatment for PPH and fibroids. Pregnancy is possible after UAE. Recurrent PPH is a serious and frequent complication. Synechia is also a potential complication. Desire of childbearing should be considered when choosing embolization or surgery and, in case of embolization, the choice of material used (Berkane and Moutafoff-Borie 2010a). Further studies on future fertility after UAE are needed as well as information on fertility after surgery have low rate of serious complications (except for a high abortion rate) (Mara et al. 2012).

Hysteroscopic examination of the uterine cavity revealed that patients previously treated for intramural myoma(s) by uterine artery embolization had a significantly higher incidence of abnormal findings compared with patients treated by laparoscopic occlusion of uterine arteries (59.5 % vs. 2.7 %). In particular, there was a higher incidence of necrosis in the uterine cavity of patients subjected to uterine artery embolization (43.2 %) compared with patients after surgical uterine artery occlusion (2.7 %) (Kuzel et al. 2011).

UAE is used to treat postpartum hemorrhage (PPH) and fibroids. This effective therapy is replacing surgery in many cases. One of the main goals of UAE is to preserve the uterus and therefore fertility (pregnancies, menses, and ovarian reserve). Pregnancies after this technique have been described. The main complications encountered during these pregnancies are not only PPH but also miscarriages and cesarean deliveries after UAE for fibroids. Conflicting results varying from completely well tolerated to serious complications such as definitive negative effect on endometrium and ovary function have been reported. Nevertheless, the series differ in that they included women of different ages and used different materials for vessel occlusion (definitive microparticles of varying sizes, temporary pledgets of gelatin sponge, etc.).

UAE is an effective treatment for PPH and fibroids. Pregnancy is possible after UAE. Recurrent PPH is a serious and frequent complication. Synechia is also a potential complication. Desire of childbearing should be considered when choosing embolization or surgery and, in case of embolization, the choice of material used. Further studies on future fertility after UAE are needed as well as information on fertility after surgery (Berkane and Moutafoff-Borie 2010b).

Another new advanced technology is ExAblate 2100 system (Insightec Ltd, Haifa, Israel) for magnetic resonance imaging (MRI)-guided focused ultrasound surgery on treatment outcomes in patients with symptomatic uterine fibroids, as measured by the nonperfused volume ratio.

A retrospective analysis of 115 women (mean age, 42 years; range, 27–54 years) with symptomatic fibroids who consecutively underwent MRI-guided focused ultrasound treatment in a single center with the new generation ExAblate 2100 system from November 2010 to June 2011. Mean ± SD total volume and number of treated fibroids (per patient) were 89 ± 94 cm and 2.2 ± 1.7, respectively. Patient baseline characteristics were analyzed regarding their impact on the resulting nonperfused volume ratio. Magnetic resonance imaging-guided focused ultrasound treatment was technically successful in 115 of 123 patients (93.5 %). In 8 patients, treatment was not possible because of bowel loops in the beam pathway that could not be mitigated ($n = 6$), patient movement ($n = 1$), and system malfunction

($n = 1$). Mean nonperfused volume ratio was 88 % ± 15 % (range, 38–100 %). Mean applied energy level was $5,400 \pm 1,200$ J, and mean number of sonications was 74 ± 27. No major complications occurred. Two cases of first-degree skin burn resolved within 1 week after the intervention. Of the baseline characteristics analyzed, only the planned treatment volume had a statistically significant impact on nonperfused volume ratio (Trumm et al. 2013).

13.6 Temporary Artery Occlusion

A new exciting device, utilizing the principle of interference with the blood circulation, has recently been developed (Vascular Control Systems, Inc., San Juan Capistrano, CA) (Flowstat) for the treatment of fibroids with non-incision, only compression. However, there were few clinical centers who managed to adopt and control the device and therefore it has been removed from the market, but still I believe it could gain some clinical application in the future.

The system consists of a guiding cervical tenaculum, a transvaginal vascular clamp with integrated Doppler ultrasound crystals, and a small, battery powered transceiver that generates audible Doppler sound (Fig. 13.5). The clamp slides along the guiding tenaculum to the level of the lateral vaginal fornices at the 9:00 and the 3:00 cervical positions. When the crystals on the arms of the clamp contact

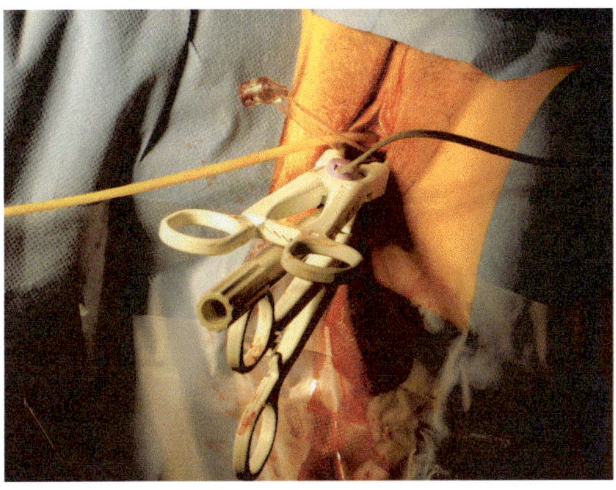

Fig. 13.5 The transvaginal vascular clamp with integrated Doppler ultrasound crystals and Doppler receiver

the vaginal mucosa, they return audible signals from the right and left uterine arteries. When the clamp is further advanced along the guiding tenaculum, the clamp displaces the uterine arteries superior to their points of insertion into the uterus. When closed, the clamp occludes the uterine arteries bilaterally by squeezing them against the lateral borders of the uterus, and the clamp is remained in place for 6 h (Fig. 13.5).

13.7 In Vitro and In Vivo Studies

After uterine artery occlusion, pH falls and when clot lyses and reperfusion occurs, pH returns to baseline. This has been investigated and monitored continuously before, during, and 24 h after laparoscopic occlusion of uterine arteries (Lichtinger et al. 2003). In patients with symptomatic fibroids, pH was measured with a catheter electrode embedded in the endometrium and in others in the myometrium. In 62 % of the patients pH dropped 0.4–0.8 units, while in 38 % the drop was greater, and the minimum was reached between 5 and 73 min. The return back to baseline was on average 5 h. After the uterine artery is occluded, blood reaches the myometrium by secondary pathways and for most women, these vascular pathways are insufficient to maintain aerobic metabolism. Until clotting occurs, blood continues to flow and supply oxygen to the myometrium, although at a new and slower speed.

13.8 Clinical Studies

We presented the first publication with this new technique in 2004 where a 43-year-old woman with menorrhagia, dysmenorrhea, and pelvic pain of several years duration with the uterus enlarged by fibroids to the size of a 16-week pregnancy was treated (Istre et al. 2004). Her uterine arteries were noninvasive transvaginally identified and occluded for 6 h with a clamp that was guided by audible Doppler ultrasound. Following removal of the clamp, blood flow in the uterine arteries returned immediately. Three

months following treatment, the uterine volume had decreased by 49 % and the dominant fibroid volume by 54 % (Fig. 13.6).

Thirty patients treated with this technique were presented in 2006. Two alternatives of analgesic was chosen (para cervical and epidural block was utilized in 17 and 13 patients, respectively), menorrhagia was reduced in both groups, however in the para cervical group fibroid reduction was 12–24 % and in the epidural group 24–45 %. Two cases of hydronephrosis were observed and they were treated successfully with a stent (Vilos et al. 2006). The explanation of additional fibroid reduction in the epidural group could be related to a more stable tenaculum placement, lesser pain, and consequently constant compression of the uterine artery during the treatment time.

13.9 Complications

A disadvantage of the noninvasively transvaginal clamping technique is fibroid location close to the cervix, in which there are some difficulties to apply the clamp location correctly. In addition, possibility of clamping the urethers with subsequent hydronephrosis and possible damage of the renal function is of concern.

Another possible application of the temporary artery uterine clamp is during and after myomectomy operations. Thereby, we can reduce peri- and postoperative bleeding. In addition, the clamping may act as adjuvant therapy of possible residual fibromas. However, few results exist so far, and further studies of this therapeutic approach are needed to prove its long-term value.

13.10 Use and Indication of Uterine Artery Techniques

The application of techniques like uterine artery occlusion is primarily for women who will avoid hysterectomy. Many women do not wish to undergo an operative procedure, as they may not accept the associated risks of the operation, and therefore prefer the less invasive procedures.

Pre–Procedure = 82cc   Post–Procedure = 38cc

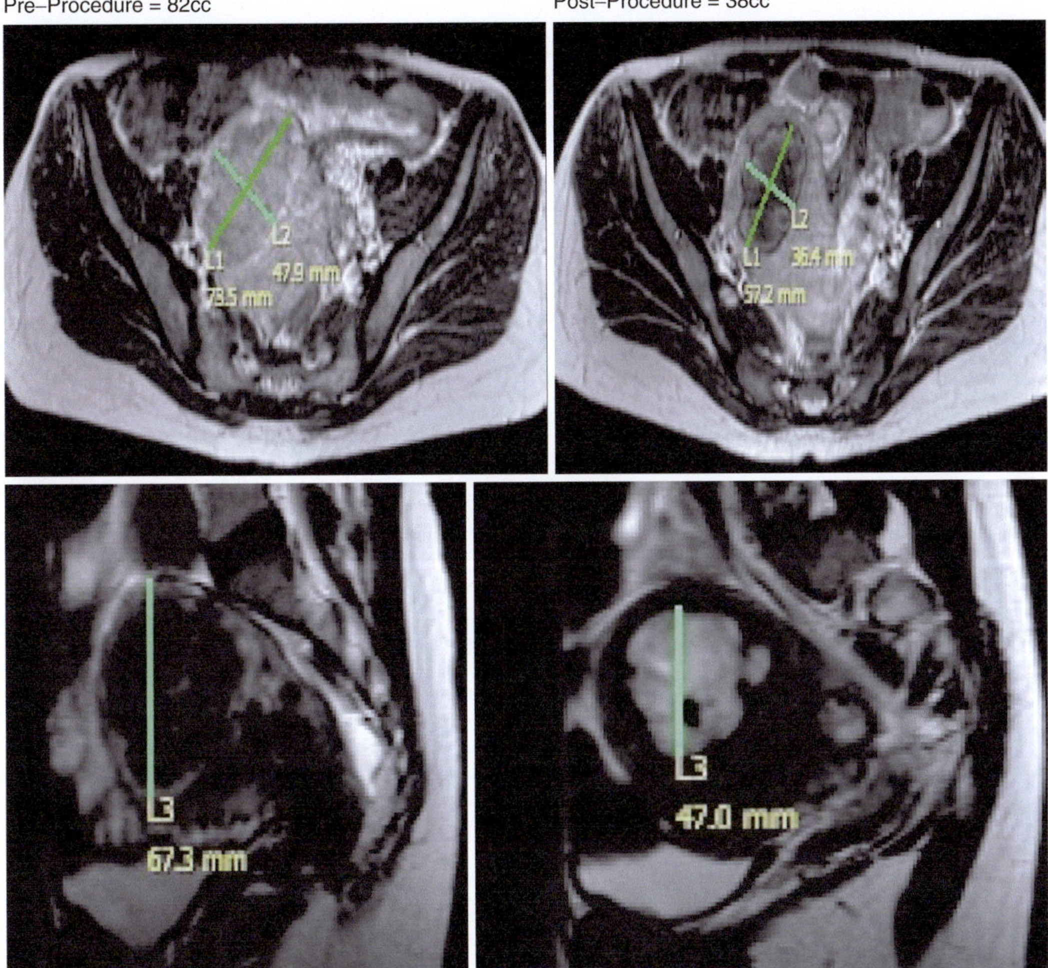

Fig. 13.6 MRI showing *Major Fibroid reduction 54 %*

Both radiological and laparoscopic occlusion techniques are potential treatment options in the treatment of fibroids. However, insufficient long-term follow-up results do not exist at present. Furthermore, both techniques are associated with a high level of skill, and consequently they should be performed only in special centers with interest in this field. Anyhow, counseling of the patients is of utmost importance before they make their own treatment choice (Hald et al. 2004).

Conclusions

Fibroids present with different symptoms in different patients, i.e., infertility, bleeding problems, pressure and pain, single or multiple, different ages, which should be treated differently. In bleeding problems, an important issue is the location of the fibroid, and in cases with submucosal fibroids hysteroscopic resection is the method of choice. In cases with intramural, subserosal, and even multiple fibroids, uterine artery therapy with embolization or laparoscopy seems to achieve good results on both bleeding problems and pressure symptoms. The temporary uterine clamp performed by general gynecologist without incision may replace the more complicated procedures like embolization performed by radiologist and laparoscopic uterine artery closure performed by skilled endoscopist.

In infertility patients, the single fibroid should be removed, while when multiple fibroids are present medical or circulation therapy may be the only option for uterus saving therapy.

References

Bateman W (1964) Treatment of intractable menorrhagia by bilateral uterine vessel interruption. Am J Obstet Gynecol 89:825–827

Berkane N, Moutafoff-Borie C (2010) Impact of previous uterine artery embolization on fertility. Curr Opin Obstet Gynecol 22(3):242–247

Burbank F (2004) Childbirth and myoma treatment by uterine artery occlusion: do they share a common biology? J Am Assoc Gynecol Laparosc 11(2):138–152

Burbank F, Hutchins FL Jr (2000) Uterine artery occlusion by embolization or surgery for the treatment of fibroids: a unifying hypothesis-transient uterine ischemia. J Am Assoc Gynecol Laparosc 7(4 Suppl):S1–S49

Chait A, Moltz A, Nelson JH Jr (1968) The collateral arterial circulation in the pelvis. An angiographic study. Am J Roentgenol Radium Ther Nucl Med 102(2): 392–400

Cramer SF, Horiszny J, Patel A, Sigrist S (1996) The relation of fibrous degeneration to menopausal status in small uterine leiomyomas with evidence for postmenopausal origin of seedling myomas. Mod Pathol 9(7):774–780

Dicker RC, Greenspan JR, Strauss LT, Cowart MR, Scally MJ, Peterson HB et al (1982) Complications of abdominal and vaginal hysterectomy among women of reproductive age in the United States. The collaborative review of sterilization. Am J Obstet Gynecol 144(7):841–848

Donnez J, Tatarchuk TF, Bouchard P, Puscasiu L, Zakharenko NF, Ivanova T et al (2012) Ulipristal acetate versus placebo for fibroid treatment before surgery. N Engl J Med 366(5):409–420

Dubuisson JB, Chapron C, Fauconnier A, Kreiker G (1997) Laparoscopic myomectomy and myolysis. Curr Opin Obstet Gynecol 9(4):233–238

Fernandez H, Sefrioui O, Virelizier C, Gervaise A, Gomel V, Frydman R (2001) Hysteroscopic resection of submucosal myomas in patients with infertility. Hum Reprod 16(7):1489–1492

Goldfarb HA (2000) Myoma coagulation (myolysis). Obstet Gynecol Clin North Am 27(2):421–430

Guarnaccia MM, Rein MS (2001) Traditional surgical approaches to uterine fibroids: abdominal myomectomy and hysterectomy. Clin Obstet Gynecol 44(2): 385–400

Hald K, Langebrekke A, Klow NE, Noreng HJ, Berge AB, Istre O (2004) Laparoscopic occlusion of uterine vessels for the treatment of symptomatic fibroids: initial experience and comparison to uterine artery embolization. Am J Obstet Gynecol 190(1):37–43

Hald K, Klow NE, Qvigstad E, Istre O (2007) Laparoscopic occlusion compared with embolization of uterine vessels: a randomized controlled trial. Obstet Gynecol 109(1):20–27

Huang SC, Yu CH, Huang RT, Hsu KF, Tsai YC, Chou CY (1996) Intratumoral blood flow in uterine myoma correlated with a lower tumor size and volume, but not correlated with cell proliferation or angiogenesis. Obstet Gynecol 87(6):1019–1024

Istre O, Hald K, Qvigstad E (2004) Multiple myomas treated with a temporary, noninvasive, Doppler-directed, transvaginal uterine artery clamp. J Am Assoc Gynecol Laparosc 11(2):273–276

Kuzel D, Mara M, Horak P, Kubinova K, Maskova J, Dundr P et al (2011) Comparative outcomes of hysteroscopic examinations performed after uterine artery embolization or laparoscopic uterine artery occlusion to treat leiomyomas. Fertil Steril 95(6):2143–2145

Laudanski T (1985) Energy metabolism of the myometrium in pregnancy and labor. Zentralbl Gynakol 107(9):568–573

Lichtinger M, Burbank F, Hallson L, Herbert S, Uyeno J, Jones M (2003) The time course of myometrial ischemia and reperfusion after laparoscopic uterine artery occlusion–theoretical implications. J Am Assoc Gynecol Laparosc 10(4):554–563

Liu WM (2000) Laparoscopic bipolar coagulation of uterine vessels to treat symptomatic leiomyomas. J Am Assoc Gynecol Laparosc 7(1):125–129

Liu WM, Ng HT, Wu YC, Yen YK, Yuan CC (2001) Laparoscopic bipolar coagulation of uterine vessels: a new method for treating symptomatic fibroids. Fertil Steril 75(2):417–422

Mara M, Kubinova K, Maskova J, Horak P, Belsan T, Kuzel D (2012) Uterine artery embolization versus laparoscopic uterine artery occlusion: the outcomes of a prospective, nonrandomized clinical trial. Cardiovasc Intervent Radiol 35(5):1041–1052

Nezhat FR, Roemisch M, Nezhat CH, Seidman DS, Nezhat CR (1998) Recurrence rate after laparoscopic myomectomy. J Am Assoc Gynecol Laparosc 5(3): 237–240

Trumm CG, Stahl R, Clevert DA, Herzog P, Mindjuk I, Kornprobst S et al (2013) Magnetic resonance imaging-guided focused ultrasound treatment of symptomatic uterine fibroids: impact of technology advancement on ablation volumes in 115 patients. Invest Radiol 48(6):359–365

Vilos GA, Hollett-Caines J, Burbank F (2006) Uterine artery occlusion: what is the evidence? Clin Obstet Gynecol 49(4):798–810

Barbed Suture Use in Minimally Invasive Gynecology: A Practical Guide

Sarah L. Cohen and Jon I. Einarsson

Contents

14.1 Introduction

Barbed suture is a novel innovation in the field of suture materials with far-reaching implications for minimally invasive gynecologic surgeons. The advantages of barbed suture include its self-anchoring feature which may enhance even distribution of tension along the length of an incision (Rodeheaver et al. 2005). Additionally, secure tissue approximation and wound holding can be achieved without knots, significantly enhancing efficiency and ease of laparoscopic suturing (Einarsson et al. 2011a, b). Although a synthetic multibarbed suture was described as early as 1967 for use in tendon repairs (McKenzie 1967), this technology did not gain regular use until the early 2000s with its application to facial plastic surgery. With the introduction of Quill™ bidirectional barbed suture (Angiotech Pharmaceuticals, Inc., Vancouver, BC, Canada) in 2004 and V-Loc™ unidirectional barbed suture (Covidien, Mansfield, MA) in 2009, barbed suture has demonstrated widespread utility in surgical fields including gynecology, urology, orthopedic surgery, and reconstructive surgery.

14.2 Available Products

Barbed suture is created by cutting barbs into a monofilament suture material in roughly 1 mm increments (Fig. 14.1). Bidirectional barbed suture (Fig. 14.2) features a needle swaged onto

S.L. Cohen, MD, MPHM (✉)
J.I. Einarsson, MD, MPH
Division of Minimally Invasive Gynecologic Surgery,
Brigham and Women's Hospital,
75 Francis Street, Boston, MA 02115, USA
e-mail: scohen20@partners.org;
jeinarsson@partners.org

O. Istre (ed.), *Minimally Invasive Gynecological Surgery*,
DOI 10.1007/978-3-662-44059-9_14, © Springer-Verlag Berlin Heidelberg 2015

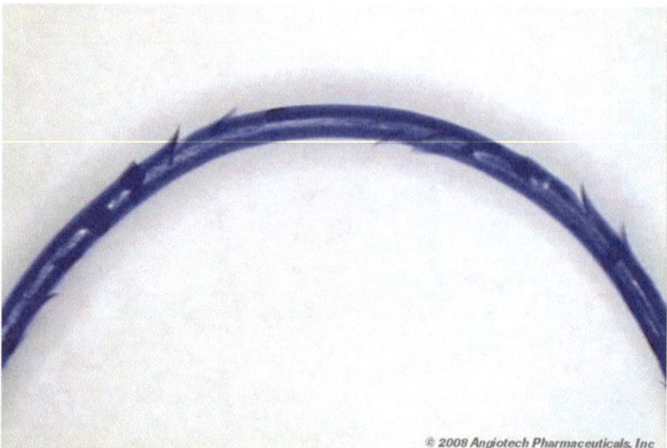

Fig. 14.1 The Barbed sutur

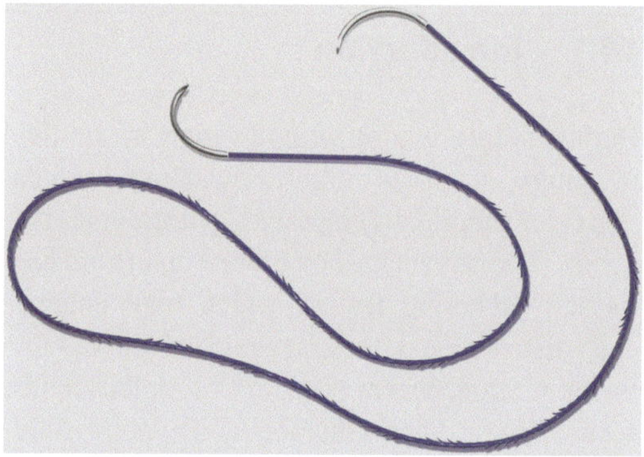

Fig. 14.2 Barbed sutur with 2 needles

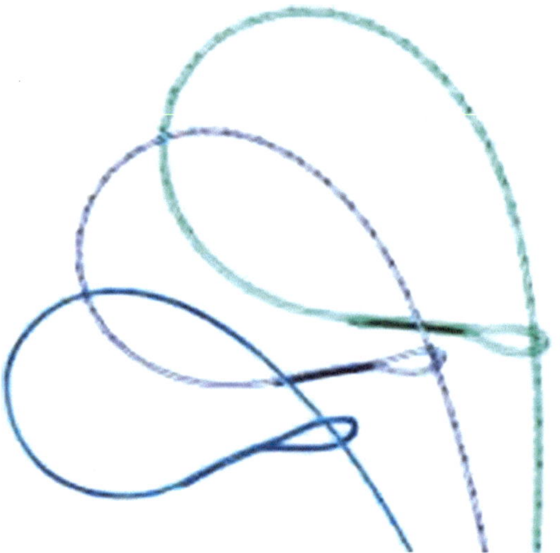

Fig. 14.3 Barbed sutur with loop

material and of equal strength as the same size smooth suture.

14.3 Tips for Use in Gynecologic Laparoscopy

both suture ends, with barbs changing direction at the mid-point of the suture. Unidirectional barbed suture (Fig. 14.3) has a needle swaged onto one end, with a loop on the trailing end; after initiating the wound closure with an initial pass through tissue, the needle is passed through the loop to anchor the suture in place.

Various combinations of suture size, length, needle type, and monofilament material (including absorbable, delayed absorbable, and permanent options) are available in both bidirectional and unidirectional form. It is important to review the grading system employed by the barbed suture manufacturer to ensure a suture of sufficient strength is selected (Greenberg 2010). Some barbed suture (for example, Quill™ or STRATAFIX™ (Ethicon, Somerville NJ) suture)) is size-rated prior to the barbs being cut, and is equivalent in strength to smooth suture of one size smaller. Other barbed suture (for example, V-Loc™) is size-rated after barbs are cut into the

Barbed suture may be particularly useful for closure of the vaginal cuff at the time of total laparoscopic hysterectomy or trachelectomy. Several options for closure technique exist, depending on whether unidirectional or bidirectional barbed suture is chosen. Utilizing unidirectional suture, the surgeon may begin at one apex, anchor the suture via the loop on the trailing end, and move toward the other apex with continuous nonlocking bites. Once the full length of the vaginal incision has been re-approximated, it may be helpful to take several back bites toward the midline in order to further anchor the suture. Additionally, one may choose to utilize two separate unidirectional sutures, beginning at each apex with an individual suture, suturing toward the midline and taking overlapping bites in the middle.

When employing bidirectional barbed suture, the surgeon may begin in the middle of the incision, taking care to pull the suture through the tissue until resistance is met, indicating the mid-point of the suture where the barbs change direction (Fig. 14.4). One needle end of the suture

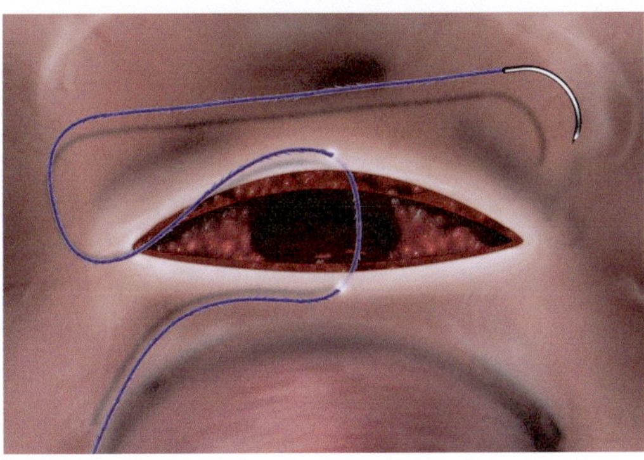

Fig. 14.4 Start in middle

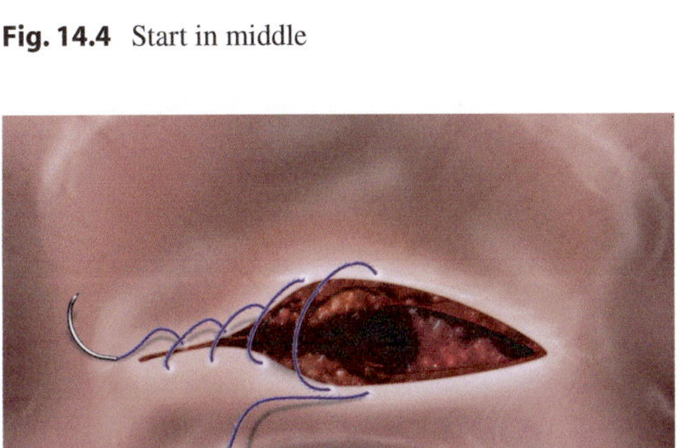

Fig. 14.5 Sutur left

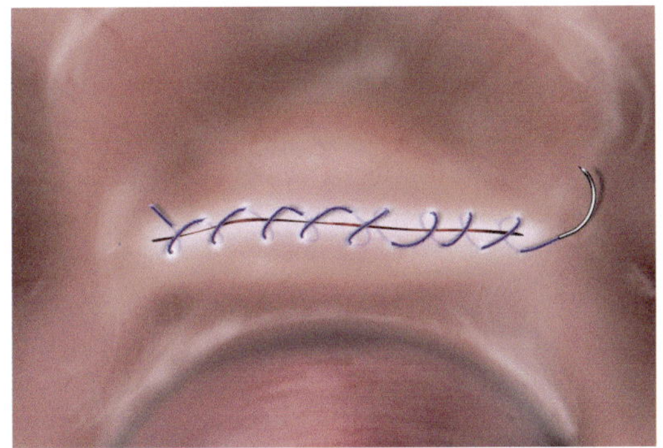

Fig. 14.6 Sutur right with the other needle

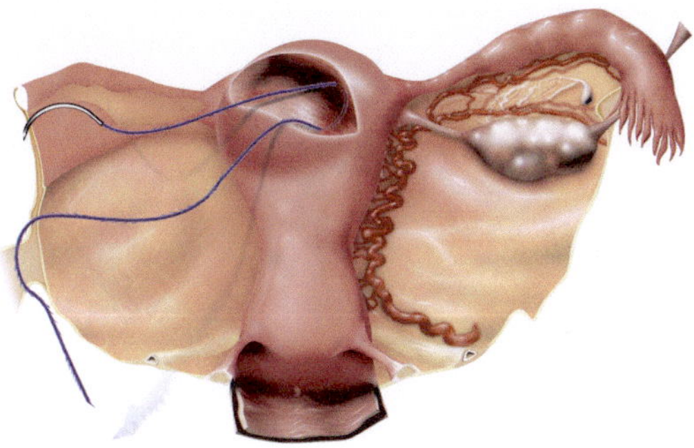

Fig. 14.7 Sutur of deep layers

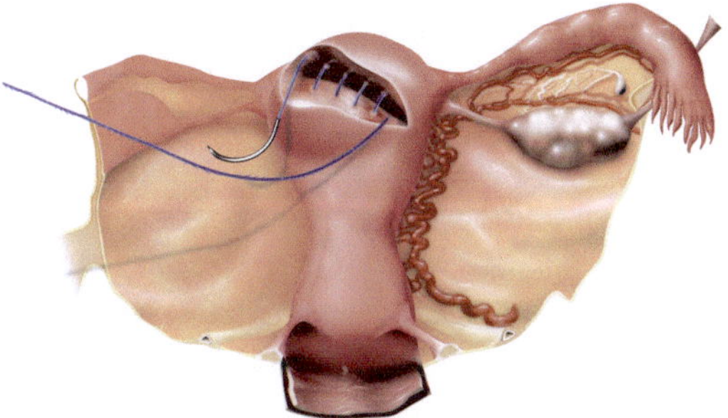

Fig. 14.8 Sutur of deep layers

is used to close toward the left of the incision, and the other to close toward the right (Figs. 14.5 and 14.6). Again, backbites may be helpful after completing closure to enhance suture anchoring. If a double-layer closure is desired, the bidirectional suturing is begun by placing the first bite at one apex, pulling the suture through until the mid-point resistance is met, and suturing in a continuous fashion toward the other apex. The second half of the suture is then utilized to work in the same direction and create an imbricating layer. Favorable outcomes have been reported with the use of barbed suture for vaginal cuff closure, including decreased incidence of cuff dehiscence, postoperative vaginal bleeding, formation of granulation tissue, and vaginal cuff cellulitis (Siedhoff et al. 2011).

During laparoscopic myomectomy, hysterotomy closure is also greatly facilitated by use of barbed suture. If a surgeon chooses unidirectional barbed suture, the defect may be closed in standard multilayer fashion by continuous suturing techniques. With bidirectional barbed suture, the first half of the suture is used to close the deepest layer, with the second half utilized for closure of the more superficial layers (Figs. 14.7, 14.8 and 14.9). It may be helpful to tack the nonworking needle to the anterior abdominal wall when using a long bidirectional suture in order to avoid tangling of the suture ends

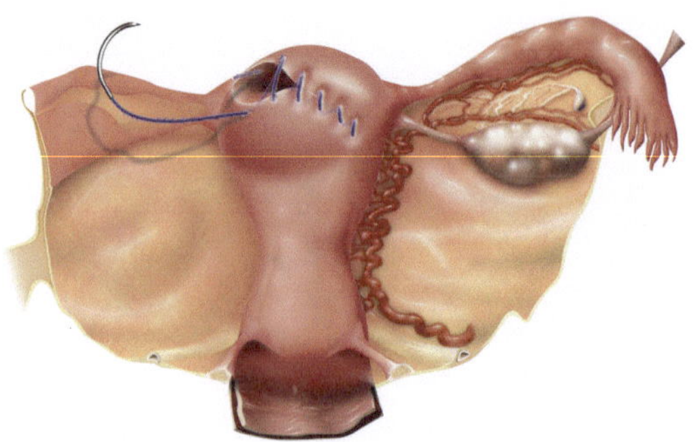

Fig. 14.9 Sutur of serosa

(Einarsson and Greenberg 2009). The use of barbed suture for laparoscopic myomectomy has demonstrated benefits including facilitating ease of a complex suturing task and decreased time required for hysterotomy closure, with variable findings regarding reduction in blood loss (Einarsson and Greenberg 2009; Allesandri et al. 2010; Angioli et al. 2012).

Use of barbed suture has also been reported in the setting of uterosacral suspension procedures or during laparoscopic sacropexy for reapproximation of peritoneum and attachment of mesh (Einarsson and Greenberg 2009; Defieux et al. 2011; Ghomi and Askari 2010). One consideration when using barbed suture to attach mesh to the cervix and/or vagina during a sacropexy is the tendency for the barbs to cause bunching of the mesh material; clinical significance of this is not known.

Conclusions

Barbed suture is a useful tool for advanced laparoscopic gynecology. As with any innovative technology, it is important to be aware of potential for unforeseen complications. Bowel obstruction has been reported in cases involving barbed suture use; this may be related to leaving a long trailing end of barbed suture in the abdomen (Buchs et al. 2011; Donnellan and Mansuria 2011; Thubert et al. 2011). Surgeons are advised to trim the ends of barbed suture short so as to avoid this potential complication. Adhesion formation due to exposed barbs has also been investigated in a sheep model; no difference was found with regard to adhesion formation with barbed compared to smooth suture (Einarsson et al. 2011a, b). Areas for further investigation include the incidence of uterine rupture during pregnancy following laparoscopic myomectomy with barbed suture and the occurrence of dyspareunia (or partner dyspareunia) following vaginal cuff closure with barbed suture.

References

Alessandri F, Remorgida V, Venturini PL et al (2010) Unidirectional barbed suture versus continuous suture with intracorporeal knots in laparoscopic myomectomy: a randomized study. J Minim Invasive Gynecol 17(6):725–729

Angioli R, Plotti F, Montera R et al (2012) A new type of absorbable barbed suture for use in laparoscopic myomectomy. Int J Gynaecol Obstet 117(3):220–223

Buchs NC, Ostermann S, Hauser J et al (2011) Intestinal obstruction following use of laparoscopic barbed suture: a new complication with new material? Minim Invasive Ther Allied Technol 2(5): 369–371

Deffieux X, Pachy F, Donnadieu AC et al (2011) Peritoneal closure using absorbable knotless device during laparoscopic sacrocolpopexy. J Gynecol Obstet Biol Reprod 40(1):65–67

Donnellan NM, Mansuria SM (2011) Small bowel obstruction resulting from laparoscopic vaginal cuff closure with a barbed suture. J Minim Invasive Gynecol 18(4):528–530

Einarsson JI, Greenberg JA (2009) Barbed suture, now in the toolbox of minimally invasive gyn surgery. OBG Manage 21(9):39–41

Einarsson JI, Chavan NR, Suzuki Y et al (2011a) Use of bidirectional barbed suture in laparoscopic myomectomy: an evaluation of perioperative outcomes, safety and efficacy. JMIG 18(1):92–95

Einarsson JI, Grazul-Bilska AT, Vonnahme KA (2011b) Barbed vs standard suture: randomized single-blinded comparison of adhesion formation and ease of use in an animal model. J Minim Invasive Gynecol 18(6): 716–719

Ghomi A, Askari R (2010) Use of bidirectional barbed suture in robot-assisted sacrocolpopexy. J Robot Surg 4:87–89

Greenberg JA (2010) The use of barbed sutures in obstetrics and gynecology. Rev Obstet Gynecol 3(3):82–91

McKenzie AR (1967) An experimental multiple barbed suture for the long flexor tendons of the palm and fingers. Preliminary report. J Bone Joint Surg Br 49(3): 440–447

Rodeheaver GT, Piñeros-Fernandez A, Salopek LS et al (2005) Barbed sutures for wound closure: In vivo wound security, tissue compatibility and cosmesis measurements. Society for biomaterials 30th annual meeting transactions 232

Siedhoff MT, Yunker AC, Steege JF (2011) Decreased incidence of vaginal cuff dehiscence after laparoscopic closure with bidirectional barbed suture. J Minim Invasive Gynecol 18(2):218–223

Thubert T, Pourcher G, Deffieux X (2011) Small bowel volvulus following peritoneal closure using absorbable knotless device during laparoscopic sacral colpopexy. Int Urogynecol J 22(6):761–763

Laparoscopic Cerclage

15

Evelien M. Sandberg, Jon I. Einarsson, and Thomas F. McElrath

Contents

E.M. Sandberg • J.I. Einarsson, MD, MPH (✉)
T.F. McElrath, MD, PhD
Brigham and women's Hospital,
Boston, MA, USA
e-mail: jeinarsson@partners.org

15.1   Introduction

Preterm delivery is the most common cause of neonatal morbidity and mortality, with reported preterm birth rates in Europe and other developed countries around 5–11 % of all deliveries (Lawn et al. 2010). Cervical insufficiency contributes to both preterm delivery and second-trimester fetal loss. It has been conservatively reported that cervical insufficiency complicates approximately 0.1–1 % of all pregnancies, and estimates suggest that 8 % of women with repeated second or early third-trimester losses may be affected (Ludmir 1988; Scarantino et al. 2000). In a normal pregnancy, the cervix stays both closed, with substantial length (>3 cm) and only toward the end of term the cervix starts to progressively shorten, become effaced in preparation for normal labor and delivery. In some cases, however, the cervix starts to shorten and dilates pathologically early in gestation (Alfirevic et al. 2012). This condition has been described as early as the seventeenth century by Riverius and was formerly termed 'cervical incompetence'. While this term has largely given way to the less pejorative, 'cervical insufficiency' they both refer to a condition where the cervix fails to maintain an intrauterine pregnancy until term (Ludmir 1988). Cervical insufficiency is characterized by painless dilation of the cervix followed by either the premature rupture or prolapse of the fetal membranes but without uterine contractions.

O. Istre (ed.), *Minimally Invasive Gynecological Surgery*,
DOI 10.1007/978-3-662-44059-9_15, © Springer-Verlag Berlin Heidelberg 2015

The pathogenesis of the cervical insufficiency has never been well understood. It has been thought to be possibly associated with everything from congenital weakness or previous cervical trauma, such as prior cone biopsy, improperly performed pregnancy terminations, or precipitous vaginal delivery. However, several recent studies have suggested that maternal and fetal inflammations are more likely key factors contributing to premature cervical effacement and dilatation (Harger 2002; Warren et al. 2009; Rust et al. 2001; McElrath et al. 2008). Work has suggested that specific cytokines present in the maternal and fetal milieu are directly correlated to premature labor causes and more specifically to cervical insufficiency (McElrath et al. 2011; Faupel-Badger et al. 2011). Moreover, the contribution of this background of biochemical, inflammatory, and immunological stimuli could explain why the ability of the cervix to remain closed varies from pregnancy to pregnancy. It is likely that cervical insufficiency is not an independent condition but one portion of a spectrum of conditions leading to spontaneous preterm birth (Lawn et al. 2010).

Nonetheless, cervical insufficiency is associated with dramatic consequences which may contribute to further morbidity including intraamniotic infection, preterm premature rupture of the fetal membranes (PPROM) and preterm labor and delivery (PTD), and fetal loss (www.uptodate.org).

To prevent the adverse effects caused by cervical insufficiency, a variety of therapies have been proposed and will be discussed briefly in this chapter. More specifically will be discussed the laparoscopic transabdominal cerclage.

15.2 Methods to Prevent Preterm Loss Associated with Cervical Insufficiency

When cervical insufficiency is suspected, a variety of diagnostic and treatment options can be considered:

Fetal fibronectin: The fetal fibronectin test is a test performed between 24 and 35 weeks gestation and measures the fibronectin protein that leaks into the vagina. If higher concentrations are noted, the risk of preterm delivery is increased. A negative test is reassuring as the possibility of preterm labor within the next 7–10 days is diminished. However, the test has a high false-positive rate. Despite this disadvantage, there is now substantial evidence that the fibronectin test is a reasonable test to reassure pregnant women (Duhig et al. 2009; Honest et al. 2009).

Progesterone: Administration of progesterone either intramuscularly or vaginally in the second and third trimester of pregnancy, depending on the indication, has been demonstrated to reduce the risk of primary or recurrent preterm birth (Berghella et al. 2010). Intramuscular progesterone has been specifically demonstrated to reduce the risk of recurrent preterm birth in women with prior history of premature birth (Berghella et al. 2010). Therefore in this group of women, it is appropriate to conduct progesterone prophylaxis between 16 weeks and 36 weeks gestation. More research is needed in terms of efficacy and the long-term consequences of progesterone use (Arisoy and Yayla 2012).

Pessary: A pessary is a silicone device that is inserted through the vagina and provides support to the cervix. It is a noninvasive, easy to apply, and cost-effective method and has been used over the past 50 years to prevent preterm birth, without gaining much popularity though. In a recent randomized control trial, however, a significant difference was found in the prolongation of pregnancy between women with cervical shortening treated with pessary and those managed expectantly. The authors concluded that the pessary is an affordable and safe alternative in a population of appropriately selected at-risk pregnant women with a cervical length of 25 mm or less (Goya et al. 2012). Pessary presents an interesting new option in the management of cervical insufficiency.

15.3 Cerclage

Considered generally, the placement of a cervical cerclage involves the circumferential suturing of the uterine cervix or lower uterine segment.

The aim is to give mechanical support and thereby maintain the cervical length and integrity. Cerclage can be placed either transvaginally or transabdominally. In 1957, Lash and Lash (1950), Shirodkar (1955), and McDonald (1957) first reported outcomes on cerclage placed transvaginally. In 1965, Benson and Durfee described the first transabdominal approach for women in whom a vaginal approach was not possible or had previously failed (Benson and Durfee 1965). More than 30 years later, in 1998, the first laparoscopically performed transabdominal cerclage was reported (Burger et al. 2011). It is currently estimated that, in the United States, cerclage is performed at a rate of 1 per every 300 pregnancies (Menacker and Martin 2008). Elsewhere in the world, cerclage placement has been reported to be higher, up to 1 per every 100 pregnancies (Al-Azemi et al. 2003). In multiple pregnancies, placement of cerclage occurs more often, up to 10 % for triplets.

15.3.1 Indication for Cerclage Placement

Historically, the indications for cerclage placement (either transabdominally or transvaginally) have been diverse and include factors such as poor obstetric history, uterine anomalies, cervical trauma, and cervical shortening seen on ultrasound examination. More recently, the Cochrane review (Alfirevic et al. 2012) divided the indications of cerclage into the following categories:

- History indicated cerclage: this type of cerclage is placed because of a perceived increased risk related to a woman's obstetric or gynecological history. The history indicated cerclage is preferably placed at 12–14 weeks of gestation, after assessment of viability and chromosomal risk. Multiple authors suggest that a history-indicated cerclage might be considered for women meeting the following three criteria (MRC/RCOG 1993; Buckingham et al. 1965; Leppert et al. 1987; Rechberger et al. 1988): (1) Two or more consecutive prior second trimester pregnancy losses or three or more early (<34 weeks) preterm births. (2) Risk factors for cervical insufficiency are present (history of cervical trauma and/or short labors or progressively earlier deliveries in successive pregnancies). (3) Other causes of preterm birth (e.g., infection, placental bleeding, multiple gestation) have been excluded.

- Ultrasound-indicated cerclage: if the cervical length decreases to less than 25 mm on screening prior to 24 weeks, placement of a transvaginal cerclage could be considered (Committee opinion no. 522: 2012; Society for Maternal-Fetal Medicine Publications Committee 2012). The efficacy of this cerclage is limited to women with a prior preterm birth who are not found to have a cervical length <2.5 cm. In a randomized control trial comparing Shirodkar cerclage to expectant management in women with short cervix, no significant differences were found with regard to perinatal or maternal morbidity (To et al. 2004).

- Exam indicated cerclage is a rare procedure in which a cervical suture is placed in women who are incidentally found to have a dilated cervix with or without prolapsed membranes. In order to perform this type of cerclage, the patient must not be in labor and not have heavy vaginal bleeding or infection (Liddiard et al. 2011). The complication rate, mainly due to the membrane ruptures, as well as the loss rate was higher than in other types of cerclage placement (Liddiard et al. 2011).

As elsewhere transvaginal cervical is the initial procedure of choice in our institution. However, for those with who have failed prior prophylactic methods designed to prevent recurrent spontaneous preterm birth, we reserve consideration of a transabdominal cerclage.

15.3.2 Transvaginal Cerclage

The transvaginal approach, which is most commonly used, has two primary placement techniques:

1. The *McDonald cerclage*, consists of placing a purse-string suture at the cervico-vaginal junction. This cerclage is typically placed between 12 and 14 weeks of pregnancy and the stitch is generally removed around the 37th week of gestation.

2. A *Shirodkar cerclage* is a similar technique, except that the sutures are placed close to the level of the internal os and are tunneled through the walls of the cervix, leaving them largely unexposed. The Shirodkar is technically more difficult than the McDonald cerclage and it involves some degree of bladder mobilization.

15.3.3 Transabdominal Cerclage

The transabdominal cerclage involves a Mersilene band (or other nonabsorbable suture material) passed around the cervicouterine isthmus at the level of the uterosacral ligament insertions with either an anterior or posterior tying of the ligature (Mingione et al. 2003). This procedure is typically reserved for patients who have failed one or more prior prophylactic techniques to prevent preterm birth (Reid et al. 2008).

Advantages of transabdominal over transvaginal cerclage are the more proximal placement of stitches (at the level of the internal os) and the ability to leave the suture in place for future pregnancies (Carter and Soper 2005). A disadvantage of this approach is the need for two surgeries during pregnancy (one to place the cerclage and a cesarean section for the delivery of the infant). Additionally, there is the possibility that additional surgery may be required in case of miscarriage or fetal demise (Lesser et al. 1998; Davis et al. 2000). In a systematic review, transabdominal cerclage was associated with a lower likelihood of perinatal death or delivery before 24 weeks of gestation (6 versus 12.5 % with repeat transvaginal cerclage), but a higher rate of serious operative complications, such as need for transfusion or organ injury (3 versus 0 %) compared with transvaginal cerclage (Zaveri et al. 2002). Subsequent studies have reported similar findings (Debbs et al. 2007). It has been suggested that the reason for the improved outcomes associated with abdominal cerclage is that the position of the cerclage at the level of the internal os (House and Socrate 2006).

The question whether cerclage should be placed via laparotomy or laparoscopy is still up for debate. In a recent systematic review comparing the effectiveness of abdominal cerclage placed via laparotomy or laparoscopy, the authors concluded that the outcomes of both methods of cerclage were excellent, with mean fetal survival rate (defined as total number of live born infants who survived the neonatal period, which is 6 weeks after delivery, divided by total number of pregnancies) between 80.9 and 90.8 %. The perioperative complication rates for both procedures were low and not significantly different, however in favor of the laparoscopic group (Burger et al. 2011).

Despite the limited available data, the present results seem to indicate that both approaches are safe and associated with good perinatal outcomes in patients with a poor obstetrical history. Therefore, it has been suggested that when possible, the abdominal cerclage should be done via laparoscopy, as this is associated with lower cost and the traditional benefits of minimally invasive surgery, such as fewer adhesions, less postoperative pain, no required hospitalization, and more timely recovery (Burger et al. 2011). However, more research with sufficient power needs to be done to define if one method is superior to the other.

15.3.4 Timing of Placement

Transabdominal cerclage placement can be performed prior to conception or, as stated by the American College of Obstetricians and Gynecologists' guideline on cervical insufficiency (2003), during early pregnancy (11–14 weeks), after ultrasound evaluation (American College of Obstetricians and Gynecologists 2003). The preconceptional approach is associated with less blood loss and avoids the risk of pregnancy-associated complications (e.g., rupture of the fetal membranes). It is also much easier to place the cerclage in a nonpregnant patient, which shortens operating time.

Placement of an abdominal cerclage late or after the first trimester is not possible since the large size of the uterus makes the procedure difficult if not impossible and is therefore associated with higher risk. At our institution, we prefer placing the cerclage prior to conception due to the greater ease of placement and the reduced risk of complications. A laparoscopic approach is also associated with minimal morbidity and therefore seems justifiable, even in the rare cases where patients are not able to conceive after the cerclage placement.

15.3.5 Contraindication of Cerclage Placement

Not all women are appropriate candidates for consideration of cerclage placement. The major contraindications are fetal anomaly incompatible with life, intrauterine infection, active uterine bleeding, uterine activity, preterm premature rupture of membranes, and fetal demise. Another relative contraindication is the presence of prolapsing fetal membranes through the external cervical os given that the risk of iatrogenic rupture of the membranes is extremely high, up to 50 % (Harger 2002; American College of Obstetricians and Gynecologists 2003). Frequently, the membranes can be reduced with maternal positioning (intraoperative Trendelenburg), back-filling the maternal bladder, decompression amniocentesis.

There is evidence that suggests that performing a cerclage in multiple pregnancies may be detrimental and is associated with an increase in preterm delivery and pregnancy loss. One randomized control trial on this subject has been published so far, comparing the effect of a cerclage versus no treatment for multiple gestations and the authors concluded that no significant additional benefit was to be found in the cerclage group (Dor et al. 1982). However, the number of study patients was limited. In a meta-analysis, outcomes were found to be even worse in the subgroup of women carrying twins, with a doubling of delivery before 35 weeks, compared to the group with expectant management (Jorgensen et al. 2007).

15.3.6 Laparoscopic Cerclage Operation Technique

In this section is presented the laparoscopic technique for cerclage placement as it is done at our institution. However, many variations of this operation have been described over time.

The placement of cerclage via laparoscopic approach is performed under general endotracheal anesthesia. After placing the patient in the modified dorsal lithotomy position, the patient is prepped and draped in the usual fashion for abdominal/vaginal procedure. A Foley catheter is inserted in the bladder and for nonpregnant women, a uterine manipulator is placed in the uterus. Then, as per author's preference, a 10 mm umbilical trocar is inserted with 5 mm accessory trocars in bilateral lower quadrants and left upper quadrant.

With the Harmonic Ace (Ethicon, Cincinnati, OH) the vesicouterine peritoneum is opened and dissected off the lower uterine segment, in order to view anteriorly on both side the uterine vessels and to expose the avascular window between the uterine artery and the uterus. A 5-mm nonabsorbable Mersilene (Ethicon Inc., Somerville, NJ) polyester suture, with adjacent straightened blunt needles to allow passage through the trocar, is then introduced into the abdominal cavity. The stitch is placed by passing each needle medial to the uterine vessels from posterior to anterior, at the level of the internal cervical os bilaterally. The uterosacral ligaments are used as reference point; a distance of 1.5 cm superior and 1 cm lateral to the insertion of the uterosacral ligament on the posterior uterus is a good initial guide for needle placement. After placing the stitch, the two needles are cut off and removed, and the Mersilene suture is then tied tightly around the cervix with six knots using intracorporeal knot tying. The ends of the stitch are trimmed and a silk suture is used to secure the knot to the lower uterine segment in an effort to minimize protrusion of the knot. Then the visceral peritoneum is closed over the cerclage with a running 2–0 Monocryl (Ethicon Inc., Somerville, NJ) suture that is tied intracorporeally.

The patient is observed in the recovery room for 3–4 h until she can tolerate oral pain medication, void spontaneously, and has adequate pain control. The patient may then be discharged home.

15.3.7 Complications

The major intraoperative complication of cerclage placement is bleeding from inadvertent damage to adjacent vessels. We feel the risk of bleeding can be minimized if the cerclage is placed prior to conception, when the pelvic vessels are smaller. Other adverse events described in case reports and case series include fetal death (defined as fetal loss during surgery or 2 weeks later) and intrauterine growth restriction (from inadvertent ligation of the uterine arteries), suture migration, infection, premature labor, premature rupture of membranes, uterine rupture, rectovaginal fistula, and maternal discomfort (www.uptodate.org). In a systematic review (Burger et al. 2011), a comparison of perioperative complications was made between women with laparotomy cerclage and laparoscopic cerclage. The conclusion of the authors was that the perioperative complications were low and not significantly different between the two groups.

15.3.8 Delivery

For women with a transabdominal cerclage in place, elective cesarean delivery at 37 weeks of gestation is advised at our institution. We prefer not to wait until 39 weeks since this may increase the risk of active labor with the cerclage in place. In our experience, laboring against an abdominal cerclage has been associated with tearing of the lower uterine segment and uterine dehiscence.

The Mersilene band can then be removed or left in place if future pregnancies are planned. Successful repeated pregnancies are routine at our institution.

In cases of a miscarriage or a fetal demise, the cervix can be dilated to accommodate the uterine evacuation and pregnancies up to 20 weeks have been successfully evacuated by appropriately trained personnel in this manner. If fetal demise occurs in the late second trimester, the cerclage may need to be taken down either transvaginally or laparoscopically in order to allow the vaginal delivery of the pregnancy and to avoid the need for a hysterotomy.

15.3.9 Outcome and Efficacy

Unfortunately the efficacy of cerclage placement for prevention of premature delivery remains uncertain, and according to the literature, the reported outcomes vary widely. Smaller observational studies have suggested that transvaginal cerclage reduces preterm birth (MacNaughton et al. 1993). More rigorous studies have been less optimistic but there does seem to be a positive effect for women with a history of prior preterm birth and newly diagnosed cervical shortening (Daskalakis 2009). Abdominal cerclage outcomes have not been rigorously tested but success rates have been reported between 85 and 90 % (Novy 1991; Witt et al. 2009) for cerclages placed via laparotomy and between 79 and 100 % for the cerclage placed laparoscopically (Al-Fadhli and Tulandi 2004; Carter et al. 2009; Whittle et al. 2009).

Although these numbers suggest very optimistic results, the use of cerclage and its efficacy still remains uncertain. At our institution, we reserve placement of an abdominal cerclage for situations where a patient has both had multiple prior preterm losses despite the concurrent use of medically indicated conventional prophylactic therapy. Given that the efficacy of abdominal cerclage has not yet been rigorously demonstrated, we hesitate to offer this as a primary prophylactic therapy to patients who have not already failed more standard treatment.

Conclusion

While the available literature on transabdominal cerclage is limited and clinical outcomes of cerclage placement remains uncertain, current experience indicates that laparoscopic cerclage is a safe and effective procedure. Studies indicate that it is comparable with the laparotomy approach or even superior in terms of surgical outcomes, cost, and postoperative morbidity (Fick et al. 2007). Furthermore, laparoscopic cerclage placement has been associated with excellent perinatal outcomes, even in patients with a poor obstetrical history (Fick et al. 2007). Further research with larger patient populations needs to be done to adequately define the appropriate indications for cerclage placement as well as the optimal choice of mode of access, i.e., vaginal vs. laparoscopic vs. abdominal, as well as the potential combination with alternative techniques.

Main Points

- Maternal and fetal inflammation may be a key factor contributing to the pathogenesis of cervical insufficiency.
- Cerclage can be placed either transvaginally or transabdominally.
- When the standard and conventional therapy fails, it has been our practice to attempt transabdominal placement.
- Laparoscopic cerclage seems to be a safe and effective procedure, comparable with the laparotomy approach or even superior in terms of surgical outcomes, cost, and postoperative morbidity.
- Further research with larger patient populations needs to be done to adequately define the appropriate indications for cerclage placement as well as the optimal choice of mode of access.

References

Al-Azemi M, Al-Qattan F, Omu A, Taher S, Al-Busiri N, Abdulaziz A (2003) Changing trends in the obstetric indications for cervical cerclage. J Obstet Gynaecol 23:507–511

Al-Fadhli R, Tulandi T (2004) Laparoscopic abdominal cerclage. Obstet Gynecol Clin North Am 31:497–504

Alfirevic Z, Stampalija T, Roberts D, Jorgensen AL (2012) Cervical stitch (cerclage) for preventing preterm birth in singleton pregnancy. Cochrane Database Syst Rev 4:CD008991

American College of Obstetricians and Gynecologists (2003) ACOG practice bulletin. Cervical insufficiency. Obstet Gynecol 102:1091

Arisoy R, Yayla M (2012) Transvaginal sonographic evaluation of the cervix in asymptomatic singleton pregnancy and management options in short cervix. J Pregnancy 4:1–10

Benson RC, Durfee RB (1965) Transabdominal cervico-uterine cerclage during pregnancy for treatment of cervical incompetency. Obstet Gynecol 25:145–155

Berghella V, Mackeen AD (2011) Cervical length screening with ultrasound-indicated cerclage compared with history-indicated cerclage for prevention of preterm birth: a meta-analysis. Obstet Gynecol 118(1):148–155

Berghella V, Figueroa D, Szychowski JM, Owen J, Hankins GD, Iams JD, Sheffield JS, Perez-Delboy A, Wing DA, Guzman ER (2010) Vaginal ultrasound trial 17-alpha-hydroxyprogesterone caproate for the prevention of preterm birth in women with prior preterm birth and a short cervical length. Am J Obstet Gynecol 202(4):351

Buckingham JC, Buethe RA Jr, Danforth DN (1965) Collagen-muscle ratio in clinically normal and clinically incompetent cervices. Am J Obstet Gynecol 91:232

Burger NB, Brolmann HA, Einarsson JI, Langebrekke A, Huirne JA (2011) Effectiveness of abdominal cerclage placed via laparotomy or laparoscopy: systematic review. J Minim Invasive Gynecol 18:696–704

Carter JF, Soper DE (2005) Laparoscopic abdominal cerclage. JSLS 9(4):491–493

Carter JF, Soper DE, Goetzl LM, Van Dorsten JP (2009) Abdominal cerclage for the treatment of recurrent cervical insufficiency: laparoscopy or laparotomy? Am J Obstet Gynecol 201:111.e1–111.e4

Committee opinion no. 522: incidentally detected short cervical length. Obstet Gynecol 2012. 119:679

Daskalakis GJ (2009) Prematurity prevention: the role of cerclage. Curr Opin Obstet Gynecol 21(2):148–152, Review

Davis G, Berghella V, Talucci M, Wapner RJ (2000) Patients with a prior failed transvaginal cerclage: a comparison of obstetric outcomes with either transabdominal or transvaginal cerclage. Am J Obstet Gynecol 183:836–839

Debbs RH, DeLa Vega GA, Pearson S, Sehdev H, Marchiano D, Ludmir J (2007) Transabdominal cerclage after comprehensive evaluation of women with previous unsuccessful transvaginal cerclage. Am J Obstet Gynecol 197(3):317

Dor J, Shalev J, Mashiach S, Blankstein J, Serr DM (1982) Elective cervical suture of twin pregnancies diagnosed ultrasonically in the first trimester following induced ovulation. Gynecol Obstet Invest 13:55–60

Duhig KE, Chandiramani M, Seed PT, Kenyon AP, Shennan AH (2009) Fetal fibronectin as a predictor of spontaneous preterm labour in asymptomatic women with a cervical cerclage. Br J Obstet Gynaecol 116(6): 799–803

Faupel-Badger JM, Fichorova RN, Allred EN, Hecht JL, Dammann O, Leviton A, McElrath TF (2011) Cluster analysis of placental inflammatory proteins can distinguish preeclampsia from preterm labor and premature membrane rupture in singleton deliveries less than 28 weeks of gestation. Am J Reprod Immunol 66(6): 488–494. doi:10.1111/j.1600-0897.2011.01023.x

Fick AL, Caughey AB, Parer JT (2007) Transabdominal cerclage: can we predict who fails? J Matern Fetal Neonatal Med 20(1):63–67

Final report of the Medical Research Council/Royal College of Obstetricians and Gynaecologists multicentre randomised trial of cervical cerclage. MRC/RCOG working party on cervical cerclage. Br J Obstet Gynaecol 1993. 100:516–23

Goya M, Pratcorona L, Merced C, Rodó C, Valle L, Romero A, Juan M, Rodríguez A, Muñoz B, Santacruz B, Bello-Muñoz JC, Llurba E, Higueras T, Cabero L, Carreras E, Pesario Cervical para Evitar Prematuridad (PECEP) Trial Group (2012) Cervical pessary in pregnant women with a short cervix (PECEP): an open-label randomised controlled trial. Lancet 379(9828): 1800–1806

Harger JH (2002) Cerclage and cervical insufficiency: an evidence-based analysis. Obstet Gynecol 100: 1313–1327

Honest H, Forbes CA, Durée KH, Norman G, Duffy SB, Tsourapas A, Roberts TE, Barton PM, Jowett SM, Hyde CJ, Khan KS (2009) Screening to prevent spontaneous preterm birth: systematic reviews of accuracy and effectiveness literature with economic modelling. Health Technol Assess 13(43):1–627

House M, Socrate S (2006) The cervix as a biomechanical structure. Ultrasound Obstet Gynecol 28(6):745–749

Jorgensen AL, Alfirevic Z, Tudur Smith C, Williamson PR, Cerclage IPD Meta-analysis Group (2007) Cervical stitch (cerclage) for preventing pregnancy loss: individual patient data meta-analysis. BJOG 114(12):1460–1476

Lash AF, Lash SR (1950) Habitual abortion: the incompetent internal os of the cervix. Am J Obstet Gynecol 59:68–76

Lawn JE, Gravett MG, Nunes TM, Rubens CE, Stanton C, GAPPS Review Group (2010) Global report on preterm birth and stillbirth (1 of 7): definitions, description of the burden and opportunities to improve data. BMC Pregnancy Childbirth 10(Suppl 1):S1

Leppert PC, Yu SY, Keller S et al (1987) Decreased elastic fibers and desmosine content in incompetent cervix. Am J Obstet Gynecol 157:1134

Lesser KB, Childers JM, Surwit EA (1998) Transabdominal cerclage: a laparoscopic approach. Obstet Gynecol 91:855–856

Liddiard A, Bhattacharya S, Crichton L (2011) Elective and emergency cervical cerclage and immediate pregnancy outcomes: a retrospective observational study. JRSM Short Rep 2(11):91, Epub 28 Nov 2011

Ludmir J (1988) Sonographic detection of cervical incompetence. Clin Obstet Gynecol 31:101–109

MacNaughton MC, Chalmers JG, Dubowitz V et al (1993) Final report of the Medical Research Council/Royal College of Obstetrics and Gynaecology multicentre randomized trial of cervical cerclage. Br J Obstet Gynaecol 100:516–523

Mcdonald IA (1957) Suture of the cervix for inevitable miscarriage. J Obstet Gynaecol Br Emp 64:346

McElrath TF, Hecht JL, Dammann O, Boggess K, Onderdonk A, Markenson G, Harper M, Delpapa E, Allred EN, Leviton A (2008) Pregnancy disorders that lead to delivery before the 28th week of gestation: an epidemiologic approach to classification. Am J Epidemiol 168(9):980–989

McElrath TF, Fichorova RN, Allred EN, Hecht JL, Ismail MA, Yuan H, Leviton A, ELGAN Study Investigators (2011) Blood protein profiles of infants born before 28 weeks differ by pregnancy complication. Am J Obstet Gynecol 204(5):418.e1–418.e12

Menacker F, Martin JA (2008) Expanded health data from the new birth certificate, 2005. Natl Vital Stat Rep 56(13):1–24, J Obstet Gynaecol 2003;23:507–511

Mingione MJ, Scibetta JJ, Sanko SR, Phipps WR (2003) Clinical outcomes following interval laparoscopic transabdominal cervico-isthmic cerclage placement: case series. Hum Reprod 18(8):1716–1719

Norwitz ER, Lee DM, Goldstein DP (1997) Transabdominal cervicoisthmic cerclage: placing the stitch before conception. J Gynecol Tech 3:53

Novy MJ (1991) Transabdominal cervicoisthmic cerclage: a reappraisal 25 years after its introduction. Am J Obstet Gynecol 164:1635–1641

Rechberger T, Uldbjerg N, Oxlund H (1988) Connective tissue changes in the cervix during normal pregnancy and pregnancy complicated by cervical incompetence. Obstet Gynecol 71:563

Reid GD, Wills HJ, Shukla A, Hammill P (2008) Laparoscopic transabdominal cervico-isthmic cerclage: a minimally invasive approach. Aust N Z J Obstet Gynaecol 48(2):185–188

Rust OA, Atlas RO, Reed J, van Gaalen J, Balducci J (2001) Revisiting the short cervix found by transvaginal ultrasound in the second trimester: why cerclage therapy may not help. Am J Obstet Gynecol 185:1098–1105

Scarantino SE, Reilly JG, Moretti ML, Pillari VT (2000) Laparoscopic removal of a transabdominal cervical cerclage. Am J Obstet Gynecol 182:1086–1088

Shirodkar VN (1955) A new method of operative treatment for habitual abortion in the second trimester of pregnancy. Antiseptic 52:299

Society for Maternal-Fetal Medicine Publications Committee, with the assistance of Vincenzo Berghella, MD (2012) Progesterone and preterm birth prevention: translating clinical trials data into clinical practice. Am J Obstet Gynecol 206:376

To MS, Alfirevic Z, Heath VC, Cicero S, Cacho AM, Williamson PR, Nicolaides KH, Fetal Medicine

Foundation Second Trimester Screening Group et al (2004) Cervical cerclage for prevention of preterm delivery in women with short cervix: randomised controlled trial. Lancet 363(9424):1849–1853

Warren JE, Nelson LM, Stoddard GJ, Esplin MS, Varner MW, Silver RM (2009) Polymorphisms in the promoter region of the interleukin-10 (IL-10) gene in women with cervical insufficiency. Am J Obstet Gynecol 201(4):372.e1-5

Whittle WL, Singh SS, Allen L et al (2009) Laparoscopic cervico-isthmic cerclage: surgical technique and obstetric outcomes. Am J Obstet Gynecol 201:364. e1–364.e7

Witt MU, Joy SD, Clark J, Herring A, Bowes WA, Thorp JM (2009) Cervicoisthmic cerclage: transabdominal vs transvaginal approach. Am J Obstet Gynecol 201:105.e1–105.e4

www.uptodate.org (Topic cerclage, June 2012)

Zaveri V, Aghajafari F, Amankwah K, Hannah M (2002) Abdominal versus vaginal cerclage after a failed transvaginal cerclage: a systematic review. Am J Obstet Gynecol 187(4):868–872

Laparoscopic Approach to Pelvic Organ Prolapse

16

Catherine Hill-Lydecker and Jon Ivar Einarsson

Contents

16.1 Introduction

Pelvic organ prolapse (POP), or pelvic relaxation, is a common condition in which the uterus or vaginal apex and/or the vaginal walls descend into the vagina. Millions of women are afflicted with POP, and one facility has reported patient populations with rates of up to 37 % in women ages 20–80 (Progetto Menopausa Italia Study Group 2000). Cases of surgical management for pelvic organ prolapse are estimated to number as many as 350,000 annually in the USA (Subak et al. 2001). Just as concerning as the high incidence of prolapse are the reported rates of recurrence, which have reported to occur in up to 50–60 % of women following pelvic surgery (Whiteside et al. 2004).

16.1.1 Diagnosis/Symptoms

While up to 40% of women with pelvic organ prolapse (Swift et al. 2005) do not manifest specific symptoms, the majority of women experience multiple symptoms including pelvic pressure, urinary retention, dyschezia, dyspareunia, and in cases of severe prolapse bulging of pelvic organs protruding from the vagina (Hirata et al. 2004; Ellerkmann et al. 2001). In these women for whom symptoms are present, conservative management such as vaginal pessary use and Kegel and pelvic floor exercises frequently fail,

C. Hill-Lydecker • J.I. Einarsson, MD, MPH (✉)
Brigham and women's Hospital,
Boston, MA, USA
e-mail: jeinarsson@partners.org

O. Istre (ed.), *Minimally Invasive Gynecological Surgery*,
DOI 10.1007/978-3-662-44059-9_16, © Springer-Verlag Berlin Heidelberg 2015

and surgical treatment is indicated. While surgery for prolapse as the primary procedure is generally not recommended for women who are asymptomatic, it may be performed concomitantly with other pelvic surgeries, such as hysterectomy, if the patient possesses risk factors that indicate future exacerbation of prolapse.

16.1.2 Subtypes

Pelvic organ prolapse is a term that can refer to relaxation in many anatomical sites within the pelvic cavity. Both surgical and conservative treatments depend on the specific type of prolapse, and therefore prolapse degree and location should be elucidated upon an initial examination.

Anterior prolapse (cystocele) refers to the relaxation of the anterior vaginal wall and may be accompanied by sagging of the urinary bladder, which often results in symptoms of frequent urination or urinary retention. Protrusion of the rectum and/or the rectosigmoid into the posterior vaginal wall is identified as posterior prolapse (enterocele) and is associated with dyschezia and constipation. Anterior and posterior prolapse result from weakening in the muscles and connective tissues of the vaginal wall or endopelvic fascia. Apical prolapse occurs when to the uterus, cervix or vaginal apex, if posthysterectomy, herniates into the vagina. Generally, women do not report symptoms of apical prolapse until the uterus or vaginal vault has descended to the level of the hymen.

16.1.3 Classification

In an effort to standardize prolapse classification, several measurement tools are used to assess the severity and source of prolapse. The Pelvic Organ Prolapse Quantitation (POP-Q), established in 1996, continues to be the most commonly used classification system (Bump et al. 1996). The POP-Q system designates nine pelvic anatomical measurements expressed in centimeters that are used to assess an overall prolapse rating which establishes stages 0 (no prolapse) through IV (complete protrusion of pelvic organs). Numerical values for each individual compartment are taken during relaxation and Valsalva to obtain the greatest severity of the prolapse. The Valsalva maneuver is a position in which the patient forces an exhale into closed airways, thereby inducing a strain that allows for maximum prolapse to be visualized. A ruler or any instrument that has discernable centimeter increments can be used to determine the measurements. Positive measurements represent points that are distal to the hymen, whereas negative values are proximal to the hymen and indicate less severe prolapse. The values can also be used to determine specific locations of the prolapse (e.g., anterior or posterior) and give stages for each location.

An alternative classification tool is the Baden–Walker Halfway Scoring System, which defines the prolapse stage of each anterior, posterior, and apical prolapse relative to the hymen. Scoring ranges from 0 to 4. Normal positioning is given a score of 0, 1 represents descent halfway to the hymen, descent to the hymen scores as 2, 3 indicates descent halfway past the hymen, and stage 4, being the most severe prolapse, is complete eversion of pelvic organs (procidentia). The Baden–Walker System can be performed with in the dorsal lithotomy position under visual examination during both relaxation and Valsalva (Baden and Walker 1972).

16.1.4 Risk Factors for Pelvic Organ Prolapse

Not surprisingly, age plays a significant role in the development of prolapse (Swift et al. 2005). Increased age is associated with breakdown in collagen, muscles, and connective tissues, which weaken the support structures within the pelvis that lead to the descent of uterus or vaginal vault (Soderberg et al. 2004). The incidence of pelvic organ prolapse has been demonstrated to increase with parity as well, with vaginal delivery placing women at a significantly higher risk than cesarean deliveries. Higher birth weights of delivered fetuses also correlate with increased severity and incidence of prolapse. Other factors contributing to pelvic organ prolapse include prior hysterectomy, chronic constipation, obesity, heavy work, and genetic predisposition (Whiteside et al. 2004).

16.2 Pre-operative Considerations

Laparoscopic repair of apical, uterine or vaginal vault, prolapse should be considered in patients with troublesome symptoms. Appropriate candidates include those who have not achieved satisfactory results via conservative methods and are appropriate candidates for abdominal surgery or have declined nonsurgical treatment and desire surgical management.

Because POP presents in such a diverse fashion, a detailed discussion with the patient to determine the most concerning and bothersome symptoms is necessary. In patients presenting with urinary symptoms, urodynamic testing may be necessary to determine if a concomitant procedure for incontinence, such as transvaginal or transobturator tape, is indicated.

16.2.1 Concomitant Hysterectomy

While the role of hysterectomy in the success and longevity of prolapse repair has not been specifically addressed in the literature, the majority of prolapse repairs continue to include concurrent hysterectomies, if the uterus is present. Preserving the uterus also a valid option, however, since there is limited long-term outcome data on prolapse repair with uterine preservation, it is uncertain what effects this may have on the durability of the repair.

Patients of reproductive age should be counseled that there is limited data available regarding fertility prospects after pelvic reconstructive surgery involving uttering preservation. Reports of successful pregnancy after prolapse repair are limited to several small case studies and one trial demonstrating five vaginal deliveries out of nineteen attempting patients after sacrospinous

uterosacral ligament suspension. Despite these studies, larger randomized trials are needed before woman can be counseled on the possibility of future fertility after prolapse repair (Kovac and Cruikshank 1993; Gadonneix et al. 2012).

16.2.2 Vaginal Mesh

Vaginal mesh kits were developed to reduce the significant prolapse recurrence rates after pelvic repair surgery with native tissue used as support and to facilitate mesh placement for the majority of practitioners. Mesh in prolapse surgery has created a significant controversy due to the serious complications reported to the Food and Drug Association and their subsequent advisory statement (Food and Drug Administration 2008). It is important to realize that the FDA advisory specifically pertains to vaginal mesh placement and is not directed at abdominal or laparoscopic mesh placement.

Some studies have reported very high success rates with use of vaginal mesh, up to 97 %, whereas others report no difference in recurrence or postoperative prolapse stage between mesh procedures and those with native tissue (Keys et al. 2012). A 2012 review demonstrated the incongruent and frequently contradictory nature of data from randomized trials that have so far looked into mesh complications and recurrence rates (Keys et al. 2012). One study suggests that mesh complication rates, including dyspareunia, occur in up to 17.6 % of patients. However, a widely accepted rate for mesh erosion and infection is between 1 and 3 % of cases (Jeon et al. 2008).

The inarguable existence of severe complications related to mesh warrants a thorough discussion, with appropriate patients, regarding the risks and benefits of vaginal mesh.

The American College of Obstetricians and Gynecologists (ACOG) and the American Urogynecologic Society (AUGS) recommend that vaginal mesh be used selectively in patients with severe cases to whom the most benefit may be conferred (Committee on Gynecologic Practice 2011).

16.3 Surgical Repair

Pelvic organ prolapse is rarely confined to one compartment, as relaxation represents weakening of connection tissue and collagen throughout the pelvis. A more common presentation is prolapse in multiple compartments, which typically necessitates one or more additional repairs. There is some question as to whether with sufficient apical repair anterior and posterior compartments may be adequately supported which may obviate multiple site repairs; however, there is little evidence to support this claim (Lowder et al. 2008).

16.3.1 Anterior and Posterior Prolapse

While typically repaired vaginally, anterior and posterior prolapse repairs can be performed laparoscopically and also concomitantly with laparoscopic apical prolapse repair, if indicated.

16.3.2 Laparoscopic Apical Prolapse Repair

Laparoscopic apical prolapse repair can be performed with or without mesh. Use of mesh is generally preferred in cases of significant prolapse, i.e., when the level of prolapse is at a stage II or higher. Sacrohysteropexy refers to support of the vaginal apex with the uterus intact. Sacrocervicopexy is support of the vaginal apex with conservation of the cervix, and sacrocolpopexy refers to suspension of the vaginal apex without a uterus or cervix in place. While the traditional proximal suspension point is described at the level of S2 on the sacrum, most surgeons will suspend the mesh to the sacral promontory due to better exposure and less risk of bleeding complications. If a concomitant hysterectomy is performed, it is preferable to conserve the cervix since this will reduce the risk of mesh erosion (Bensinger et al. 2005; Warner et al. 2012). There are some relative contraindications to preserving the cervix, which include cervical dysplasia and cervical elongation.

16.3.2.1 Procedure Summary

Following peritoneal insufflation and insertion of trocars, the peritoneum over the promontory is opened exposing the anterior longitudinal ligament. The incision is then carried into the pelvis along the right pelvic sidewall midway between the ureter and the rectosigmoid. The bladder is dissected anteriorly off the cervix and upper vagina. This dissection can be carried all the way down to the bladder trigone, but practices vary greatly and the extent of dissection may depend on the level of prolapse. Posteriorly, the rectum is dissected away from the cervix and vagina and this dissection can be taken all the way down to the levator ani. Again, the extent of the dissection may vary depending on physician preference and level of prolapse. An important guide to the correct dissection is to remember that fat belongs to the rectum and the bladder. Therefore, the surgeon should consider an alternative plane of dissection if fat is encountered. In addition, the correct plane of dissection should be relatively avascular and therefore if bleeding is encountered, the surgeon is probably either too close to the rectum, vagina, or bladder. A Y-shaped polypropylene mesh is then inserted and attached to the anterior and posterior aspect of the cervical stump and the upper vagina. The type of suture material varies greatly as does the suturing. Commonly used suture materials include prolene, Ethibond® (Ethicon Endo-Surgery, Cincinnati, OH, USA), and Gore-tex® (W. L. Gore & Associates, Inc., Flagstaff, Arizona, USA), although some surgeons prefer the use of delayed absorbable materials such as PDS. Sutures can be placed with extracorporeal or intracorporeal knot tying, or with the assistance of a suturing device. The number of fixation points also varies greatly; with most surgeons placing at least four to six fixation points on each portion of the mesh. The tail end of the mesh is then fastened to the sacral promontory with either tacks or sutures. Using tacks expedites the process, although some concerns have been raised on the risk of the development of osteomyelitis (Nosseir et al. 2010). In cases with limited exposure to the promontory, it may be advisable to avoid the use of mesh since visual exposure may be limited due the mesh and a vascular injury may result. The middle sacral vessels can be fulgurated prior to fastening of the mesh to decrease the risk of bleeding. In addition, the location of the left common iliac vein is highly variable and it sometimes lies fairly close to the promontory of the sacrum (Flynn et al. 2005; Wieslander et al. 2006). It is therefore mandatory to know the location of the common iliac vein prior to the placement of mesh at the sacral promontory. The tension on the mesh should be enough to retain the vaginal apex in its correct anatomic position, but the mesh should not be placed on too much tension as this can result in back pain and potential tearing of the mesh off the apical segment of the vagina. The peritoneum is generally closed overlying the mesh and reapproximating the anterior peritoneum and the posterior peritoneum from the cervicovaginal dissection, as well as the lateral sidewall peritoneum. Although there is no evidence to support this practice, it makes sense that it may reduce the risk of hernia formation and potentially bowel adhesions to the mesh.

16.3.3 Uterosacral Ligament Suspension

Uterosacral ligament suspension is an effective procedure for apical prolapse repair. It has the advantage of no risk of mesh exposure and associated complications and is generally considered to be effective in the long run, although there are no comparative studies available comparing long-term outcomes of uterosacral ligament suspension and apical suspensions using mesh (Margulies et al. 2010; Silva et al. 2006; Diwan et al. 2006). The use of uterosacral ligament suspension is often limited to milder forms of apical prolapse (stages I and II) or as a prophylactic procedure in an attempt to prevent the development of future prolapse.

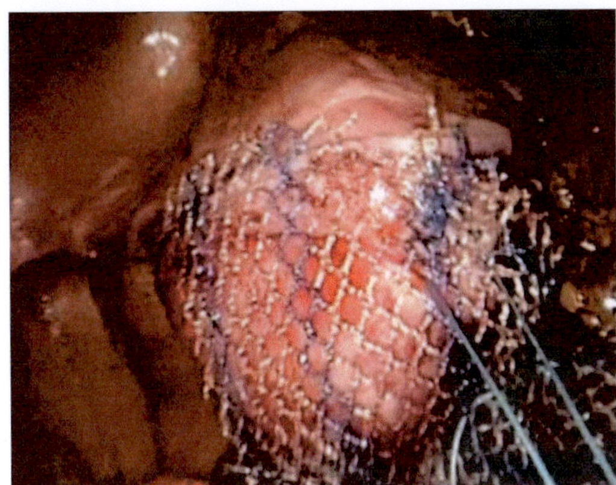

Fig. 16.1 Suturing mesh to vaginal apex

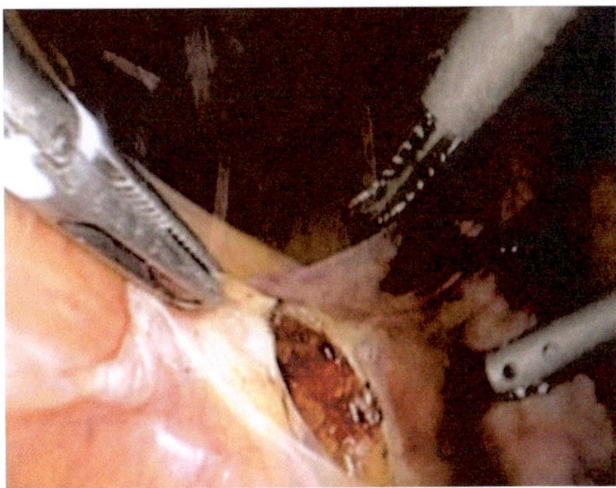

Fig. 16.2 Opening peritoneum over the sacral promontory

16.3.3.1 Procedure Summary

A concomitant hysterectomy may or may not be performed. The uterosacral ligaments and the ureters must be identified. It is very important to delineate the ureter during the dissection and if it is in close proximity to the uterosacral ligament, a relaxing peritoneal incision may be required. A suture is then taken through the uterosacral ligament at the level of the ischial spine and this is in turn attached to the ipsilateral vaginal apex. The choice of suture material varies greatly, but most commonly a permanent suture such as prolene or ethibond is utilized. The sutures are then tied using either extracorporeal or intracorporeal suturing or with the assistance of a suturing device (Fig. 16.1, 16.2, 16.3, and 16.4).

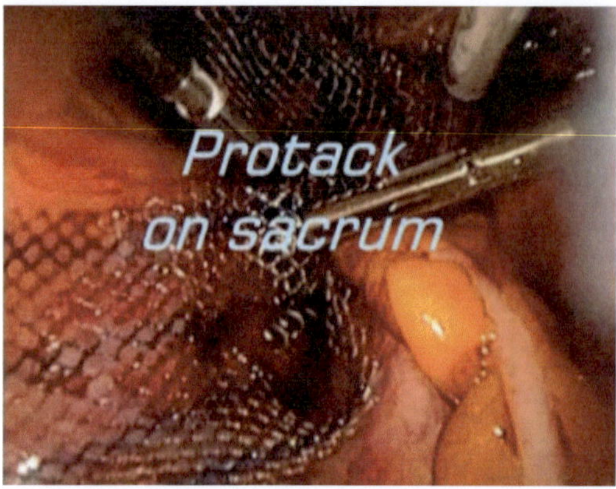

Fig. 16.3 Fastening the mesh to the sacral promontory with tacks

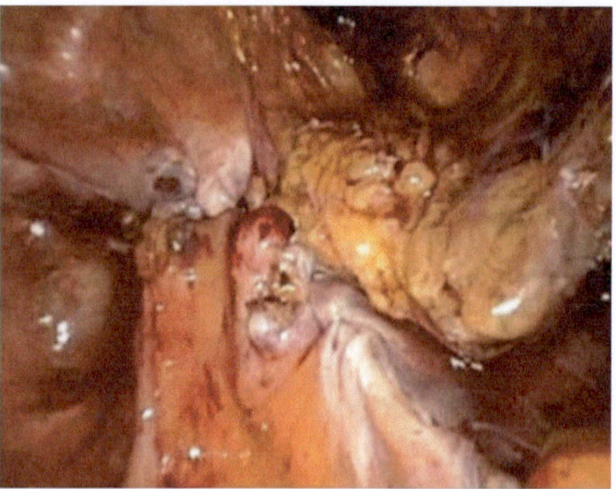

Fig. 16.4 End of the procedure with mesh covered by peritoneum

16.4 Urinary Tract Considerations

Cystoscopy should be routinely performed in pelvic organ prolapse repair surgery to ensure excellent ureteral flow at the end of surgery. However, cystoscopy is not a perfect indicator of bladder injury; a reassuring cystoscopy does not guarantee the absence of bladder injury, especially in the case of thermal injury. The possibility of injury must not be ruled out if symptoms present postoperatively. Isolation of the ureters prior to initiating any energy sources as well as maintaining direct visualization throughout the procedure are key factors in avoiding bladder injury (Jabs and Drutz 2001).

16.5 Postoperative Management

Postoperatively, the majority of patients have an uneventful recovery. Following laparoscopic prolapse repair, patients receive nonsteroidal anti-inflammatory medications along with narcotics by mouth as needed. They are generally ready for discharge the following morning. A vaginal pack may be placed over night and a Foley catheter left in place until the following morning. It is good practice to perform a voiding trial the morning after surgery prior to discharge as there is a small risk of urinary retention in these patients. It is important to remain vigilant for possible urinary tract injuries and mesh-related complications. Complications resulting from mesh use may present as fever, infection, dyspareunia, and chronic bloody vaginal discharge, and exposed mesh may be visible if erosion has taken place.

Conclusions

Laparoscopic treatment of pelvic organ prolapse is a viable option for patients desiring minimally invasive surgical management of their symptoms while also achieving optimal long-term results. More research is needed to better determine the surgical procedures and techniques of choice for various clinical scenarios.

References

Baden WF, Walker TA (1972) Statistical evaluation of vaginal relaxation. Clin Obstet Gynecol 15(4): 1070–1072

Bensinger G, Lind L, Lesser M et al (2005) Abdominal sacral suspensions: analysis of complications using permanent mesh. Am J Obstet Gynecol 193(6): 2094–2098

Bump RC, Mattiasson A, Bo K et al (1996) The standardization of terminology of female pelvic organ prolapse and pelvic floor dysfunction. Am J Obstet Gynecol 175(1):10–17

Committee on Gynecologic Practice (2011) Committee opinion no. 513: vaginal placement of synthetic mesh for pelvic organ prolapse. Obstet Gynecol 118(6): 1459–1464

Diwan A, Rardin CR, Strohsnitter WC et al (2006) Laparoscopic uterosacral ligament uterine suspension compared with vaginal hysterectomy with vaginal vault suspension for uterovaginal prolapse. Int Urogynecol J Pelvic Floor Dysfunct 17(1):79–83

Ehsani N, Ghafar MA, Antosh DD et al (2012) Risk factors for mesh extrusion after prolapse surgery: a case-control study. Female Pelvic Med Reconstr Surg 18(6):357–361

Ellerkmann RM, Cundiff GW, Melick CF et al (2001) Correlation of symptoms with location and severity of pelvic organ prolapse. Am J Obstet Gynecol 185(6):1332–1337

Flynn MK, Romero AA, Amundsen CL et al (2005) Vascular anatomy of the presacral space: a fresh tissue cadaver dissection. Am J Obstet Gynecol 192(5):1501–1505

Food and Drug Administration (2008) FDA public health notification: serious complications associated with transvaginal placement of surgical mesh in repair of pelvic organ prolapse and stress urinary incontinence. http://www.fda.gov/MedicalDevices/Safety/AlertsandNotices/PublicHealthNotifications/ucm061976.htm. Accessed 6 Jun 2012

Gadonneix P, Campagna G, Villet R (2012) Pregnancy after laparoscopic sacral colpopexy: a case report. Int Urogynecol J 23(5):651–653

Hirata H, Matsuyama H, Yamakawa G et al (2004) Does surgical repair of pelvic prolapse improve patients' quality of life? Eur Urol 45(2):213–218

Jabs CF, Drutz HP (2001) The role of intraoperative cystoscopy in prolapse and incontinence surgery. Am J Obstet Gynecol 185(6):1368–1371

Jeon MJ, Jung HJ, Choi HJ et al (2008) Is hysterectomy or the use of graft necessary for the reconstructive surgery for uterine prolapse? Int Urogynecol J Pelvic Floor Dysfunct 19(3):351–355

Keys T, Campeau L, Badlani G (2012) Synthetic mesh in the surgical repair of pelvic organ prolapse: current status and future directions. Urology May 23 [Epub ahead of print] 80(2):237–243

Kovac SR, Cruikshank SH (1993) Successful pregnancies and vaginal deliveries after sacrospinous uterosacral fixation in five of nineteen patients. Am J Obstet Gynecol 168:1778–1783

Lowder JL, Park AJ, Ellison R et al (2008) The role of apical vaginal support in the appearance of anterior and posterior vaginal prolapse. Obstet Gynecol 111(1):152–157

Maher CM, Feiner B, Baessler K et al (2011) Surgical management of pelvic organ prolapse in women: the updated summary version cochrane review. Int Urogynecol J 22(11):1445–1457

Margulies RU, Rogers MA, Morgan DM (2010) Outcomes of transvaginal uterosacral ligament suspension: systematic review and metaanalysis. Am J Obstet Gynecol 202(2):124–134

Nosseir SB, Kim YH, Lind LR, Winkler HA (2010) Sacral osteomyelitis after robotically assisted laparoscopic sacral colpopexy. Obstet Gynecol 116(Suppl 2):513–515

Paraiso MF, Falcone T, Walters MD (1999) Laparoscopic surgery for enterocele, vaginal apex prolapse and rectocele. Int Urogynecol J Pelvic Floor Dysfunct 10(4):223–229

Progetto Menopausa Italia Study Group (2000) Risk factors for genital prolapse in non-hysterectomized women around menopause. results from a large cross-sectional study in menopausal clinics in Italy. Eur J Obstet Gynecol Reprod Biol 93(2):135–140

Silva WA, Pauls RN, Segal JL et al (2006) Uterosacral ligament vault suspension: five-year outcomes. Obstet Gynecol 108(2):255–263

Soderberg MW, Falconer C, Bystrom B et al (2004) Young women with genital prolapse have a low collagen concentration. Acta Obstet Gynecol Scand 83(12):1193–1198

Subak LL, Waetjen LE, van den Eeden S et al (2001) Cost of pelvic organ prolapse surgery in the United States. Obstet Gynecol 98:646–651

Swift S, Woodman P, O'Boyle A et al (2005) Pelvic organ support study (POSST): the distribution, clinical definition, and epidemiologic condition of pelvic organ support defects. Am J Obstet Gynecol 192(3):795–806

Whiteside JL, Weber AM, Meyn LA, Walters MD (2004) Risk factors for prolapse recurrence after vaginal repair. Am J Obstet Gynecol 191(5):1533–1538

Wieslander CK, Rahn DD, McIntire DD et al (2006) Vascular anatomy of the presacral space in unembalmed female cadavers. Am J Obstet Gynecol 195(6):1736–1741

Henrik Halvor Springborg
and Amanda Nickles Fader

Contents

H.H. Springborg, MD (✉)
Division of Minimally Invasive Gynecologic Surgery,
Aleris-Hamlet Hospital, Copenhagen, Denmark
e-mail: Henrik.springborg@aleris-hamlet.dk

A.N. Fader, MD
Division of Gynecologic Oncology,
Department of Gynecology and Obstetrics,
Greater Baltimore Medical Center/Johns Hopkins
Medical Institutions, Baltimore, MD, USA
e-mail: amandanfader@gmail.com

17.1 Introduction

Laparoscopic surgery has gained increasing acceptance as a preferred surgical modality for the performance of a variety of gynecologic procedures, due to its many advantages, including shorter hospital stay, less pain, more rapid postoperative recovery, and better cosmetic results compared with traditional laparotomy.

In an effort to reduce abdominal wall trauma and obtain better cosmetic results, reduction in port size and optic and instrument diameter has been employed. In most procedures however, morcellator and/or specimen extraction are required; therefore, a minimum one port of 10–20 mm is needed in most gynecologic procedures. Specimen extraction through the umbilicus leads to less pain than extraction via a lateral port (Cho et al. 2012), and the umbilicus is the thinnest part of the abdominal wall and is relatively avascular.

Special access devices and special optics and instruments have now made it possible to perform laparoendoscopic single-site (LESS) surgery through the umbilical incision alone. The total length of the umbilical incision required to perform LESS surgery is often the same as the incision needed to perform specimen extraction in traditional laparoscopy. In these cases, two or three ports are avoided by using the LESS technique.

This LESS technique is cosmetically preferable to the multiple incisions associated with conventional laparoscopy, since the only scar

O. Istre (ed.), *Minimally Invasive Gynecological Surgery*,
DOI 10.1007/978-3-662-44059-9_17, © Springer-Verlag Berlin Heidelberg 2015

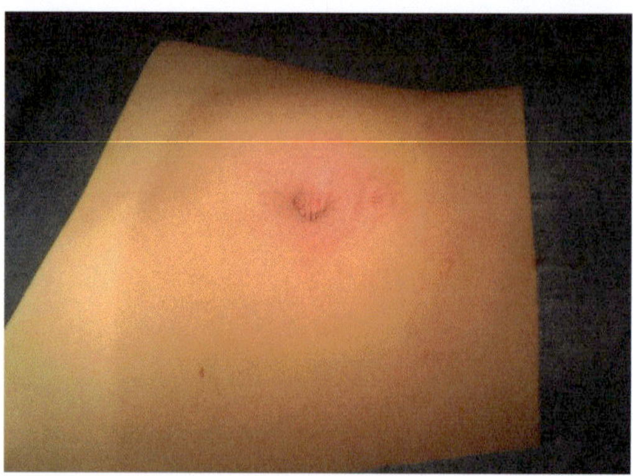

Fig. 17.1 Cosmetic result immediately after surgery

is concealed within the umbilicus (Fig. 17.1). Reports in the gynecology literature have demonstrated the feasibility and safety of the procedure, and if these findings are confirmed, LESS may, in accordance with "the spirit of minimally invasive gynecology," become an alternative standard of care in the treatment of several benign and oncologic gynecologic conditions. In this chapter, laparoendoscopic single-site surgery will be described in more detail. In Chap. 20, the safety of the procedure, learning curve, and future directions of LESS will be described.

17.2 Terminology

Various terminologies have been used to describe laparoscopic surgical procedures performed through a single incision or surgical site. In 2008, an international consortium of minimally invasive experts (the Laparoscopic Single-Site Surgery Consortium for Assessment and Research) met, with the goal of standardizing the terminology for academic communications and to avoid using industry and trade names. More than 10 terms to describe surgery through a single incision were identified (Table 17.1). The conclusion of this consortium was to utilize the term "LESS surgery" to describe all procedures performed in a minimally invasive manner through a single incision.

Table 17.1 Categorization for laparoendoscopic single site

Acronym	Full procedure name
LESS	Laparoendoscopic single-site surgery
Opus	One-port umbilical surgery
NOTES	Natural orifice transluminal endoscopic surgery
RSP	Robotic single-port surgery
SILS	Single-incision laparoscopic surgery
SIMIS	Single-incision minimally invasive surgery
SLIT	Single laparoscopic incision transabdominal surgery
SPA	Single-port access
SPL	Single-port laparoscopy
SPICES	Single-port incisionless conventional equipment-utilizing surgery
U-LESS	Umbilical laparoendoscopic single-site surgery

Universal term selected by the international consortium the Laparoendoscopic Single-Site Surgery Consortium for Assessment and Research—LESSCAR in 2008

17.3 History of LESS

Simple gynecological procedures have been performed via the LESS approach for more than four decades. Three thousand six hundred cases of laparoscopic sterilization using LESS technique were reported by Wheeless et al. as early as 1973. The first hysterectomy was reported in 1991, but not until 2008 was a subsequent series of LESS gynecologic procedures reported in the literature. Since then, the number of procedures performed and described has grown exponentially (Fader et al. 2010; Escobar et al. 2010a, b; Chen et al. 2011; Cho et al. 2012; Fanfani et al. 2010; Yim et al. 2010), and in the last 2 years, several randomized trials have been published (Chen et al. 2011; Cho et al. 2012; Fagotti et al. 2011; Li et al. 2012).

A similar trend has been seen in general surgery. The first series of LESS cholecystectomy was described in 1997 and appendectomy in 2007. In urology, the first small series of nephrectomies were described in 2007. Randomized trials have now been performed.

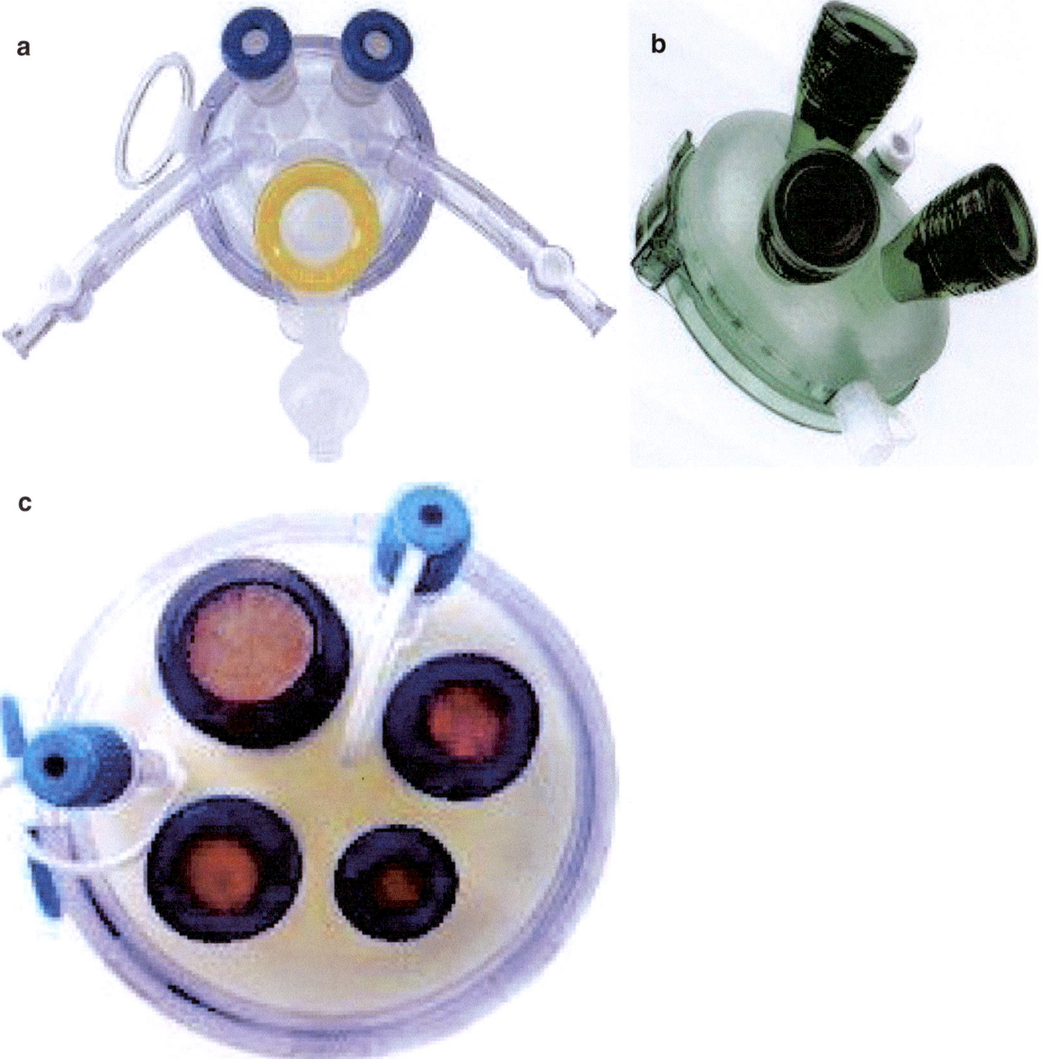

Fig. 17.2 (**a**) TriPort 15. (**b**) QuadPort. (**c**) GelPOINT

17.4 LESS Instruments and Technology

17.4.1 Access Devices

The development of access devices, allowing passage of three or more instruments through a single small incision, together with channels for CO_2 insufflation and smoke evacuation, has been the key to the fast development of this novel laparoscopic surgical modality.

Minimally invasive surgery requires an access device which allows passage of instruments and gas using the smallest possible incision. Devices using a retracting component consisting of an inner and outer ring with a thin plastic sleeve obtain this goal optimally since all space created by the incision can be used for instruments and specimen removal (TriPort 15, QuadPort, GelPOINT (Fig. 17.2)). In the newest devices, the valve system allows passage of the optic and instruments, comparable to standard trocars, and accommodates 5–15 mm instruments, including morcellator. Reusable devices on the market consist of a solid casing, enabling the optic and instruments to pass, which requires a relatively larger fascial incision.

17.4.2 Optics

LESS surgery can be performed with several types of optics. However, a small diameter scope (5 mm or smaller) reduces the abdominal trauma and enhances surgeon ergonomics by reducing the required length of the umbilical incision and limiting the extracorporeal instrument "sword fighting" that occurs with an "in-line" surgical approach. Conventional laparoscopes have a large extracorporeal profile with light cable perpendicular to the telescope, and this increases the risk of instrument clashing. This problem can be reduced with a 90° angle on the tip of the light cable. To further avoid instrument crowding and in-line visualization and increase the overview of the operative field, using a rotatable 30 or 45° laparoscope, preferably with a flexible tip, is critical. However, if accessible, a 5 mm, angled lower-profile camera system, with light cable in line with the shaft of the telescope, is also available (EndoEYE laparoscope (Olympus Germany/America) (Fig. 17.3).

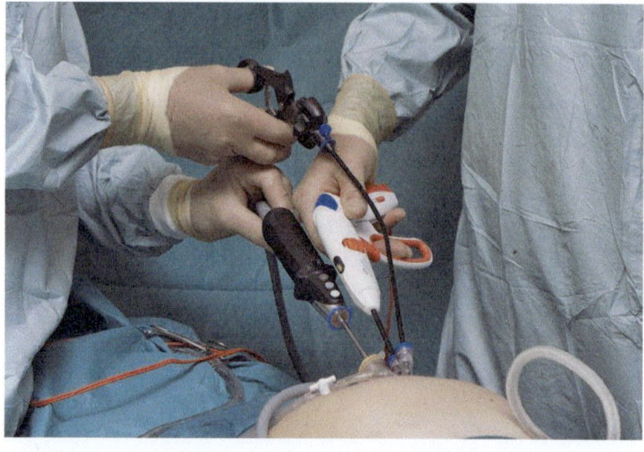

Fig. 17.3 EndoEYE 5 mm with light cable in line and cutting forceps in "gangsta" position

17.4.3 Active Instruments and Graspers

Special single-site instruments have been introduced, including curved and/or flexible instruments. These instruments, principally 5 mm, allow for intracorporeal triangulation, which provides the illusion of extracorporeal triangulation that is the tenet in traditional laparoscopy. Several single-site graspers are on the market, and in combination with an angled optic and a uterine manipulator, a traditional straight active instrument offers the best performance and is recommended in most cases.

17.5 Essentials in the Procedure of Laparoendoscopic Single-Site Surgery

Most single-port devices must be placed by an open access technique. The Hasson technique or a modification of this is recommended. The Hasson technique has been proven safe. After a 1.5–2.0 cm longitudinal transumbilical skin incision is made, the subcutaneous fat is opened, and the fascia elevated upward with two Kocher clamps. The fascia is incised between the clamps, and a blunt retractor is inserted through the peritoneum into the peritoneal cavity. The final placement of the port differs between the different devices. In order to avoid lesions of the bowel, an ultrasound over the umbilicus preoperatively during deep inspiration and expiration may be helpful in evaluating the presence of umbilical adhesions.

Instrument crowding and external instrument clashing may occur due to several instruments being passed through a single port. As mentioned above, unique single-port curved instruments are available, and utilization of a curved grasper and an angled optic, combined with a straight (or curved) active instrument, reduces this problem significantly and even makes triangulation possible. It is important to maintain the laparoscope and surgical instruments in different horizontal planes (Fig. 17.4),

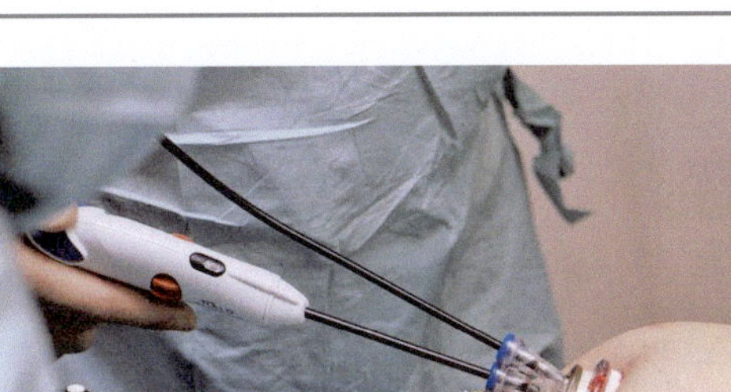

Fig. 17.4 Camera, cutting forceps, and grasper in three different planes during operation

with attention to keeping at least one of the instrument handles horizontal and parallel to the floor ("gangsta") to reduce the problem of instrument clashing further (Fig. 17.3). It is recommended to place the grasper in correct position and then consider whether the active instrument has to pass over or under the grasper, before it is introduced. In gynecology, one grasper is often sufficient due to the possibility of utilizing a high-quality uterine manipulator, which is highly recommended and provides additional adequate traction-countertraction during pelvic procedures.

Multifunctional instruments, which grasp, coagulate, and cut, reduce the number of instrument movements and exchanges and are especially helpful in LESS surgery.

Closure of the umbilical incision must be meticulous and is usually easy, because the minimum length of the incision, about 1.5 cm, makes visualization of the fascia possible in nearly all cases. Continuous or interrupted sutures can be used, and reattachment of the umbilical stalk has been recommended. It is our recommendation to consider closing with a 1-0 delayed absorbable suture in a running "mass closure" fashion. In order to avoid infection and development of granulation tissue in the umbilical scar, antibiotic prophylaxis is proposed, and a thorough skin closure, avoiding inversion of skin edges, is recommended.

Training in a dry lab or enrolling in a training course is highly recommended in order to become familiar with the LESS technology. To work with and observe an experienced LESS surgeon is also very helpful when beginning to perform LESS surgery.

17.6 Status of LESS in Gynecology

In the last few years, several prospective studies have described LESS in adnexal surgery for benign pathologies, including unilateral or bilateral salpingo-oophorectomy, adhesiolysis, and excision of endometriosis. These investigations suggest good results in terms of safety, cosmetics, and postoperative pain. Ovarian cystectomy is, however, technically challenging due to difficulty in achieving the optimal traction-countertraction required for this procedure. These difficulties might be solved by using an additional 2 mm miniport.

LESS in total laparoscopic hysterectomy (TLH), supracervical hysterectomy (LSH), and laparoscopic-assisted vaginal hysterectomy (LAVH) have been described and demonstrated safe and feasible. Case-control studies in LAVH have shown improved blood loss, hospital stay, and pain scores (all $p < 0.001$) in women who had LESS performed, compared to conventional multipuncture surgery. In total laparoscopic hysterectomy, suturing of the vaginal cuff can be a difficult and time-consuming task which may be eased by the use of a laparoscopic suturing device or a vaginal approach to close the cuff.

In gynecological oncology, a minimally invasive technique, resulting in the fastest possible recovery, is often essential in order to achieve more timely administration of adjuvant therapies. One center has published several reports demonstrating feasibility, safety, and reproducibility of the LESS approach for treatment of select early-stage endometrial or ovarian cancers and pelvic masses and for risk-reducing salpingo-oophorectomy (Fader and Escobar 2009; Fader et al. 2010).

More complicated procedures in gynecological oncology have been performed. Pelvic and para-aortic lymphadenectomy have been demonstrated safe and feasible with comparable nodal counts to open or conventional laparoscopic surgery (Escobar et al. 2010a, b). In patients with truncal adiposity, reduced access to the left para-aortic nodal region has been experienced. One possible solution to this limitation is to position the patient in a lateral position with the left flank elevated in order to facilitate exposure of the left para-aortic lymph nodes, a technique used in urology when performing laparoscopic nephrectomy.

Learning curve and complications associated with LESS will be described in Chap. 20.

17.7   Indications for LESS

LESS generally improves the cosmetic benefits of minimally invasive surgery by providing only one incision and a relatively hidden umbilical scar. Further research will likely confirm the initial studies, reporting low complication rates, fast recovery times, less pain, and high patient satisfaction. Most studies have, however, been performed by experts in laparoscopic surgery. The routine application of LESS in gynecology not only requires evaluation of safety but also of cost-effectiveness since the use of single-use devices is high.

Conclusion

Minimally invasive surgery has become a standard of care for the treatment of many benign and malignant gynecological conditions. LESS represents the newest frontier in minimally invasive surgery. Comparative data and prospective trials are required in order to determine the clinical utility and impact of LESS in treatment of gynecological conditions. Future directions are associated with laparoendoscopic single-site surgery, including minimization of ports and instruments and the possibility of merging this technology with da Vinci robotic systems.

References

Chen YJ, Wang PH, Ocampo EJ, Twu NF, Yen MS, Chao KC (2011) Single-port compared with conventional laparoscopic-assisted vaginal hysterectomy: a randomized controlled trial. Obstet Gynecol 117:906–912

Cho YJ, Kim ML, Lee SY, Lee HS, Kim JM, Joo KY (2012) Laparoendoscopic single-site surgery (LESS) versus conventional laparoscopic surgery for adnexal preservation: a randomized controlled study. Int J Womens Health 4:85–91

Chou LY, Sheu BC, Chang DY, Huang SC, Chen SY, Hsu WC, Chang WC (2010) Comparison between transumbilical and transabdominal ports for the laparoscopic retrieval of benign adnexal masses: a randomized trial. Eur J Obstet Gynecol Reprod Biol 153(2):198–202

Escobar PF, Bedaiwy MA, Fader AN, Falcone T (2010a) Laparoendoscopic surgery in patients with benign adnexal disease. Fertil Steril 93:2074

Escobar PF, Fader AN, Rasool N, Espaliliat LR (2010b) Single-port laparoscopic pelvic and para-aortic lymph node sampling or lymphadenectomy. Int J Gynecol Cancer 20:1268–1273

Fader AN, Escobar PF (2009) Laparoendoscopic single-site surgery in gynecologic oncology: technique and initial report. Gynecol Oncol 16:589–591

Fader AN, Rojas-Espaillat L, Ibeanu O, Grumbine FC, Escobar PF (2010) Laparoendoscopic single-site surgery (LESS) in gynecology: a multi-institutional evaluation. Am J Obstet Gynecol 203:501

Fagotti A, Bottoni C, Vizzielli G, Alletti SG, Scambia G, Marana E, Fanfani F (2011) Postoperative pain after conventional laparoscopy and laparoendoscopic single site surgery (LESS) for benign adnexal disease: a randomized trial. Fertil Steril 96:255–259

Fanfani F, Fagotti A, Scambia G (2010) Laparoendoscopic single-site surgery for total hysterectomy. Int J Gynecol Obstet 109:76–77

Gill IS, Advincula AP, Aron M, Caddedu J, Canes D, Curcillo PG 2nd et al (2010) Consensus statement of the consortium for laparoendoscopic single-site surgery. Surg Endosc 24:762–768

Li M, Han Y, Feng YC (2012) Single-port laparoscopic hysterectomy versus conventional laparoscopic hysterectomy: a prospective randomized trial. J Int Med Res 40:701–708

Wheeles CR, Thompson BH (1973) Laparoscopic sterilization. Review of 3600 cases. Obstet Gynecol 42:751–758

Yim GW, Jung YW, Paek J, Lee SH, Kwon HY, Nam EJ et al (2010) Transumbilical single-port access versus conventional total laparoscopic hysterectomy: surgical outcomes. Am J Obstet Gynecol 203:26

Learning Curve and Perioperative Outcomes Associated with Laparoendoscopic Single-Site Surgery

Camille Catherine Gunderson
and Amanda Nickles Fader

Contents

C.C. Gunderson, MD (✉)
Department of Gynecology and Obstetrics,
Johns Hopkins Medical Institutions,
Baltimore, MD, USA

325 NE 4th Street #1,
Oklahoma City, OK 73104, USA
e-mail: ccgunder@gmail.com

A.N. Fader, MD
Department of Gynecology and Obstetrics,
Johns Hopkins Medical Institutions,
Baltimore, MD, USA

Department of Gynecology and Obstetrics,
Division of Gynecologic Oncology, Greater
Baltimore Medical Center/Johns Hopkins Medical
Institutions, Baltimore, MD, USA
e-mail: amandanfader@gmail.com

18.1 Introduction

Single-port laparoscopic surgery is a novel minimally invasive technique that is being increasingly utilized in gynecologic surgery. Although numerous terms are associated with this technique, it was recently determined that the most accurate and scientific terminology is laparoendoscopic single-site surgery (LESS) (Gill et al. 2010). This approach involves performing a surgical procedure through a single, small umbilical incision (1.5–2.5 cm) employing specialized multichannel, single-port technology. Published reports in the general surgery, urologic, and gynecologic literature demonstrate safe and reproducible results with LESS utilized for a variety of procedures including cholecystectomy, nephrectomy, splenectomy, hysterectomy, and adnexal surgery, among others (Fader et al. 2010; Desai et al. 2009; White et al. 2009; Froghi et al. 2010; Fumagalli et al. 2010). Initial reports in the gynecologic literature have demonstrated the feasibility of LESS for the performance of a variety of benign and oncologic procedures with excellent clinical outcomes and overall low rates of major perioperative morbidity, ranging from 1 to 3 % (Fader et al. 2010; Lee et al. 2010; Kim et al. 2009; Fader and Escobar 2009; Escobar et al. 2009; Escobar et al. 2010; Cho et al. 2007; Kalogiannidis et al. 2007).

O. Istre (ed.), *Minimally Invasive Gynecological Surgery*,
DOI 10.1007/978-3-662-44059-9_18, © Springer-Verlag Berlin Heidelberg 2015

18.1.1 Pain Associated with LESS

For abdominal or pelvic procedures, LESS is performed exclusively through the base of the umbilicus. Thus, in theory, the single incision should yield less pain than conventional laparoscopy as it utilizes the privileged location of the umbilicus: the relatively avascular, thinnest portion of the anterior abdominal wall. Prior studies have demonstrated that in conventional laparoscopy, specimen extraction through an umbilical port leads to less postoperative pain than extraction via a lateral port (Chou et al. 2010). There is a paucity of high-quality data evaluating postoperative pain associated with LESS as it is a relatively new technique. In one of the larger series of women undergoing gynecologic single-port laparoscopic surgery, 38 % did not require narcotic use as an outpatient (Fader et al. 2010). Retrospective data has demonstrated decreased pain with single-port laparoscopic hysterectomy as compared to conventional total laparoscopic hysterectomy (TLH) (Yim et al. 2010; Kim et al. 2010). Furthermore, a recent randomized controlled trial reported decreased pain scores on a visual analog scale and lesser analgesia requirements with single-port laparoscopic-assisted vaginal hysterectomy (LAVH) as compared to conventional LAVH (Chen et al. 2011). Fagotti et al. also demonstrated decreased immediate postoperative pain and less postoperative analgesia requirements in another randomized prospective study including women undergoing surgery for benign adnexal disease (Fagotti et al. 2011). However, other prospective studies have not found a difference in postoperative pain scores and analgesia requirements with LESS (Jung et al. 2011; Li et al. 2012). At this time, the available data suggest similar or better pain profiles with LESS as compared to conventional laparoscopy for gynecologic procedures (Table 18.1).

18.1.2 Infection Associated with LESS

The incidence of incisional cellulitis or wound infection with LESS appears to be at least comparable to that of conventional laparoscopy. In a large multi-institutional series of women undergoing LESS for a gynecologic procedure, 5.2 % of women developed umbilical cellulitis. None of these patients required readmission or an additional procedure to manage this minor complication, and obesity was found to be significantly associated with umbilical morbidity (Gunderson et al. 2012). However, some reports have actually concluded lower rates of infection with LESS. In a prospective randomized trial of 108 women undergoing hysterectomy via LESS or conventional total laparoscopic hysterectomy (TLH), Li et al. reported a 1.9 % infection rate with LESS versus 8.9 % with TLH ($p = 0.03$) (Li et al. 2012).

Concern rightfully exists regarding the occult bacteria that the umbilicus may harbor, even after a sterilizing prep is applied. The American College of Obstetricians and Gynecologists does not routinely recommend antibiotic prophylaxis for adnexal surgery without hysterectomy (ACOG 2009). However, we propose consideration of antibiotic use with any LESS procedure in concordance with the individual's umbilical anatomy, planned procedure, and underlying comorbidities.

18.1.3 Hernia Associated with LESS

Given the larger size of the umbilical incision required for LESS as compared to conventional laparoscopy, there is a theoretically increased risk of umbilical hernia formation. Furthermore, it is well understood that the incidence of hernia formation correlates with incision size, complexity and length of procedure, and underlying comorbidities (Kadar et al. 1993; Boike et al. 1995). However, the available data encompassing LESS in gynecology actually suggests a comparable rate of hernia formation to that of conventional laparoscopy. In a series of 211 women undergoing LESS for a variety of gynecologic procedures, Gunderson et al. noted a 2.4 % incidence of umbilical hernia formation when utilizing a 1.5–2.5 cm umbilical incision (Gunderson et al. 2012). It should be noted that the authors of

Table 18.1 Comparison of outcomes with LESS in gynecology (as compared to conventional laparoscopy when applicable)

Study	Pain	Infection	Hernia	Convalescence	Complications
Chen et al.	*VAS:* 24 h postop: 3.6±2.8 vs. 5.1±2.8, *p=0.011* 48 h postop: 1.9±2.3 vs. 2.8±2.1, *p=0.043* *Analgesia usage:* Total meperidine dosage (mg): 74.4±24.3 vs. 104.8±57.1, *p=0.001* Total NSAID dosage (mg): 16.0±13.4 vs. 33.6±28.7, *p<0.001*	NR	NR	NR	2 % (vs. 4 %) *p>0.999*
Cho et al. (2012)	*VAS:* After 24 h: 3.3±1.9 vs. 3.5±2.0, *p=*NS After 48 h: 2.3±1.4 vs. 2.2±1.6, *p=*NS *Analgesia usage:* Intramuscular use within 24 h: 0.4±0.7 vs. 0.3±0.5, *p=*NS Oral use after discharge: 1.3±1.8 vs. 0.9±1.5, *p=*NS	NR	NR	Return to work (days): 7.4±3.8 vs. 6.4±3.5, *p=*NS	
Fader et al. (2010)	38 % did not require outpatient narcotic usage	1.4 %	NR	NR	4 %
Fagotti et al.	*VAS:* 2 h postop: *p=0.02* 4 h postop: *p=0.004* Upon discharge: *p=*NS *Analgesia usage:* 8 vs. 21 of paracetamol, *p=0.001*	NR	NR	NR	3 % vs. 0 %, *p=0.5*
Gunderson et al.	NR	5.2 %	2.4 %	NR	2.4 %
Kim et al. (2010)	*VAS:* After 24 h: 2.5±0.7 vs. 3.5±0.8, *p=0.01* After 36 h: 1.7±1.2 vs. 2.9±1.1, *p=0.01*	0 % vs. 0 %	NR	NR	0 % vs. 0 %
Lee et al.	*Request for additional analgesic medications:* 7 patients vs. 19 patients, *p=0.597*	0 % vs. 0 %	NR	NR	0 % vs. 0 %
Li et al.	*Patients requiring postop analgesics: 7.7 % vs. 10.7 %, p=*NS	1.9 % vs. 8.9 %, *p=0.03*	0 % vs. 0 %	Duration of immobilization (h): 14.6±2.1 vs. 15.7±2.3, *p=0.01*	0 % vs. 0 %

NR not recorded, *LESS* laparoendoscopic single-site surgery, *VAS* visual analog scores, *NSAID* nonsteroidal anti-inflammatory drugs, *NS* not significant this study used a meticulous incisional closure technique to reapproximate the fascia in a "mass closure" fashion and reattach the fascia to the umbilical stalk. Prospective studies are warranted to further validate these findings.

18.1.4 Cosmesis Associated with LESS

Advocates of the LESS approach deem that the single umbilical incision is cosmetically preferable to the multiple smaller incisions associated with conventional laparoscopy. The single central incision is relatively "scarless" as it may be easily concealed within the umbilicus. Several years ago, it was proposed that this predilection was purely surgeon speculation and was not based on objective information regarding actual patient preferences (Ramirez 2009). However, data have subsequently emerged which dispute this claim. Park et al. surveyed patients undergoing urologic surgery and found that they favored the cosmetic outcomes of LESS as compared to conventional laparoscopy or laparotomy (Park et al. 2011). This validation has also been recognized within the gynecologic surgery literature. Higher patient satisfaction scores were reported with LESS hysterectomy as compared to TLH (Li et al. 2012). Additionally, a recent randomized controlled trial noted a statistically significant higher rate of satisfaction by both the patient and the surgeon with the cosmetic result of LESS for benign adnexal surgery as compared to conventional laparoscopy. The improved satisfaction scores were noted both upon discharge from the hospital and 30 days postoperatively (Fagotti et al. 2011).

18.1.5 Convalescence Associated with LESS

The single incision and seemingly decreased pain associated with LESS may yield quicker convalescence. Yim et al. retrospectively reported earlier diet intake ($p < 0.001$) and shorter hospital stay ($p = 0.001$) with LESS hysterectomy as compared to TLH (Yim et al. 2010). However, other studies have demonstrated no difference in length of postoperative hospital stay (Li et al. 2012; Fagotti et al. 2011). With the current available data, it seems that convalescence after LESS is at least as rapid as that of conventional laparoscopy.

18.1.6 Learning Curve Associated with LESS

There is an undeniable learning curve associated with any new surgical technique. LESS imposes unique challenges as it precludes the triangulation which a surgical team utilizes with conventional multiport laparoscopy. Instrument collision ("sword fighting") and difficulty with overcoming in-line visualization are perhaps two of the greatest challenges. The use of flexible tip laparoscopes and articulating instruments can assist in restoring the typical intracorporeal triangulation to maximize exposure and allow for countertraction.

Efficiency has become a topic of interest as technology has allowed minimally invasive approaches to become more widely embraced. This is paramount considering the risk and cost incurred while under general anesthesia. Several retrospective studies in the gynecology literature have noted similar operative times for LESS as compared to conventional laparoscopy. Bedaiwy et al. studied a group of 78 women and reported a 1 min difference in operative time with LESS versus conventional laparoscopy for adnexectomy ($p = 0.08$) (Bedaiwy et al. 2012). Furthermore, Yim et al. reported 117 min for LESS hysterectomy versus 110 min with TLH ($p = 0.924$) (Yim et al. 2010). A randomized controlled trial by Cho et al. further supports similar operative times with LESS and conventional laparoscopy (Cho et al. 2012).

Fader et al. reported the first learning curve analysis for LESS hysterectomy and bilateral salpingo-oophorectomy (BSO). Therein, the authors described a dramatic reduction in operative time between the tenth and twentieth cases (Figs. 18.1 and 18.2). The results did achieve statistical significance, both with time for entry and port insertion ($p < 0.001$) and for total operative time ($p = 0.002$). This trend applied to both cancer staging and benign procedures. The decrease in operative time stabilized after 20 cases were

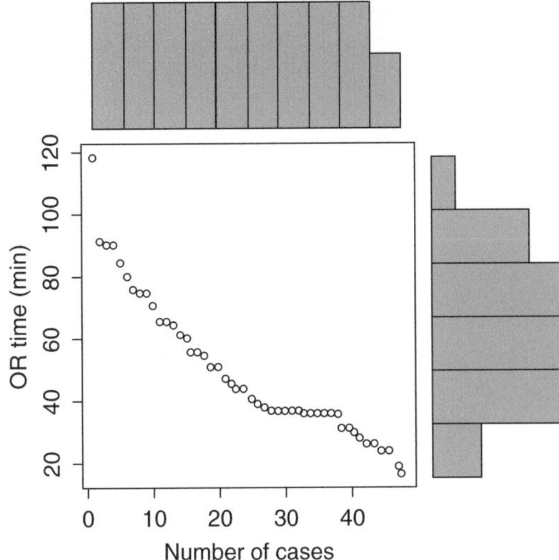

Fig. 18.1 Learning curve of LESS with benign procedures

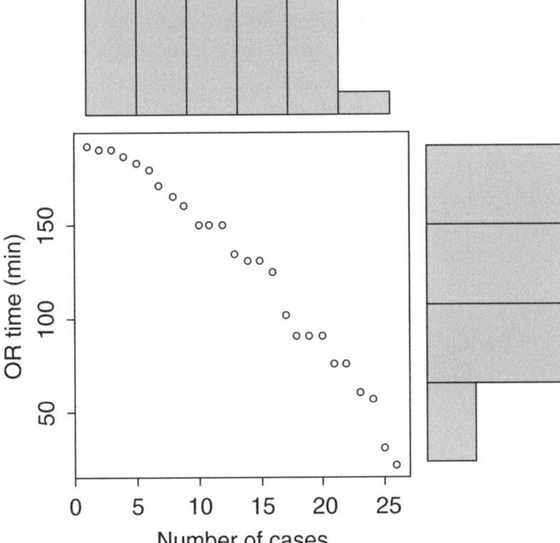

Fig. 18.2 Learning curve of LESS with cancer staging procedures

performed by a uniform team; these results suggest performance of a minimum of 20 cases for proficiency (Fader et al. 2010).

18.1.7 Future Directions Associated with Laparoendoscopic Single-Site Surgery

As we continue to embrace new minimally invasive approaches, it is crucial to ensure safety and efficacy in order to minimize morbidity. As with the introduction of any new technique, the initial data is largely retrospective and involves relatively small cohorts of subjects. Well-designed larger and randomized trials are required to validate the results of the early studies and to effectively compare LESS to other minimally invasive surgical approaches.

Another exciting innovation will be the merger of LESS is with the da Vinci robotic system (Intuitive Surgical, Sunnyvale, CA, USA). Escobar and Fader et al. reported the first successful robotic-assisted LESS hysterectomy/BSO in 2009; this was performed as a risk-reducing procedure in a woman with a *BRCA* mutation. The procedure was performed with the da Vinci S robot utilizing a GelPort (Applied Medical, Rancho Santo Margarita, CA) through which a 30°, 12-mm robotic laparoscope was inserted, along with two standard 8 mm robotic trocars (Escobar et al. 2009). Since then, Escobar et al. have described a cadaveric model to apply robotic-assisted LESS to perform several gynecologic oncology procedures (Escobar et al. 2011). The da Vinci single-port surgery adaptation is currently undergoing investigation and FDA approval, and its emergence on the market is eagerly anticipated.

Conclusion

Although once developed as an extension of conventional laparoscopy, LESS has now established itself as an independent surgical approach with its own unique benefits and indications. The goals in employing LESS technology are to minimize postoperative pain and complications, decrease convalescence time, and optimize cosmetic results. Although initial studies in the gynecologic and nongynecologic surgical literature have demonstrated the feasibility, safety, and reproducibility of this approach, these results must be validated. Additionally, further questions remain to be answered including the long-term risks and benefits as well as the cost-effectiveness of LESS. In the process of collecting data to address these crucial uncertainties, more information can be gathered regarding the learning curve and optimal setting for the application of LESS.

References

ACOG Committee on Practice Bulletins (2009) Antibiotic prophylaxis for gynecologic procedures. ACOG Practice Bulletin

Bedaiwy MA, Starks D, Hurd W, Escobar PF (2012) Laparoendoscopic single-site surgery in patients with benign adnexal disease: a comparative study. Gynecol Obstet Invest 73:294–298

Boike GM, Miller CE, Spirtos NM et al (1995) Incisional bowel herniations after operative laparoscopy: a series of nineteen cases and review of the literature. Am J Obstet Gynecol 172:1726–1731

Chen YJ, Wang PH, Ocampo EJ, Twu NF, Yen MS, Chao KC (2011) Single-port compared with conventional laparoscopic-assisted vaginal hysterectomy: a randomized controlled trial. Obstet Gynecol 117:906–912

Cho YH, Kim DY, Kim JH, Kim YM, Kim YT, Nam JH et al (2007) Laparoscopic management of early uterine cancer: 10-year experience in Asian Medical Center. Gynecol Oncol 106:585–590

Cho YJ, Kim ML, Lee SY, Lee HS, Kim JM, Joo KY (2012) Laparoendoscopic single-site surgery (LESS) versus conventional laparoscopic surgery for adnexal preservation: a randomized controlled study. Int J Women's Health 4:85–91

Chou LY et al (2010) Comparison between transumbilical and transabdominal ports for the laparoscopic retrieval of benign adnexal masses: a randomized trial. Eur J Obstet Gynecol Reprod Biol 153(2):198–202

Desai MM, Berger AK, Brandina R, Aron M, Irwin BH, Canes D et al (2009) Laparoendoscopic single-site surgery: initial hundred patients. Urology 74:805–812

Escobar PF, Fader AN, Paraiso MF, Kaouk JH, Falcone T (2009) Robotic-assisted laparoendoscopic single-site surgery in gynecology: initial report and technique. J Minim Invasive Gynecol 16:589–591

Escobar PF, Bedaiwy MA, Fader AN, Falcone T (2010) Laparoendoscopic surgery in patients with benign adnexal disease. Fertil Steril 93:2074

Escobar PF, Kebria M, Falcone T (2011) Evaluation of a novel single-port robotic platform in the cadaver model for the performance of various procedures in gynecologic oncology. Gynecol Oncol 120:380–384

Fader AN, Escobar PF (2009) Laparoendoscopic single-site surgery in gynecologic oncology: technique and initial report. Gynecol Oncol 16:589–591

Fader AN, Rojas-Espaillat L, Ibeanu O, Grumbine FC, Escobar PF (2010) Laparoendoscopic single-site surgery (LESS) in gynecology: a multi-institutional evaluation. Am J Obstet Gynecol 203:501

Fagotti A, Bottoni C, Vizzielli G, Alletti SG, Scambia G, Marana E, Fanfani F (2011) Postoperative pain after conventional laparoscopy and laparoendoscopic single site surgery (LESS) for benign adnexal disease: a randomized trial. Fertil Steril 96:255–259

Froghi F, Sodergren MH, Darzi A, Paraskeva P (2010) Single-incision Laparoscopic Surgery (SILS) in general surgery: a review of current practice. Surg Laparosc Endosc Percutan Tech 20:191–204

Fumagalli U, Verrusio C, Elmore U, Massaron S, Rosati R (2010) Preliminary results of transumbilical single-port laparoscopic cholecystectomy. Updates Surg 62:105–109

Gill IS, Advincula AP, Aron M, Caddedu J, Canes D, Curcillo PG 2nd et al (2010) Consensus statement of the consortium for laparoendoscopic single-site surgery. Surg Endosc 24:762–768

Gunderson CC, Knight J, Ybanez-Morano J, Ritter C, Escobar PF, Ibeanu O et al (2012) The risk of umbilical hernia and other complications with laparoendoscopic single-site surgery. J Minim Invasive Gynecol 19(1):40–45

Jung YW et al (2011) A randomized prospective study of single-port and four-port approaches for hysterectomy in terms of postoperative pain. Surg Endosc 25(8)2462–9.

Kadar N, Reich H, Liu CY, Manko GF, Gimpelson R (1993) Incisional hernias after major laparoscopic gynecologic procedures. Am J Obstet Gynecol 168:1493–1495

Kalogiannidis I, Lambrechts S, Amant F, Neven P, Van Gorp T, Vergote I (2007) Laparoscopy-assisted vaginal hysterectomy compared with abdominal hysterectomy in clinical stage I endometrial cancer: safety, recurrence, and long-term outcome. Am J Obstet Gynecol 196:248

Kim TJ, Lee YY, Kim MJ, Kim CJ, Kang H, Choi CH et al (2009) Single port access laparoscopic adnexal surgery. J Minim Invasive Gynecol 16:612–615

Kim TJ, Lee YY, Cha HH, Kim CJ, Choi CH, Lee JW, Bae DS, Lee JH, Kim BG (2010) Single-port-access laparoscopic-assisted vaginal hysterectomy versus conventional laparoscopic-assisted vaginal hysterectomy: a comparison of perioperative outcomes. Surg Endosc 24:2248–2252

Lee YY, Kim TJ, Kim CJ, Park HS, Choi CH, Lee JW et al (2010) Single port access laparoscopic adnexal surgery versus conventional laparoscopic adnexal urgery: a comparison of peri-operative outcomes. Eur J Obstet Gynecol Reprod Biol 151:181–184

Li M, Han Y, Feng YC (2012) Single-port laparoscopic hysterectomy versus conventional laparoscopic hysterectomy: a prospective randomized trial. J Int Med Res 40:701–708

Park SK, Olweny EO, Best SL, Tracy CR, Mir SA, Cadeddu JA (2011) Patient-reported body image and cosmesis outcomes following kidney surgery: comparison of laparoendoscopic single-site, laparoscopic, and open surgery. Eur Urol 60:1097–1104

Ramirez PT (2009) Single-port laparoscopic surgery: is a single incision the next frontier in minimally invasive gynecologic surgery? Gynecol Oncol 114:143–144

White WM, Haber GP, Goel RK, Crouzet S, Stein RJ, Kaouk JH (2009) Single-port urological surgery: single-center experience with the first 100 cases. Urology 74:801–804

Yim GW, Jung YW, Paek J, Lee SH, Kwon HY, Nam EJ et al (2010) Transumbilical single-port access versus conventional total laparoscopic hysterectomy: surgical outcomes. Am J Obstet Gynecol 203:26

Per Lundorff

Contents

19.1   Epidemiology

The SCAR study (Surgical and Clinical Adhesion Research Study) from 1999 was the first study to verify the extent of problems after open surgery in terms of adhesions. This Scottish database showed that about one-third of almost 30,000 patients who underwent open surgery were readmitted a mean of 2.1 times for complications related to adhesions over a 10-year period. Of all readmissions, 22 % occurred within the first year, but the readmissions continued over the next 10 years of the study period. So adhesions are a consequence of an iatrogenic disease (Ellis et al. 1999).

The SCAR-2 study revealed the overall extent of adhesion-related readmissions following open and laparoscopic gynecological procedures. In this study, it was shown that certain surgical sites are associated with increased risk of adhesions. Also, that adhesion formation results in a large number of readmissions following both open surgery as well as laparoscopy and that risk for adhesion formation and related complications can be seen many years after the surgical procedure (Hawthorn et al. 2003).

19.2   Clinical Aspects

Adhesions develop as a response to a trauma to the peritoneum. This trauma can be induced either after inflammation or after surgery.

P. Lundorff
Private Hospital Mølholm, DK-7100, Vejle, Denmark
e-mail: d191167@dadlnet.dk

O. Istre (ed.), *Minimally Invasive Gynecological Surgery*,
DOI 10.1007/978-3-662-44059-9_19, © Springer-Verlag Berlin Heidelberg 2015

Concomitant factors to increase risk of developing adhesions are inflammation, abrasion, desiccation, ischemia, heat, light, electrocautery, and suturing. Furthermore, bleeding and leaking of plasma proteins can lead to fibrin deposits and concomitant adhesion formation.

Adhesions can have serious consequences as bowel obstruction (Menzies 1993), chronic pelvic pain (Duffy and diZerega 1996), and fertility-related adhesions (Hershlag et al. 1991). It has been shown that the vast majority of small bowel obstructions are related to adhesions, 40 % of patients with chronic pelvic pain are related to adhesions, and 15–20 % of women with secondary infertility are adhesion related (Menzies et al. 2001). Adhesions make reoperation more difficult and may increase complication rate (Coleman et al. 2000). Operating time may be prolonged and risk of bowel or bladder injury may increase. Each additional laparotomy induces de novo adhesion and thereby increases the risk of enterostomy at future surgery.

Some operative procedures are related with greater risk of adhesion developing and consequently reoperation.

In ovarian surgery, 75 of 100 procedures will be readmitted during the first year (Lower et al. 2000), and in myomectomy, 41 of 100 procedures will be readmitted during the first year (Dubuisson et al. 1998).

19.3 Economy

Readmissions due to adhesion-related complications have a major impact on healthcare, and in UK, bed stay for these women represents 2 % of the total bed occupancy per year (Mentiez et al. 2001). The costs of all UK hospital readmissions involved treatment with adhesiolysis are estimated at about 24 million pounds 1 year after surgery and about 95 million pounds 10 years after surgery (Wilson et al. 2002).

To reduce these costs, surgeons should focus upon the surgical procedures with optimizing the techniques and further apply adhesion-preventing adjuvants available for the management and prevention of adhesions.

19.4 Adhesion Prevention

19.4.1 Surgical Techniques

A number of adhesion prevention strategies and techniques were reviewed in 1997 by Risberg, and among these, two strategies were identified (1) good surgical technique and (2) use of antiadhesive adjuvants.

As to good surgical techniques, several factors have been highlighted to illustrate the relationship between adhesion formation and surgery.

First of all, laparoscopy rather than laparotomy is associated with less postoperative adhesions (Mais et al. 1996). In a randomized trial by Lundorff et al. (1991), surgery for ectopic pregnancy by laparotomy showed a significant larger proportions of postoperative adhesions compared with laparoscopy revealed at second-look surgery few months later.

Careful surgical techniques can minimize factors that increase risk for adhesion formation. Well-known factors are ischemia, infection, or serosal trauma associated with increased adhesion formation due to decreased fibrinolytic activity during the postoperative 3–5 days. These factors include traction of the peritoneum, drying of the serosal surface, excessive use of suturing material, or retention of blood clots. The result is increased fibroblast activity with formation of adhesions (Ellis 1971).

Molinas et al. have demonstrated that the use of carbon dioxide (CO_2) during laparoscopic surgery can cause peritoneal hypoxia and thus induce respiratory acidosis leading to metabolic acidosis and metabolic hypoxia (Molinas et al. 2004).

High peritoneal temperature and the use of dry gases can be potential cofactors in adhesion formation, and hypothermia can reduce the toxic effects of hypoxia in mice.

Furthermore, the use of humidified gases has been demonstrated to minimize adhesion formation induced by desiccation. So the combination of controlled intraperitoneal cooling with a rigorous prevention of desiccation can be important for adhesion prevention (Binda et al. 2004); (Binda et al. 2006).

Other animal studies have demonstrated that the addition of 3 % oxygen to the CO_2

pneumoperitoneum further decreases adhesion formation (Elkelani et al. 2004).

Further improvement in adhesion prevention during surgery should always be based upon the use of good surgical techniques, using newly developed instruments, based on the basic principles of microsurgery, liberal irrigation of the abdominal cavity and may be installation of large amount of Ringer's lactate or saline at the end of the surgical procedure (Tulandi 1997).

19.4.2 Antiadhesive Adjuvants

A number of antiadhesive adjuvants are increasingly available, and especially in high-risk procedures, precautions should be taken.

Procedures at high risk for developing postoperative adhesions are as follows:

- Ovarian surgery
- Endometriosis surgery
- Tubal surgery
- Myomectomy
- Adhesiolysis

Several agents have been tested to decrease adhesion formation after surgery.

19.4.3 Anti-inflammatory Drugs

NSAIDs interferes the postsurgical inflammatory response by affecting the metabolism of arachidonic acid, prostaglandins, and thromboxane. Animal studies have shown that NSAIDs administered intraperitoneally are effective, yet not proven in clinical studies. In an animal model, the agents must be administered continuously for 2–3 days with a miniosmotic pump to be efficient (Gomel et al. 1996).

However, there is no significant evidence from any published study to recommend their use in humans (Wiseman 1994).

19.4.3.1 Corticosteroids

Immunosuppression and prolonged healing of wound are the backgrounds for using corticosteroids. Older studies show mixed results and are difficult to interpret, as it is often used parallel with antihistamine. Serious side effects minimize the use for the prevention of adhesions (Swolin 1967; Querleu et al. 1989).

As a conclusion, corticosteroids show poor efficacy, delayed wound healing, do not remain in the body during the process of wound healing (4–5 days).

19.4.4 Fibrinolytics

It has been hypothesized that an imbalance between fibrin-forming and fibrin-dissolving activities in the peritoneum is a major pathogenetic factor in adhesion formation in animals (diZerega and Campeau 2001).

Fibrinolytic agents act by reducing the fibrinous mass directly and indirectly by stimulating the plasminogen activator (PA) activity and thereby have been suggested to reduce adhesion formation (Hellebrekers et al. 2000).

Studies to reveal safety and side effects are still awaiting.

19.4.5 Anticoagulants

In animal studies, heparin has been widely used for the purpose of adhesion prevention. Nevertheless, no study has been able to demonstrate reduced adhesion formation when heparin was administered alone or in combination with other agents such as Interceed TC7 barrier (Jansen 1988; Reid et al. 1997).

Furthermore, compared to Ringer's lactate no significant reduction in adhesion formation was found (Fayez and Schneider 1987).

19.4.6 Barriers Adjuvants

19.4.6.1 Preclude and Seprafilm

Preclude Peritoneal membrane (Goretex) 0.1-mm thin membrane consisting of polytetrafluorethylene. The microporous structure inhibits the ingrowth of cells and thus convenient as a barrier method. It is not absorbed and gives no inflammatory response. Not easy to handle, should be sutures in place, and removed later. Studies show reduction of de novo adhesions as well as reformation of adhesions (Goldberg et al. 1987; The Surgical Membrane Study Group 1991).

19.4.6.2 Seprafilm II

Is a derivate of hyaluronic acid and carboxymethylcellulose. The membrane separates the injured surfaces during the first day of wound healing and is resorbed within 7 days. Promising results have been described (Diamond 1996; Becker et al. 1996).

19.4.6.3 Interceed

Interceed (Gynecare, Johnson & Johnson) is an oxidized regenerated cellulose woven into a special net. When the net has been applied to the peritoneal surface, it adheres without sutures and turns into a gel within few hours, thus serving as a barrier between two surfaces. It has been shown to reduce adhesion formation, both in animal studies and in human studies (Marana et al. 1997; Franklin 1995).

The efficacy of Interceed is reduced in an environment of blood and liquid and is only effective when a good hemostasis has been obtained.

Several clinical studies have demonstrated the positive effect of Interceed [Sekiba 1992; Nordic Adhesion Prevention Study Group 1995; Interceed (TC7) Adhesion Barrier Study Group II 1993; Adhesion (TC7) Barrier Study Group 1989].

19.4.6.4 Spray Gel (Confluent Surgical, Waltham, MA, USA)

Is a solid polymer, acting as an adhesion barrier. It consists of two synthetic liquid precursors that rapidly cross-link to form an absorbable, flexible hydrogel, when it is applied and mixed during laparoscopy. No reports so far have shown evidence that there is decreased adhesion formation using Spray Gel Specialist equipment and technique (Dunn et al. 2001; Mettler et al. 2004).

19.4.6.5 Oxiplex/AP Gel (FzioMed, San Louis Obispo, CA, USA)

Is a viscoelastic gel composed of polyethylene oxide and carboxymethyl cellulose stabilized with calcium chloride. Preclinical studies were encouraging (Berg et al. 2003).

In a randomized multicenter European trial, the results concluded that the viscoelastic gel significantly reduced adnexal adhesions in patients undergoing gynecologic laparoscopic surgery (Lundorff et al. 2005).

Furthermore, another prospective randomized trial evaluated efficacy of Oxiplex/QP gel and could conclude that the gel was easy to use, safe, and reduce adhesion scores (Young et al. 2005).

Recently approved as site-specific agent.

19.4.6.6 Crystalloids (LRS)

Rapidly reabsorbed, ineffective in reducing adhesions.

Crystalloids, including saline solution and Ringers acetate solution, have been widely used to minimize the risk of postoperative adhesion formation. Yet, no significant improvement can be shown in clinical studies (diZerega 1994; Gomel et al. 1996).

As peritoneal healing takes place within 5–7 days after surgery, crystalloids are absorbed long ago. The peritoneal surface absorbs 15–30 ml of crystalloids per hour, so even if you leave 1 l of crystalloids, it will be absorbed within 24 h.

19.4.6.7 Hyscon

Hyscon is a 32 % solution of Dextran 70. It creates an osmotic gradient in the peritoneal cavity, producing transient ascites. Adverse results, and serious side effects such as anaphylaxis, coagulopathy and vulvar edema have disqualified the agent (Adhesion Study Group 1983).

19.4.6.8 Icodextrin (Adept, Baxter, USA)

Is a glucose polymer of high molecular weight, rapidly metabolized to glucose but slowly absorbed by the peritoneal cavity. Because the 4 % Icodextrin solution has a longer resorption time from the peritoneal cavity (>4 days) compared to crystalloids, it will give the internal organs a longer hydroflotation time and thereby theoretical a better adhesion protection after surgery.

Animal studies have shown a decreased reformation of adhesions and decreased de novo adhesion formation postoperatively after irrigation with Icodextrin 4 % (Verco et al. 2000).

A randomized pilot study and later a clinical trial have confirmed these observations (diZerega et al. 2002; Brown et al. 2007).

Geneva study (Gynaecological ENdoscopic EValuation of Adept), a double-blind randomized study with 25 European centers enrolling patients to assess the safety and efficacy of Adept compared with lactated ringers solution when used as an intraoperative irrigation solution. Safety of Adept was confirmed, but overall there was no evidence of clinical effect (Trew et al. 2011).

19.4.7 Hyaloronic Acid

Hyaluronan (HA) is a naturally occurring component of the extracellular matrix and peritoneal fluid that has received much attention because of its possible application as an adhesion–prevention adjuvant in a variety of surgical procedures. Indeed, several authors in different experimental and clinical settings have proposed that deposition of HA around surgically treated tissues reduces postoperative adhesion formation (Chen and Abatangelo 1999). Moreover, native HA has a high degree of biocompatibility and a favorable safety profile (Laurent and Fraser 1992).

19.4.8 Hyalobarrier

A highly viscous gel of HA derivatives obtained through an autocross-linking process that does not introduce foreign bridge molecules, namely Hyalobarrier®, has recently been developed. The autocross-linked polymer is an inter and intramolecular ester of HA in which a proportion of the carboxyl groups are esterified with hydroxyl groups belonging to the same and/or different molecules of the polysaccharide, thus forming a mixture of lactones and intermolecular ester bonds. The level of cross-linking can be varied by modulating the reaction conditions. The absence of foreign bridge molecules ensures the release of native HA only during degradation, while the autocross-linking process improves the viscoelastic properties of the gel compared with unmodified HA solutions of the same molecular weight (Renier et al. 2005).

Preclinical trials in animal models have shown that Hyalobarrier® gel reduces the incidence and severity of postoperative adhesions (Belluco et al. 2001; Pucciarelli et al. 2003; Mais et al. 2006).

Moreover, preliminary clinical studies in hysteroscopic surgery as well as laparotomic and laparoscopic myomectomy have suggested that Hyalobarrier® gel may reduce the incidence and severity of postoperative adhesions in pelvic surgery (Pellicano et al. 2003; Guida et al. 2004) with improvement in the pregnancy rate in infertile patients who were submitted to laparoscopic myomectomy (Pellicano et al. 2005).

For a clinical point of view, recommendations for the use of antiadhesion agents can be summarized as:

Site-specific agent (Intercoat, Interceed, Hyalobarrier), to be used preferably in connection with:

- Ovarian surgery
- Tubal surgery
- Minor endometriotic lesions
- Myomectomy

Nonsite-specific agent (Adept), to be used preferably in connection with:

- Major endometriosis surgery
- Adhesiolysis
- Myomectomy

References

Adhesion (TC7) Barrier Study Group (1989) Prevention of postsurgical adhesions by Interceed (TC79, an absorbable adhesion barrier: a prospective, randomised multicenter clinical study. Fertil Steril 51:933–938

Adhesion Study Group (1983) Reduction of post operative pelvic adhesions with intraperitoneal 32 % dextran 70: a prospective randomized clinical study. Fertil Steril 40:612–619

Becker JM, Dayson MT, Fazio VW, Beck DE, Stryker SJ, Wexner SD, Wolff BG, Roberts PL, Smith

LE, Sweeney SA, Moore M (1996) Prevention of postoperative abdominal adhesions by sodium hyaluronate-based bioabsorbable membrane: a prospective randomized, double-blind multicenter study. J Am Coll Surg 183:297–306

Belluco C, Meggiolaro F, Pressato D, Pavesio A, Bigon E, Dona M, Forlin M, Nitti D, Lise M (2001) Prevention of postsurgical adhesions with an autocrosslinked hyaluronan derivative gel. J Surg Res 100:217–221

Berg RA, Rodgers KE, Cortese S et al (2003) Postsurgical adhesion reformation is inhibited by Oxiplex adhesion barrier gel. In: Marana R, Busacca M, Zupi E (eds) International proceedings. World meeting on Minimal invasive surgery in gynecology, Rome, pp 17–21

Binda MM, Molinas CR, Mailova K et al (2004) Effect of temperature upon adhesion formation in a laparoscopic mouse model. Hum Reprod 19:2626–2632

Binda MM, Molinas CR, Hansen P et al (2006) Effect of desiccation and temperature during laparoscopy on adhesion prevention in mice. Fertil Steril 86:166–175

Brown CB, Luciano AA, Martin D, Peers E, Scrimgeour A, diZerega GS (2007) Adept (icodextrin 4% solution) reduces adhesions after laparoscopic surgery for adhesiolysis: a double-blind, randomized, controlled study. Fertil Steril 5:1413–1426, Epub 26 Mar 2007

Chen WY, Abatangelo G (1999) Functions of hyaluronan in wound repair. Wound Repair Regen 7(2):79–89

Coleman MG, McLain AD, Moran BJ (2000) Impact of previous surgery on time taken for incision and division of adhesions during laparotomy. Dis Colon Rectum 43:1297–1299

Diamond MP, Seprafilm Adhesion Study Group (1996) Reduction of adhesions after uterine myomectomy by Seprafilm membrane (Hal-F), a blinded, prospective, randomized, multicenter clinical study. Fertil Steril 66(6):904–910

diZerega GS (1994) Contemporary adhesion prevention. Fertil Steril 64:219–235

diZerega GS, Campeau JD (2001) Peritoneal repair and postsurgical adhesion formation. Hum Reprod Update 7:547–555

diZerega GS, Verco SJ, Young P et al (2002) A randomized, controlled pilot study of the safety and efficacy of 4% icodextrin solution in the reduction of adhesions following laparoscopic gynaecological surgery. Hum Reprod 17:1031–1038

Dubuisson JB, Fauconnier A, Chapron C, Kreiker G, Norgaard C (1998) Second look after laparoscopic myomectomy. Hum Reprod 13:2102–2106

Duffy DM, diZerega GS (1996) Adhesion controversies: pelvic pain as a cause of adhesions, crystalloids in preventing them. J Reprod Med 41:19–26

Dunn R, Lyman MD, Edelman PG et al (2001) Evaluation of SprayGel adhesion barrier in the rat cecum abration and rabbit uterine horn adhesion models. Fertil Steril 75:411–416

Elkelani OA, Binda MM, Molinas CR et al (2004) Effect of adding more that 3% of oxygen to carbon dioxide pneumoperitoneum upon adhesion formation in a laparoscopic mouse model. Fertil Steril 82:1616–1622

Ellis H (1971) The cause and prevention of postoperative intraperitoneal adhesions. Surg Gynecol Obstet 133:497–511

Ellis H, Moran BJ, Thompson JN, Parker MC, Wilson MS, Menzies D et al (1999) Adhesion-related hospital readmissions after abdominal and pelvic surgery: a retrospective cohort study. Lancet 353:1476–1480

Fayez JA, Schneider PJ (1987) Prevention of pelvic adhesion formation by different modalities of treatment. Am J Obstet Gynecol 157:1184–1188

Franklin RR, Ovarian Adhesion Study Group (1995) Reduction of ovarian adhesions by the use of Interceed. Obstet Gynecol 86:335–340

Goldberg JM, Toledo AA, Mitchell PE (1987) An evaluation of the Goretex surgical membrane for the postoperative peritoneal adhesions. Obstet Gynecol 70:846–848

Gomel V, Urman B, Gurgan T (1996) Pathology of adhesion formation and strategies for prevention. J Reprod Med 41:35–41

Guida M, Acunzo G, Di Spiezio Sardo A, Bifulco G, Piccoli R, Pellicano M, Cerrota G, Cirillo D, Nappi C (2004) Effectiveness of auto-crosslinked hyaluronic acid gel in the prevention of intrauterine adhesions after hysteroscopic surgery: a prospective, randomized, controlled study. Hum Reprod 19:1461

Hawthorn RJS, Lower A, Clark D, Knight AD, Crowe AM (2003) Adhesion-related readmissions following gynaecological laparoscopy in Scotland, an epidemiological study of 24,046 patients. Rev Gynaecol Pract 3(1) Supplement:1

Hellebrekers BW, Trimbos-Kember TC, Trimbos JB et al (2000) Use of fibrinolytic agents in the prevention of post-operative adhesion formation. Fertil Steril 74:203–212

Hershlag A, Diamond MP, DeCherney AH (1991) Adhesiolysis. Clin Obstet Gynecol 34:395–402

Interceed (TC7) Adhesion Barrier Study Group II (1993) Pelvic sidewall adhesion reformation: microsurgery alone or with Interceed absorbable adhesion barrier. Surg Gynecol Obstet 177:135–139

Jansen RP (1988) Failure of peritoneal irrigation with heparin during pelvic operations upon young women to reduce adhesions. Surg Gynecol Obstet 166:154–160

Laurent TC, Fraser JR (1992) Hyaluronan. FASEB J 6:2397–2404

Lower AM, Hawthorn RJS, Ellis H, O'Brien F, Buchan S, Crowe AM (2000) The impact of adhesions on hospital readmissions over ten years after 8849 open gynaecological operations: an assessment from the Surgical and Clinical Adhesions Research Study. BJOG 107:855–862

Lundorff P, Hahlin M, Kallfelt B et al (1991) Adhesion formation after laparoscopic surgery in tubal pregnancy: a randomized trial versus laparotomy. Fertil Steril 55:911–915

Lundorff P, Donnez J, Korell M et al (2005) Clinical evaluation of a viscoelastic gel for reduction of adhesions following gynaecological surgery by laparoscopy in Europe. Hum Reprod 20:514–520

Mais V, Ajossa S, Mascia M et al (1996) Laparoscopy versus abdominal muomectomy: a prospective randomized trial to evaluate benefits on early outcome. Am J Obstet Gynecol 174:654–658

Mais V, Bracco GL, Litta P, Gargiulo T, Melis GB (2006) Reduction of postoperative adhesions with an auto-crosslinked hyaluronan gel in gynaecological laparoscopic surgery: a blinded, controlled, randomized, multicentre study. Hum Reprod 21(5): 1248–1254

Marana R, Catalano GF, Caruana P et al (1997) Postoperative adhesion formation and reproductive outcome using Interceed after ovarian surgery: a randomized trial in the rabbit model. Hum Reprod 12:1935–1938

Menzies D (1993) Postoperative adhesion: their treatment and relevance in clinical practive. Ann R Coll Surg Engl 75:147–153

Mentiez D, Parker M, Hoare R, Knight A (2001) Small bowel obstruction due to postoperative adhesions: treatment patterns and associated costs in 110 hospital admissions. Ann R Coll Surg Engl 83:40–46

Mettler L, Audeberg A, Lehmann-Willenbrock E et al (2004) A randomized, prospective, controlled, multicenter clinical trial of a sprayable, site-specific adhesion barrier system in patients undergoing myomectomy. Fertil Steril 82:398–404

Molinas CR, Tjwa M, Vanacker B et al (2004) Role of CO_2 pneumoperitoneum-induced acidosis in CO_2 pneumoperitoneum-enhanced adhesion formation in mice. Fertil Steril 81:708–711

Nordic Adhesion Prevention Study Group (1995) The efficacy of Interceed (TC7) for prevention of reformation of postoperative adhesions on ovarie, fallopian tubes and fimbriae in microsurgical operations for fertility: a multicenter study. Fertil Steril 63:709–714

Pellicano M, Bramante S, Cirillo D, Palomba S, Bifulco G, Zullo F, Nappi C (2003) Effectiveness of autocrosslinked hyaluronic acid gel after laparoscopic myomectomy in infertile patients: a prospective, randomized, controlled study. Fertil Steril 80:441–444

Pellicano M, Guida M, Bramante S, Acunzo G, Di Spiezio Sardo A, Tommaselli GA, Nappi C (2005) Reproductive outcome after autocrosslinked hyaluronic acid gel application in infertile patients who underwent laparoscopic myomectomy. Fertil Steril 83:498

Pucciarelli S, Codello L, Rosato A, Del Bianco P, Vecchiato G, Lise M (2003) Effect of antiadhesive agents on peritoneal carcinomatosis in an experimental model. Br J Surg 90:66

Querleu D, Vankeerberghen DF, Deffense F, Boutteville C (1989) The effect of noxytiolin and systemic corticosteroids in infertility surgery; a prospective randomised study. J Gynecol Obstet Biol Reprod 18:935–940

Reid RL, Hahn PM, Spence JE et al (1997) A randomized trial of oxidized regenerated cellulose adhesion barrier (Interceed TC7) alone or in combination with heparin. Fertil Steril 67:23–29

Renier D, Bellato P, Bellini D, Pavesio A, Pressato D, Borrione A (2005) Pharmacokinetic behaviour of ACP gel, an autocrosslinked hyaluronan derivative, after intraperitoneal administration. Biomaterials 26: 5368–5374

Risberg B (1997) Adhesions: preventive strategies. Eur J Surg Suppl 163:32–39

Sekiba K, The Obstetrics and Gynecology Adhesion Prevention Commiteé (1992) Use of Interceed (TC7) absorbable adhesion barrier to reduce post operative adhesion reformation in infertility and endometrioses surgery. Obstet Gynecol 79:518–522

Swolin K (1967) Die Einwirkung von Grossen Intraperitonealen Dosen Glucocorticoid auf die Bildung von Postoperative Adhaisionen. Acta Obstet Gynecol Scand 46:204–209

The Surgical Membrane Study Group (1991) Prophylaxis of pelvic sidewall adhesions with Gore-Tex surgical membrane; a multicenter clinical investigation. Fertil Steril 57:921–923

Trew J, Pistofides G, Pados G et al (2011) Gynaecological endoscopic evaluation of 4 % icodextrin solution: a European, multicentre, double-blind, randomized study of the efficacy and safety in the reduction of de novo adhesions after laparoscopic gynaecological surgery. Hum Reprod 26:2015–2027

Tulandi T (1997) How can we avoid adhesions after laparoscopic surgery? Curr Opin Obstet Gynecol 9:239–243

Verco SJ, Peers EM, Brown CB et al (2000) Development of a novel glucose polymer solution (Icodextrin) for adhesion prevention: preclinical studies. Hum Reprod 15:1764–1772

Wilson MS, Menzies D, Knight AD, Crowe AM (2002) Demonstrating the clinical and cost effectiveness of adhesion reduction strategies. Colorectal Dis 4:355–360

Wiseman DM (1994) Polymers for the prevention of surgical adhesions. In: Domb AJ (ed) Polymeric site-specific pharmacotherapy. Wiley, Chichester, pp 369–421

Young P, Johns A, Templeman C et al (2005) Reduction of post-operative adhesions after laparoscopic gynaecological surgery with Oxiplex/AP gel: a pilot study. Fertil Steril 84:1450–1456

Complications

20

Frank Willem Jansen

Contents

20.1   Introduction

In the past decades, an enormous increase in number of laparoscopic approaches in surgery is observed at debit of the conventional open procedures. Furthermore, in gynecology, a shift from diagnostic procedures to therapeutic interventions is perceived. Despite the great enthusiasm at the introduction of this surgical technique, in both within the field of gynecology and general surgery, one should not lose sight of the fact that complications can also occur during this surgical approach and even during (simple) procedures where they are not expected.

The incidences of complications in literature are generally collected from retrospective obtained data. Whereas approximately half of all complications in laparoscopy are a result of the introduction of the Veress needle or the blind insertion of the first trocar and are therefore inherently an *entry-related* complication. The other half is a result of the applied surgical technique and is similar to the conventional approach operating technique related. Entry-related complications are however mainly vascular and/or gastrointestinal lesions. To define a complication as a result of a surgical intervention, one has to be aware that there has to be similarity in definition and severeness. Some authors classify for example complications in minor and major. The latter are complications that need a laparotomy or when mortality occurs. Minor complications are classified as lesions or problems which can

F.W. Jansen, MD, PhD
Department of Gynaecology,
Leiden University Medical Center,
9600, 2300RC Leiden, The Netherlands
e-mail: f.w.jansen@lumc.nl

O. Istre (ed.), *Minimally Invasive Gynecological Surgery*,
DOI 10.1007/978-3-662-44059-9_20, © Springer-Verlag Berlin Heidelberg 2015

be solved during the regular laparoscopic procedure. This classification has the disadvantage that there is an under classification of some complications, which are classified as "minor" although they can lead to subsequent morbidity, both intra- and postoperatively. Therefore, it is of utmost importance to specifically define a complication so that its definition can be applied at the exact same way and everywhere. Currently, an internationally accepted definition of a (surgical) complication is: a complication is an unintended and undesirable event or condition during or following medical intervention, to such an extended disadvantage to the patient's health condition that adjustment of medical intervention is necessary, and/or irreparable damage has occurred. The results of the actual medical intervention, the probability of the complication, and the possible presence or absence of human error are of no concern. Responsibility period ranges from the (first) day of admission until 6 weeks after discharge. Furthermore, the severity or impact of the complication has to be weighted. The latter varies from no surgical reintervention (grade A), surgical reintervention (grade B), everlasting damage (grade C) to death (grade D).

When we use this internationally accepted definition, more unity on incidences and prevalence on complications can be collected.

A number of complications can be avoided by a consistent application of the preoperative protocols (e.g., catheterization of the bladder for each procedure). As proclaimed by Nezhat: *an ounce of prevention is worth a pound of cure.* Unfortunately, complications may occur in relatively 'simple' procedures when they are least expected. Negligence may be the cause of these complications and can be blamed.

In literature, conversion to laparotomy is usually used as the indicator for the severity of the complication. However, converting to a laparotomy does not necessarily mean that the procedure failed. Most of the time, the patients (as well as the surgeon) have a better clinical outcome when the operation is converted to the conventional procedure as per laparotomy, instead of persisting in the original laparoscopic surgical procedure leading to a complicated postoperative course.

In this chapter, risk factors which lead to complications are discussed. Intraoperative and postoperative complications as a result of laparoscopic procedure are highlighted.

20.2 Risk Factors

Beside a critical look at the indication for the surgical laparoscopic intervention, several risk factors for a laparoscopic procedure have to be considered. They can be classified as:

1. Surgeon's experience
2. Patient characteristics
3. Type of procedure
4. Equipment and instruments
5. Anesthesia

20.2.1 Surgeon's Experience

It is well established that the experience of the surgeon is related to the good clinical outcome of the procedure and is directly correlated to the occurrence of complications. However, it is also known that most complications occur in the learning phase. The training situation, where the resident is trained to learn diagnostics and simple laparoscopic procedures is at highest risk for a complication. However, this phase is usually performed under strict and skilled supervision. Unfortunately, there are hardly any good studies on this laparoscopic learning curve available. Just one study in the 1970s of the past century showed that the percentage of complications decreased from 14.7 (promille) to 3.8 (promille) when about 100 laparoscopies in total were performed by the surgeon concerned. Therefore, it is important that gynecologists in training perform these number of procedures under direct supervision during residency. In this way complications associated with inexperience of the surgeon can be reduced to a minimum. Furthermore, the laparoscopic surgeon has to be familiarized with the instruments he/she has to be trained in the basic skills preferably on an endotrainer in a skills laboratory and has to be familiar with the applied surgical techniques by observing the surgeon (*preceptorship*). Finally, he/she has to perform the first procedures under direct supervision (*proproctorship*) before starting to perform operations independently. Also, working in accordance to a protocol, results in a considerable reduction of complications. This was already described in 1973. A tenfold reduction of the number of complications in laparoscopic sterilization was noticed when the gynecologists started to work according to a standard protocol. Finally, a 3–4 times lower complication incidence was observed when the surgeon attended a course on specific operations and skills obtained at an animal laboratory.

In this context, recently studies came available on experience of the surgeon toward laparoscopic hysterectomy. This advanced surgical procedure is usually learned after obtaining enough experience with the basic skills for laparoscopic surgery. Nevertheless, these studies showed that the skills factor of the surgeon concerned was an independent predictor toward the occurrence of adverse events. That means not only experience counts as prevention to complications but also dealing with a skilled surgeon is a preventive item toward the occurrence of these side effects.

20.2.2 Patient Characteristics

In the past decades, a shift was observed from absolute to relative contraindications for a laparoscopic procedure. In the past century, oncology was considered an absolute contraindication for this approach due to the fear of spillage. Nowadays, this indication has changed to a relatively contraindication when spillage of content is expected. Only severe heart failure (class IV) has to be considered an absolute contraindication for laparoscopy. The latter is, however, also for the conventional open approach a relative contraindication. In general, all patients who have additional comorbidity do have a higher risk for an operation (e.g., diabetes mellitus, long failure, etc.), whether for the laparoscopic as the conventional approach. In this context, we

have to consider that the laparoscopic approach has the disadvantages during its procedure (e.g., Trendelenburg position gives lung compression, prolonged operating time, etc.), whereas the conventional approach has usually negative impact on the postoperative phase (more postoperative infections, thrombosis, etc). Obesity and older age are not contraindications any more for a laparoscopic approach. Even a better clinical outcome has to be expected for this group of patients when compared to the conventional approach. Especially since the obese patient has a longer postoperative recovery time than those who have a normal BMI. The same trend is seen for elderly patients compared to their younger peers.

20.2.3 Type of Procedure

A higher complication rate can be expected, when more technically difficult laparoscopic procedures are performed. This is the reason that international societies [e.g., Royal College of Obstetricians and Gynaecologists (RCOG) and the Council on Residents Education in Obstetrics and Gynecology (CREOG)] developed guidelines and levels of difficulty for laparoscopic procedures. In summary, four levels are distinguished and shown in Table 20.1.

It is advised that the relatively simple procedures (level 1 and a part of level 2) can generally be performed by all credentialed gynecologists, whereas more difficult procedures (levels 3 and 4) have to be performed by gynecologists with a special interest and experience in laparoscopic surgery. For the level 4 procedures, it is advised to centralize these procedures in specialized institutions because of the multidisciplinary approach with general surgeons and urologists (e.g., severe endometriosis cases).

Data in scientific literature expose that both complication rate and conversion rate increase when the laparoscopic procedure turns to be more difficult. However, we have to take into account that the incidence of complications is also higher for these procedures when they are performed primarily by laparotomy.

Table 20.1 Gynecologic laparoscopic surgery classified in difficulty in accordance with the ESGE (http://www. esge.org/sl_laparoscopy.htm)

1st level: Basic level
  Diagnostic laparoscopy
  Sterilization
  Needle aspiration of simple cysts
  Ovarian biopsy

2nd level: Intermediate level (normal training during specialization in obs/gyn)
  Salpingostomies for ectopic pregnancy
  Salpingectomies
  Salpingo-oophorectomies
  Ovarian cystectomies
  Adhesiolysis, including moderate bowel adhesions
  Treatments of mild or moderate endometriosis—salpingostomy and salpingo-ovariolysis

3rd level: Advanced level (advanced procedures requiring extensive training)
  Hysterectomy
  Myomectomy
  Treatment of incontinence
  Surgery for severe endometriosis
  Extensive adhesiolysis including bowel and ureter
  Repair of simple intestinal or bladder injuries

4th level: (procedure under evaluation or practised in specialized centers)
  Pelvic floor defects
  Oncology procedures: lymphadenectomy, radical hysterectomy, and axilloscopy
  Rectovaginal nodules
  Other procedures not yet described

20.2.4 Equipment and Tools

Due to the often 'blind' insertion of sharp instruments at laparoscopy (Veress needle and first trocar), this inherently can lead to complications which are not completely avoidable. To decrease the chance of such a complication, a number of standard precautionary measures have to be made.

(a) At each laparoscopic procedure the bladder has to be emptied. When a longer procedure is expected, a *catheter à demeure* has to be applied.

(b) The stomach preferably has to be emptied before the Veress needle is applied. Anxiety or a difficult intubation may result in aerophagia with probably a dilatation of the stomach below the level of the umbilicus. Furthermore, a dilated stomach can push the transverse colon below the umbilical level as well. These two occasions may result in visceral laceration when the Veress needle or first trocar is applied.

(c) At introduction of the Veress needle, the patient should be in a horizontal position. If this position is altered (too early Trendelenburg position), the angle of application to Veress needle or first trocar might be changed as well. This will result in less angling with the chance of injury to the aorta. The application of the first trocar after applying pneumoperitoneum is also advised to be performed when the patient is placed in a horizontal position. Figure 20.1 shows this preventable situation.

(d) Testing of the Veress needle with an aspiration test or drop test gives relative information about the correct position of the Veress needle. In the past, these tests provided us with the best information about the position of the Veress needle. However, more recent data in literature showed us the relative value of these tests. A pressure level below 10 mmHg is the best informant of the position of the Veress needle tip. However, still relatively good information is obtained by the aspiration test to assure that the tip of the Veress needle is not applied intravascular or in a gastrointestinal organ.

A low initial abdominal pressure (<10 mmHg), followed by a free influx of CO_2, is a reliable indicator of correct intraperitoneal Veress needle placement. Still, however, there are only insufficient high-quality comparative studies available on safety and effectiveness of the different aspects in these specific open- and closed-entry techniques. Furthermore, the peritoneal hyper distention has only been studied and found to be safe in healthy female patients with low ASA score (e.g., score 1 or 2). The latter technique (application of an intra-abdominal pressure of 20–24 mmHg) results in an increase size of the gas bubble and creates more distance between the abdominal wall and the organs at risk.

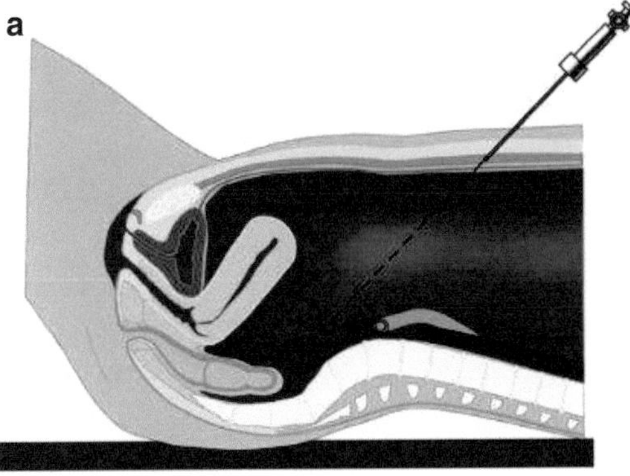

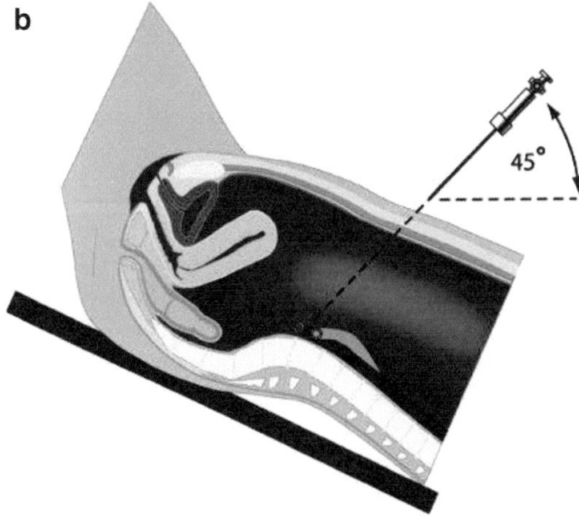

Fig. 20.1 Too early placement in Trendelenburg position and the angle consequences of the introduced Veress needle

An internationally adapted open Hasson technique is an alternative for the closed entry technique. However, the number of specific entry complications has not been diminished with either approach. Both, the number of vascular and gastrointestinal injuries are equal at each technique applied.

20.2.5 Anesthesia and Pneumoperitoneum

Due to the relatively high intra-abdominal CO_2 pressure and the (steep) Trendelenburg position, inherently anesthesiological problems may occur. Furthermore, the extensive use of cold fluids intra-abdominally can lower the patient's temperature with its consequences.

20.3 Intraoperative Complications

20.3.1 Abdominal Wall Bleeding

A lesion of an epigastric vein or artery is the most common observed complications of a bleeding of the abdominal wall. The given incidence in literature varies between 0.17 and 6.4 per 1,000. This large range can to be explained to the fact that most studies on this subject are of retrospective origin and no discrimination is made between a superficial abdominal wall bleeding and an intra-abdominal bleeding.

20.3.1.1 Prevention

Most bleedings of the epigastric veins are caused as a result of blind insertion of the additional side trocars. Precautions to avoid this complication are relatively simple. Knowledge of the anatomy of the abdominal wall veins (Fig. 20.2), transillumination of the abdominal wall by the laparoscope, and insertion of the secondary side trocars only under direct vision is one of them. However, an abdominal wall bleeding is not always directly recognizable due to the tamponade of the trocar during the surgical procedure. If this trocar is accidentally removed during the operation, a bleeding or the development of a hematoma could originate. Securing of the trocar with a screw (cave: diameter of the incision is enlarged) or a stitch can prevent the unintended removal of the trocar during the procedure.

20.3.1.2 Treatment

Usually, a reactive policy is recommended for an abdominal wall bleeding, especially since the trocar tamponades the manifestation of the bleeding. However, when the bleeding persists and is visible by dripping of blood into the abdomen, besides the trocar, this is usually a result of a lesion of the epigastric inferior vein. Several ways are described to stop the bleeding from the trocar side. First, the vein can be coagulated by bipolar coagulation. However, when the bleeding persists it is advised to leave the trocar in situ and apply a Foley catheter into the trocar, remove the trocar and clamp it at the abdominal side. Tamponade with a catheter balloon (filled with saline) tamponades the bleeding

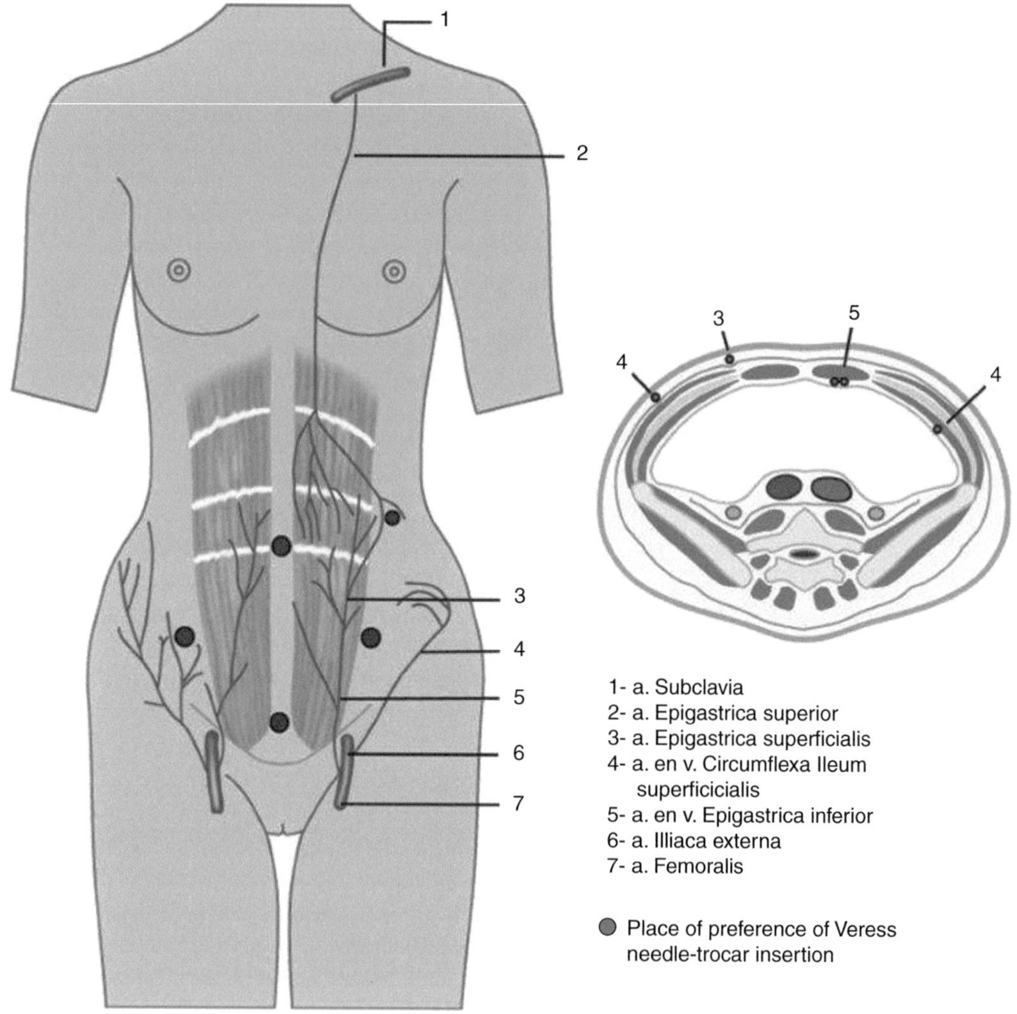

Fig. 20.2 Anatomical pathway of arteries and veins in the abdominal wall

by pressure from the inside of the balloon toward the peritoneal side of the abdominal wall. Other alternatives are by applying a laparoscopic stitch to the abdominal wall or enlarging the incision to locate the bleeding and then the vein can be stitched in a conventional way.

20.3.2 Intra-abdominal Bleeding

In general, intra-abdominal bleeding is a result of the applied technique or, similar to conventional surgery, a result of 'bad' luck during the procedure. The incidence of this complication as a result of the blind insertion of Veress needle or first trocar is 2.7/1,000 or 2.4–2.7/1,000, respectively. Sometimes, an intra-abdominal bleeding is not visible or manifest during the procedure because of a combination of factors. The Trendelenburg position and the high intra-abdominal pressure (14–16 mmHg) give a relative supine hypotension. At the end or after the procedure, when this combination of factors is dissolved, intra-abdominal bleeding can become manifest.

20.3.2.1 Prevention

Apart from the application of general preoperative precautions, there are not many means to prevent a bleeding. Like in conventional surgery, one surgical procedure has more bloody course than the other. Some preventive measurements to comply within laparoscopic surgery are that at the end of the operation the intra-abdominal overpressure as well as the Trendelenburg position have to be released. By inspecting the operating field, an intra-abdominal bleeding can be seen and arrangements for stopping the bleeding can be made. One has to be aware that a manual overshoot during the blind insertion of either the Veress needle or the first trocar can occur. Precaution to overshoot is that when the Veress needle has passed the peritoneum (after two clicks), no further application is necessary intra-abdominally. The same is applicable for the first trocar. The extreme thin patient (BMI < 18) and children are especially at risk for lesions of aorta and vena cava because these structures are situated just under the skin. Also, the angle in which the instruments are applied is of importance. The fatter the patient, the more at 90° angle the instruments have to be introduced.

20.3.2.2 Treatment

The occurrence of an intra-abdominal bleeding does not mean that the planned laparoscopic procedure has to be abandoned. Many bleedings can primarily be treated and stopped with bipolar coagulation. Also, clips or stitches can be used to stop the bleeding as well as the application of an endoloops. Furthermore, a sterile gauze can be applied toward the diffuse bleeding surface to tamponade the bleeding for a while. Lastly, there are several hemostatic products available which are laparoscopically applicable.

20.3.3 Gastrointestinal Lesions

Gastrointestinal lesions can be a result of the blind insertion of the Veress needle or the first trocar and are therefore entry-related complications. Furthermore, gastrointestinal lesions can occur due to the technique used in the procedure. One of the biggest problems of gastrointestinal lesions is that they are not always immediately noticed. Some described that only in 1/3 of cases these lesions are observed intraoperatively. When, after the operation, abdominal pain occurs as a result of generalized peritonitis, the lesion becomes manifest. When the lesion is a result of a sharp trauma (e.g., Veress needle, trocar or laceration during sharp adhesiolysis), clinical signs will be manifest within 72 h. In contrast, thermo damage due to electric coagulation or laser coagulation are manifest sometimes just after 4 or 10 days. At reintervention, it is from macroscopic point of view difficult to distinguish if the lesion is a result of a sharp or a coagulation trauma. In both cases, the perforation has a macroscopic whitish area of necrosis at the lesion. At microscopic level, however, a distinction between lesions can be made. At electrocoagulation trauma, dead amorphous tissue without polymorphic core infiltration is visible. Perforation lesion as a result of sharp trauma shows capillary ingrowth, leukocyte infiltration, and fibrin deposition at the edges of the wound.

Gastrointestinal lesions can occur both on the small intestine and on the colon. Small intestinal lesions usually occur as a result of a trauma by the first trocar, usually in patients with a history of prior laparotomy. However, also blunt dissection of small intestines may result in lesions of these organs. Colon lesions usually occur as a result of introducing too blunt trocars with too much force, usually in absence of an adequate pneumoperitoneum.

20.3.3.1 Prevention

An adequate pneumoperitoneum (>20 mmHg) ensures that the gastrointestinal organs are located far from the abdominal wall. This decreases the risk that these gastrointestinal organs can be damaged. The stomach has to be emptied before the operation starts. In this context, it is interesting to see that gastrointestinal lesions at the open-entry technique usually are recognized earlier than in blind technique. In general, it is found that patients with a prior laparotomy have a higher incidence of gastrointestinal lesions and operations where extensive adhesiolysis is performed are at risk.

When, during the closed entry, a bowel lesion occurs or is suspect, it is advised to leave the Veress needle or trocar in situ to identify the lesion during laparotomy. Finally, at the end of the laparoscopic procedure, trocars have to be removed under direct vision in order to prevent slippage of the small gastrointestinal organs in the abdominal defect due to the evolved negative abdominal pressure. At removing the trocars, this can lead to herniation and incarceration of the bowels or omentum.

20.3.3.2 Treatment

Instantly noticed perforation of small intestines or colon can be repaired immediately by stitching the defect. It is well established that bowel preparation does not play a role anymore for the clinical results after repairing a gastrointestinal lesion. However, when a bowel lesion has to be repaired after a longer period of time, this preparation is debatable. When at the fifth or sixth postoperative day, a patient reports abdominal tenderness, slight fever, nausea and/or vomiting with diminished appetite, and a progression in these symptoms, it is suspect for an (unnoticed) gastrointestinal lesion. Lesions with a later manifestation have a higher morbidity and are usually treated by laparotomy. Small intestine lesions are usually treated with an end-to-end anastomosis. However, the latter depends if the blood supply is not damaged. Treatment of lesions of the colon, recognized at a later date, depends on the stage of the peritonitis and will still be treated in the conventional way with a Hartman procedure.

20.3.4 Bladder Lesions

The occurrence of a lesion of the bladder is rare and usually occurs only when a patient had prior abdominal surgery (e.g., a Caesarean section) or when the bladder is preoperatively not emptied. Furthermore lesions can also occur after coagulation. Operations at risk for the occurrence of bladder lesions are the treatment of endometriosis (ablation), adhesiolysis, bladder suspension operations, and the laparoscopic hysterectomy.

The incidence found in literature varies between 0.06 and 1.2 %, which includes the occurrence of fistulas postoperatively. For many years, the laparoscopic hysterectomy (LH) was considered at risk for bladder lesions. For the latter, a recently published study from Finland showed that when experience with this surgical procedure increases, a decrease of these lesions was found. Nowadays, an incidence of 0.34 % is given for lesions at the urogenital tract including bladder and ureter lesions. This is at the same level as given for the abdominal or vaginal hysterectomy. Specifically for bladder lesions, they can stay unnoticed. However, in most cases (90 %) these lesions are directly recognized. This is in contrast with ureter lesions, which become manifest in most cases (80 %) after initial operation.

20.3.4.1 Prevention

For gynecological laparoscopic procedures, it is mandatory to empty the bladder before the procedure starts. Long-lasting procedures require a catheter a demeure. A procedure, very close to the bladder, or when there is doubt about the exact location of the boundary of the bladder a retrograde filling of the bladder is optional. With 350 cc saline solution the edges of the bladder are easily found. When secondary trocars are removed, it is important to visualize intra-abdominally if there is no leakage of urine. Tamponade of the lesion intraoperatively holds the lesion occult. When after a procedure hematuria is found, or gas (CO_2) is seen in the catheter bag, this could direct to a bladder lesion.

20.3.4.2 Treatment

Treatment options depend on the size of the lesion. When the lesion is very small (<5 mm), a catheter can be put into the bladder for 5–7 days and a spontaneous healing can occur. However, when a big laceration is found this can be stitched laparoscopically. This stitching can be done in one layer with continuous running sutures. Some advise to control the stitch with cystoscopy, especially to evaluate the orifices of the ureter. Drainage for 7 days and antibiotic prophylaxis followed by a cystogram postoperatively after 7 days are advised. The latter option depends on the severeness of the lesion and its location.

20.3.5 Ureter Injuries

Ureter lesions are usually a result of the laparoscopic applied technique (technique related) and not a result of the laparoscopic approach (entry related). Although the incidences are low, it is expected to increase in the future when more complex laparoscopic procedures will be performed. Especially the LH is the operation at risk not only for injury of the ureter, but also the laparoscopic sacrocolpopexy and procedures to extensive endometriosis treatment. The ureter is anatomically located close to the sacrouterine ligament and is therefore inherently at risk at this stage of the procedure. Ureter injury can be a result of direct (e.g., cutting, stitching, coagulating, and stapling) or indirect (e.g., coagulating near the ureter and kinking) application of used techniques. Coagulating a bleeding or endometriosis near the anatomical location of the ureter is often not only the cause of the injury, but also the use of staplers and laser in that field is risk factors.

20.3.5.1 Prevention

Anatomical knowledge of the course of the ureter in the pelvis as well as knowledge of the moments when the ureter is at risk for injury during the surgical steps is of importance (Table 20.2). Especially when additional (occult) diseases are present (e.g., endometriosis may thicken the peritoneum locally and make the ureter hard to locate) and anatomical awareness of the course of the ureter is important. Endometriosis, adhesions, and prior surgery are pitfalls during the surgery. When the procedure takes place at a risky location and it is not possible to explore the ureter, a retroperitoneal dissection might enable this. This can be succeeded through hydrodissection. In this way, the ureter can be moved to a more lateral position or by positioning the ureter further away from the operating field. At adnexexttirpation or ovariectomy, usually bipolar coagulation is used to coagulate the ligamentum infundibulo pelvicum. During this step is important that the ligament has to be moved under traction to median. Herewith, it is possible to visualize the ureter and to prevent lateral thermal injuries toward the structure.

Table 20.2 Laparoscopic procedures at risk for ureter injury

1. *Infundibulo-pelvicum ligament and fossa ovarica*	Oöphorectomy
Adhesions at pelvic side wall	
Presacral neurectomy	
Ablation or vaporization of endometriosis	
Extended bowel adhesions	
2. *Ureter*	Hysterectomy
Sacrouterine ligaments	
Transection of uterosacral nerve	
3. *Cardinal ligament*	Hysterectomy
Vaginal cuff closure	

The use of ureter catheters is debatable. These catheters have to be applied preoperatively and due to transillumination the course of the ureter can be visualized during the procedure. A disadvantage of the use of catheters is that a specialized and skilled gynecologist or urologist has to be present to introduce these catheters. Furthermore, they give additional expenses to the surgical procedure.

20.3.5.2 Treatment

Early recognition of the injury is important. One has to be aware that ureter injuries can be suspected when leakage of the urine is seen in the abdomen, bloody urine is found in the catheter bag, or when leakage is found in intravenously applied indigo carmin. Injuries are usually repaired by the urologists with an ureteroureterostomy or an ureteroneocystostomy. Usually these procedures are still performed by laparotomy. However, conservative and laparoscopic procedures are also performed to handle these injuries. Sometimes, thermal injuries can be handled with expectant management without any side effects.

20.3.6 CO_2 Insufflation Complications

Subcutaneous emphysema and CO_2 embolism can be a result of misplacing the Veress needle. Also, overpressure of CO_2 can penetrate in the tissues or by (extensive) manipulation of the trocars during the operation. CO_2 causes subcutaneous emphysema. Continuous reintroduction of the trocar during the operation may also cause application of CO_2 at the wrong places (subcutaneous). Furthermore, at manipulating the diaphragm (e.g., cholecystectomy), a pneumomediastinum can occur. In this line also the occurrence of a pneumothorax is described.

The incidence of this side effect (incidences 0.43–2 %) is considered to be rare. However, from daily practice it is actually the most observed side effect of laparoscopic surgery. On the other hand, the CO_2 embolism is the most dangerous complication, but given as very rare event. The mechanism of CO_2 embolism by insufflating CO_2 in the venous circulation is described as follows. When a CO_2 embolus enters the central (venous) circulation, this will cause a gas lock in the right cardiac atrium. When this gas lock has enough volume, the whole venous circulation toward the heart will be blocked with a total cardiovascular collapse as a result. Also due to this gas lock, a block of the pulmonary outflow in the right cardiac ventricle occurs with a pulmonal hypertension as a result. Due to this mechanism, a lowering of the pressure in the left ventricle and aorta occurs with a chance of a myocardial infarction. The clinical signs are acute hypotension, cardiac arrhythmia, tachycardia, or supraventricular tachycardia, which result in a cardiac arrest and breath arrest. Due to the blending of CO_2 in the blood during auscultation, millstone murmurs are heard. When the pCO_2 is measured, it is found that this starts to decrease first and higher up afterwards. The oxygen saturation lowers.

20.3.6.1 Prevention

After placement of the Veress needle and before starting to insufflate, it has to be proven that the needle is correctly placed. Several tests such as the Palmer test, drop test, etc. give relative information about the placement. By aspirating the Veress- needle after placement, it can be found if it is placed intravenously/arterially. It is shown in literature that the best option is that the CO_2 flow has to be <10 mmHg to give the prediction of the best placement of the Veress- needle.

20.3.6.2 Treatment

In case of occurrence of subcutaneous and/or mediastinal emphysema, expectant management is advised since the CO_2 will be absorbed by the body itself. However, in case of a CO_2 embolism, CO_2 application has to be stopped immediately, the pneumoperitoneum has to be released, and the patient has to be placed in a left tilted lateral position. The latter position is expected to advance the removal of the gas bubble from the right ventricle. Also, it is advised to suspend the general anesthesia and to apply 100 % oxygen and to perform heart massage.

20.4 Postoperative Complications

Gastrointestinal injuries, bleeding, bladder and ureteral injuries are prone to become manifest in the postoperative course. Especially the coagulation injuries occurring during the procedure are notorious for their late manifestation. One has to realize that even mortality may occur from this complication (incidence 4–8/100,000), which is described after a laparoscopic complication full course. Other most found postoperative complications are hernias, infection (abscesses, salpingitis, and peritonitis) thrombosis, lung embolism, and emphysema.

20.4.1 Postoperative Hernia

Although the incidence of occurrence of postoperative hernia, through a trocar scar, is low, the literature gives a diversity of incidences. This varies between 0 and 0.21/1,000. The use of different trocars (sharp versus blunt) and due to the removal of larger specimen (e.g., myomas), it is imaginable that in the near future an increase of postoperative herniation is found. It is observed that the use of blunt tip trocars and/or expending trocar systems gives less tissue damage of the abdominal wall and is therefore less at risk to give a herniation afterward. However, hernias may occur more often than diagnosed. This is due to the fact that the follow-up period after the procedure is usually not more than 6 weeks and a hernia does not always give clinical signs and complaints within that given timeframe. Patients at risk are, similar to conventional surgery, the very thin patient (especially the elderly), asthma patients, patients with a history of herniation, or patients with an inactive tissue ailment. Lastly, patients who have endured a wound infection postoperatively are at risk to develop a hernia. A hernia only causes trouble when small intestine, colon, or omentum slips into the hernia and get incarcerated. Hernias without clinical complaints do not need a surgical intervention.

20.4.1.1 Prevention

It is well established that the use of smaller trocars (<5 mm) reduces the chance that a hernia occurs. However, several case reports describe even herniation after the use of trocars <5 mm. To prevent slippage of intra-abdominal structures in the opening of the trocar after the procedure, it is mandatory to remove all the trocars postoperatively under direct vision. Also, the first trocar has to be removed under direct vision with an open valve of the trocar to prevent negative pressure to which intra-abdominal structures can be slipped into the opening. It is not exactly established at what size of the trocar used the abdominal wall defect has to be closed. Latest consensus shows that trocar defects >10 mm have to be closed to prevent herniation.

There are two preventive methods to close the defect. First, the defect of the fascia can be closed with a simple Z-figure stitch with a conventional round needle. Second, both the peritoneum and the fascia can be closed with a J-needle. In both cases, the skin is not to be stitched into the thread. Furthermore, one has to be aware that the skin is loosened from the thread to prevent the development of worse cosmetic results. Final, it is mandatory to control the sewing inside abdominally to prevent slippage of gastrointestinal organs or omentum into the tread.

20.4.1.2 Treatment

For the treatment of hernias, the conventional surgical procedure of hernia correction has to be applied, either by the gynecologist or by the general surgeon.

20.4.2 Infection

Postoperative infections after laparoscopic surgery are rare. However, there are no extensive comparable studies available. The risk of an infection increases if the procedure takes more time and when there are more trocars applied in the abdominal wall. Usually most infections are limited to the trocar sides which can be infected. Sometimes, a more fulminate infection occurs (peritonitis/salpingitis) usually after an operation or a diagnostic procedure with chromotubation. These infections may be a flare up because of a pre-existing infection (e.g., Chlamydia infection). The combination of extensive tissue destruction and necrosis with bacterial contamination (e.g., laparoscopic hysterectomy where the vagina is opened and endometriosis cases) is proned for secondary infection where a peritonitis may occur. Also, the spillage of cystic content can give (sterile) infection symptoms. Dermoid cysts are especially at risk for this clinical sign. The chemical peritonitis which occurs is a breeding ground for postoperative adhesion formation.

20.4.2.1 Prevention

The application of antibiotic prophylaxis at an uncomplicated relatively simple laparoscopic procedure is not mandatory. When chromotubation or a tuboplasty for fertility reasons is performed, prophylaxis is dependent on the result of the Chlamydia screening. To prevent chemical peritonitis due to spillage of content of the cyst, it is advised to use laparoscopic endobags. Furthermore, extensive rinsing of the abdomen is advised at the end of the procedure. Spillage of content of the removed tissue can have severe consequences. Not only spillage of carcinoma with its adverse effects has been described, but also materials of ectopic pregnancy can give chorionic nestling of tissue elsewhere. Also, gallbladders stones which are not removed after spillage at the cholecystectomy are described to give afterward the signs of ovarian pathology. The spillage of myoma content after morcellation may give implants. In case of (occult) malignancy this may worsen the clinical outcome and need to be prevented.

20.4.2.2 Treatment

When infectious contamination is expected, antibiotic prophylaxis is mandatory. This is similar to the conventional procedures. When, after the surgical procedure a salpingitis is diagnosed or an infection is manifest secondary treatment with antibiotics is mandatory.

20.4.3 Thrombosis

At average, a patient undergoing a laparoscopic gynecological procedure is a relatively young and healthy person. However, the combination of pneumoperitoneum, Trendelenburg position, and a relatively time-consuming surgical procedure introduces metabolic and hemodynamic changes and is therefore at risk for thrombosis. Hemodynamic changes are caused by the diminishing venous return of the blood supply from the pelvis with an increase of the central venous pressure and a dilatation of the distal veins. These factors predisposes for venous thrombosis, especially when the operation has a prolonged character.

20.4.3.1 Prevention

Thrombosis prophylaxis has to be applied as the usual hospital and (inter-) national protocol describes. When prolonged laparoscopic procedures are performed, it is mandatory to give special attention to the position of the legs in the stirrups. These can disturb the venous return from the legs with an increased risk for venous thrombosis. Stirrups with massage abilities or the French position may diminish the chance of thrombosis in the legs.

20.4.3.2 Treatment

When thrombosis occurs, this has to be treated as described in the standard protocol which is applicable in the (inter-)national guideline and adapted in every institute.

20.4.3.3 Conversion

Inherent to each laparoscopic procedure, there is a chance for conversion to a conventional laparotomy. The risk to convert depends on a combination of factors such as indication, patient characteristics, experience, and skills of the surgeon. Hence, in the past, the rate of conversions was used to determine the feasibility of the laparoscopic approach. Nowadays, it could more specifically be used as a means of evaluation.

In general, compared to a totally performed laparoscopic procedure, conversion is associated with worse outcome measures such as a longer length of surgery, more postoperative adverse events, and a prolonged hospital stay. Additionally, the reason for conversion is also of importance. The outcomes after a conversion due to an adverse event (defined as 'reactive' conversion) are significantly worse in comparison to those after a 'strategic' reason to convert in order to prevent an intraoperative adverse event in case of operative difficulty. Therefore, it is mandatory in the registration of conversions that this distinction between strategic and reactive conversions is made.

Interestingly, also laparoscopic-assisted procedures in which only a small-target incision for specimen retrieval is made show a significantly higher postoperative morbidity and prolonged hospital stay compared to a total laparoscopically performed procedure. Although this type of procedures should not be regarded as a conversion, ideally they should also be registered separately from total laparoscopically performed procedures. With respect to the associated morbidity, this will allow adequate comparison between totally laparoscopic, laparoscopically assisted, strategically converted, and reactively converted procedures. Finally, conversion rate can be used as a quality parameter tool to evaluate surgical performance. However, precautions have to be made toward the correct definition and the mentioned distinction of this phenomenon.

Suggested Reading

Aksu T, Coskun F (2004) Complications of gynaecological laparoscopy—a retrospective analysis of 3572 cases from a single institute. J Obstet Gynaecol 24:813–816

Bishoff JT, Allaf ME, Kirkels W et al (1999) Laparoscopic bowel injury: incidence and clinical presentation. J Urol 161:887–890

Blikkendaal MD, Twijnstra AR, Stiggelbout AM, Beerlage HP, Bemelman WA, Jansen FW (2013) Achieving consensus on the definition of conversion to laparotomy: a Delphi study among general surgeons, gynecologists, and urologists. Surg Endosc 27(12):4631–4639

Boike GM, Miller CE, Spirtos NM et al (1995) Incisional bowel herniations after operative laparoscopy: a series of nineteen cases and review of the literature. Am J Obstet Gynecol 172:1726–1731

Brosens I, Gordon A, Campo R, Gordts S (2003) Bowel injury in gynecologic laparoscopy. J Am Assoc Gynecol Laparosc 10(1):9–13

Brummer TH, Seppälä TT, Härkki PS (2008) National learning curve for laparoscopic hysterectomy and trends in hysterectomy in Finland 2000–2005. Hum Reprod 23:840–845

Chan JK, Morrow J, Manetta A (2003) Prevention of ureteral injuries in gynecologic surgery. Am J Obstet Gynecol 188:1273–1277

Chapron C, Querleu D, Mage G et al (1992) Complications of gynecologic laparoscopy. Multicentric study of 7,604 laparoscopies. J Gynecol Obstet Biol Reprod 21:207–213

Childers JM, Aqua KA, Surwit EA et al (1994) Abdominal-wall tumor implantation after laparoscopy for malignant conditions. Obstet Gynecol 84:765–769

Garry R, Fountain J, Mason S et al (2004) The eVALuate study: two parallel randomized trials, one comparing laparoscopic with abdominal hysterectomy, the other comparing laparoscopic with vaginal hysterectomy. BMJ 328:1229–1236

Gordon AG, Lewis BV (1995) Complications of laparoscopy. In: Gordon AG, Lewis BV, DeCherney AH (eds) Atlas of gynecologic endoscopy. Mosby-Wolfe, New York, pp 136–142

Härkki-Siren P, Sjoberg J, Kurki T (1999) Major complications of laparoscopy: a follow-up Finnish study. Obstet Gynecol 94:94–98

Hasson HM, Parker WH (1998) Prevention and management of urinary tract injury in laparoscopic surgery. J Am Assoc Gynecol Laparosc 5:99–114

Hasson HM, Rotman C, Rana N et al (2000) Open laparoscopy: 29-year experience. Obstet Gynecol 96:763–766

Hurt WG, Jones CM III (1993) Intraoperative ureteral injuries and urinary diversion. In: Nichols DH (ed) Gynecologic and obstetric surgery. Mosby, Baltimore, pp 900–910

Jansen FW, Kapiteyn K, Trimbos-Kemper T et al (1997) Complications of laparoscopy: a prospective multicenter observational study. Br J Obstet Gynaecol 104:595–600

Kadar N, Reich H, Liu CY et al (1993) Incisional hernias after major laparoscopic gynecologic procedures. Am J Obstet Gynecol 168:1493–1495

Kalhan SB, Reaney JA, Collins RL (1990) Pneumomediastinum and subcutaneous emphysema during laparoscopy. Cleve Clin J Med 57:639–642

Karaman Y, Bingol B, Günenç Z (2007) Prevention of complications in laparoscopic hysterectomy: experience with 1120 cases performed by a single surgeon. J Minim Invasive Gynecol 14:78–84

la Chapelle CF, Bemelman WA, Rademaker BM, van Barneveld TA, Jansen FW; on behalf of the Dutch Multidisciplinary Guideline Development Group Minimally Invasive Surgery (2012) A multidisciplinary evidence-based guideline for minimally invasive surgery.: Part 1: entry techniques and the pneumoperitoneum. Gynecol Surg 9(3):271–282

Leron E, Piura B, Ohana E, Mazor M (1998) Delayed recognition of major vascular injury during laparoscopy. Eur J Obstet Gynecol Reprod Biol 79(1):91–93

Li TC, Saravelos H, Richmond M et al (1997) Complications of laparoscopic pelvic surgery: recognition, management and prevention. Hum Reprod Update 3:505–515

Magrina JF (2002) Complications of laparoscopic surgery. Clin Obstet Gynecol 45:469–480

Mäkinen J, Brummer T, Jalkanen J, Heikkinen AM, Fraser J, Tomás E, Härkki P, Sjöberg J (2013) Ten years of progress–improved hysterectomy outcomes in Finland 1996–2006: a longitudinal observation study. BMJ Open 3(10):e003169

Munro MG (2002) Laparoscopic access: complications, technologies, and techniques. Curr Opin Obstet Gynecol 14:365–374

Murdock CM, Wolff AJ, Van Geem T (2000) Risk factors for hypercarbia, subcutaneous emphysema, pneumothorax, and pneumomediastinum during laparoscopy. Obstet Gynecol 95:704–709

Nagarsheth NP, Rahaman J, Cohen CJ et al (2004) The incidence of port-site metastases in gynecologic cancers. JSLS 8:133–139

Nezhat C, Childers J, Nezhat F et al (1997) Major retroperitoneal vascular injury during laparoscopic surgery. Hum Reprod 12:480–483

Nieboer TE, Johnson N, Lethaby A, Tavender E, Curr E, Garry R, van Voorst S, Mol BW, Kluivers KB (2009) Surgical approach to hysterectomy for benign gynaecological disease. Cochrane Database Syst Rev (3):CD003677

Oh BR, Kwon DD, Park KS et al (2000) Late presentation of ureteral injury after laparoscopic surgery. Obstet Gynecol 95:337–339

Ostrzenski A, Ostrzenska KM (1998) Bladder injury during laparoscopic surgery. Obstet Gynecol Surv 53:175–180

Ostrzenski A, Radolinski B, Ostrzenska KM (2003) A review of laparoscopic ureteral injury in pelvic surgery. Obstet Gynecol Surv 58:794–799

Pados G, Vavilis D, Pantazis K et al (2005) Unilateral vulvar edema after operative laparoscopy: a case report and literature review. Fertil Steril 83:471–473

Peterson HB, DeStefano F, Rubin GL et al (1983) Deaths attributable to tubal sterilization in the United States, 1977 to 1981. Am J Obstet Gynecol 146:131–136

Pillet MCL, Leonard F, Chopin N (2009) Incidence and risk factors of bladder injuries during laparoscopic hysterectomy indicated for benign uterine pathologies: a 14.5 years experience in a continuous series of 1501 procedures. Hum Reprod 24:842–849

Ramirez PT, Frumovitz M, Wolf JK et al (2004) Laparoscopic port-site metastases in patients with gynecological malignancies. Int J Gynecol Cancer 14:1070–1077

Reich H, McGlynn F, Budin R (1991) Laparoscopic repair of full-thickness bowel injury. J Laparoendoscopic Surg 1:119–122

Rodrigues SP, Wever AM, Dankelman J, Jansen FW (2012) Risk factors in patient safety: minimally invasive surgery versus conventional surgery. Surg Endosc 26(2):350–356

Saidi MH, Vancaillie TG, White AJ et al (1994) Complications and cost of multipuncture laparoscopy: a review of 264 cases. Gynecol Endosc 3:85–90

Soderstrom RM (1993) Bowel injury ligation after laparoscopy. J Am Assoc Gynecol Laparosc 1:74–77

Swank HA, Mulder IM, la Chapelle CF, Reitsma JB, Lange JF, Bemelman WA (2012) Systematic review of trocar-site hernia. Br J Surg 99(3):315–323

Tanaka Y, Asada H, Kuji N et al (2008) Ureteral catheter placement for prevention of ureteral injury during laparoscopic hysterectomy. J Obstet Gynaecol Res 34:67–72

Thompson JD (1992) Vesicovaginal fistulas. In: Thompson JD, Rock JA (eds) Te Linde's operative gynecology, 7th edn. JB Lippincott, Philadelphia, p 788

Twijnstra AR, Blikkendaal MD, van Zwet EW, van Kesteren PJ, de Kroon CD, Jansen FW (2012) Predictors of successful surgical outcome in laparoscopic hysterectomy. Obstet Gynecol 119(4):700–708

Twijnstra AR, Blikkendaal MD, van Zwet EW, Jansen FW (2013) Clinical relevance of conversion rate and its evaluation in laparoscopic hysterectomy. J Minim Invasive Gynecol 20(1):64–67

Vilos GA, Ternamian A, Dempster J et al (2007) Laparoscopic entry: a review of techniques, technologies, and complications. The Society of Obstetricians and Gynaecologists of Canada. J Obstet Gynaecol Can 29:433–465

Zaki H, Penketh R, Newton J (1995) Gynaecological laparoscopy audit: Birmingham experience. Gynecol Endosc 4:251–257

Marc Possover

Contents

21.1 Introduction

The pelvis is not only the anatomical site of various organs such as the bladder, the rectum, and the reproductive organs, but also contains the pelvic nerves. Only the pelvic nerves and plexuses enable the central nervous system the necessary control to the sexual functions, storage and elimination of urine and feces, and movement and sensation in the pelvis and the legs. Therefore, damages to these nerves lead to multiple following conditions:

- Sexual dysfunction (e.g., impotence), digestive disorders (especially constipation), and bladder dysfunction (especially overactive bladder).
- Difficulty walking and standing and difficulty moving the toes.
- Nerve disorders such as sciatica (pain that radiates from the buttocks to the toes), vulvodynia, vaginal pain, pudendal neuralgia, prostate pain, chronic prostatitis, penile and testicular pain, coccygodynia (tailbone pain), abdominal pain, and pain on urination.

Awareness that pathologies of the pelvic nerves may exist is still lacking and incidences are widely underestimated. Many patients suffering from pelvic nerve conditions only receive medication to treat the symptoms. Consequently, treatment frequently fails to address the root cause of the problems. Neurophysiological investigations to the pelvic nerves and plexuses are not especially developed. Neurosurgical

M. Possover
Possover International Medical Center,
Zuerich (CH), Switzerland

Division of Gynecology & Neuropelveology,
University of Aarhus, Aarhus, Denmark
e-mail: m.possover@possover.com

O. Istre (ed.), *Minimally Invasive Gynecological Surgery*,
DOI 10.1007/978-3-662-44059-9_21, © Springer-Verlag Berlin Heidelberg 2015

instruments and classical surgical microscopy have been introduced but are unsuitable for surgical interventions performed deep in the pelvis. The posterior surgical approach used by neurosurgeons is not suitable for the treatment of pelvic nerve disorders; in fact, they may result in even more nerve damage. Most medical specialties often neglect the pelvic nerves and a medical specialty devoted exclusively to pelvic nerve disorders has been lacking until now. The neuropelveology— the medical specialty that deals with the pathologies and functional disorders of the pelvic nerves and plexuses—closes this gap (Possover 2010a, 2011).

21.2 The Neuropelveological Diagnosis: A Combination of Different Knowledge (Possover and Forman)

In most pelvic pain syndromes, the main symptom is low abdominal pain and the main objective of treatment is to control it. Not only gynecologic, dermatologic, or urological conditions may induce pelvic pain but also central or peripheral neuropathic conditions. Patient's history and clinical examination must combine gynecological, urological, and neurological aspects of pain. The way of thinking for a proper neuropelveological diagnosis does not focus first on diagnosis of possible pelvic pathology, but on neurologic pathways of pain information to the central nervous system. The second step consists of determination of the level of the lesion (below, in, or above the pelvis), whereas the last step focuses on the determination of a possible etiology. Because several parallel nerve systems do exist, an absolute knowledge of pelvic neuroanatomy is mandatory. Pathologies of the sympathetic systems may induce visceral pelvic pain, whereas pelvic somatic nerve conditions may induce neuropathic pains. Sacral radiculopathies may induce abnormal sensation not only in the posterior surfaces of the lower limb, the pudendal (=genito–perineo–anal areas) areas, the vulva (vulvodynia), the tailbone (coccygodynia), and the buttock according with the sacral dermatomes (Fig. 21.1), but also dysfunctions of the lower limb, bladder, terminal intestine, and

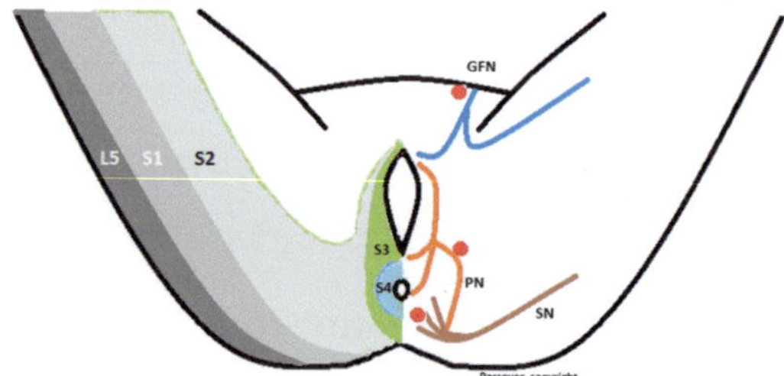

Fig. 21.1 Neuropelveologic assessment of dermatomes and trigger points of the pelvic nerves. *L5* fifth lumbar root, *S* sacral nerve root, *PN* pudendal nerve, *SN* sacral nerve roots, *GFN* genitofemoral nerve

sexual functions. In massive neurogenic lesions of the sacral plexus, loss of strength in hip extension, knee flexion, and dorsal plantar flexion of the foot can also be detected. A precise anamnesis, with a clinical examination that includes a neurologic, gynecologic, urologic, and proctologic examination, permits determination of the neurologic level of the lesion in the majority of patients. A key in neuropelveological diagnosis are the external genital organs: deep vaginodynia correspond to irritation of the inferior hypogastric plexus and have therefore characters of visceral pain accompanied by vegetative symptoms. Combination of anterior vulvodynia with groin pain (with or without irradiations in the tight) orients the diagnosis to pathology of the genitofemoral nerve (or of the lumbar plexus). A pathology of the pudendal nerve (Alcock's canal syndrome) always combined vulvodynia, perineal and perianal pain. The combination of pudendal pain with "nongynecological pains," such as sciatica, gluteal, and low-back pains, orients the diagnosis to a pathology of the sacral plexus—sacral radiculopathy. Further pain irradiations in the anterior part of the tight (lumbar dermatomes) correspond generally to pathology of the spinal cord and/or column.

21.3 The Laparoscopy: The Tool of Choice in Neuropelveology

Because of the anatomical location of the nerves within the pelvis (near major pelvic blood vessels), classical pelvic nerve surgery is very invasive and risky, especially for massive blood loss

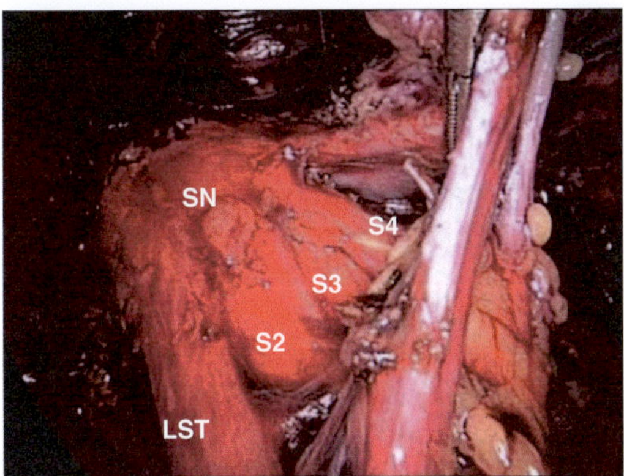

Fig. 21.2 Laparoscopic dissection of the left sacral plexus (supracardinal portion). *SN* sciatic nerve, *LST* lumbo-sacral trunk, *S* sacral nerve root

and nerves damages. Open pelvic surgery is laborious and cumbersome. Laparoscopy overcomes all of the limitations. High-resolution video cameras provide necessary magnification and microneurofunctional procedures. Thanks to these developments, all pelvic nerves and plexuses are now easily accessible for morphologic (Possover 2004a; Possover et al. 2007a) and functional (Possover et al. 2004) exploration by laparoscopy (Fig. 21.2). In addition to evaluating the disease status and making functional assessments, laparoscopic examination of the pelvic nerves also makes it possible to identify and to treat potential causes of functional disorders and neuropathic pain (Possover 2010b): neurofunctional procedures, such as nerve decompression (relief of pressure), neurolysis (release of a nerve sheath), nerve reconstruction, or implantation of stimulation electrodes in direct contact to nerves for postoperative neuromodulation (Possover et al. 2007b, c), can be done in optimal conditions by laparoscopy.

21.4 Control to Sensoric Functions of the Pelvic Nerves and Plexuses: New Therapeutic Options for Urge Amount of Patients

Pudendal pain, proctalgia, coccygodynia, vulvodynia, and pudendal neuralgia are all pain situations reported as "chronic pelvic pain". All these pain situations occur in 7–24 % of the population and are associated with impaired quality of life and high healthcare costs. Anoperineogenital pain are frequent complaint usually not only as a result of common and easily recognizable organic disorders such as anal fistula, thrombosed hemorrhoids, genitoanal cancer, or other dermatologic pathologies but can also occur under circumstances in which no organic cause can be found. Such pain syndromes are then poorly understood, with little research evidence available to guide their diagnosis and treatment. Also, lumbar pain with irradiations in the legs without any real spinal etiology is frequently treated by medical treatments on long-term or unnecessary surgeries; pelvic origins of such pain are very rarely evocated. Endopelvic lesions are less well known and because their diagnosis is difficult and surgical approach remained difficult and invasive, these etiologies are mostly managed by symptomatic treatments. In general, the number of patients suffering from pelvic nerve disorders is grossly underestimated. In the international literature, also the prevalence of pelvic nerve damage is estimated to be low. This is in stark contrast to clinical reality: both bladder and bowel dysfunctions and neurogenic pain after pelvic surgeries are seen every day in many doctors' offices around the world. This may be due to a lack of awareness of the existence of such diseases and to the complexity of the pelvic nerve anatomy. In our experience, the most frequent etiologies for pelvic nerve irritation or even damages are:

- Deeply infiltrative sciatic nerve (plexus sacralis endometriosis as part of a parametric endometriosis or as an isolated condition) (Possover et al. 2011)
- Surgical nerves damages, especially surgeries with mesh implantation (Possover 2009; Possover and Lemos 2011)
- Vascular compression syndrome of the pelvic nerves
- More seldom, pelvic nerve conditions such as schwannomas (Possover 2013a) and pathologies of the sacral bone

Procedures of laparoscopic nerve decompression have proven safe and effective. They are reported to achieve remarkable pain relief in 62 % of patients with postoperative nerve damage, in 78 % of patients with endometriosis involving the pelvic nerves, and in more than

80 % of patients with pelvic nerve compression by varicose veins in the pelvic area.

In axonal nerve pathologies, or in event of failure of the classical peripheral nerve surgical techniques, the neuromodulation is a well-known option to control both neural pain and dysfunctions of the lower intestinal and urinary tract. The surgical procedure is designed to implant an electrode in contact to the injured nerve proximal to the lesion, which is connected to a pacemaker that produces continuous low-level electrical current. The LION procedure to pelvic nerves in pain situation is only indicated in neurogenic nerves damages (axonal lesion) that represent only a small percent of indications.

21.5 The LION Procedure to the Pudendal Nerve to Treat Motor Pelvic Dysfunctions

Urinary and fecal dysfunctions affects millions of women and men all over the world and this condition encompasses overactive bladder, urinary/fecal incontinence, chronic constipation, and urination difficulties due to obstructions of the urinary tract or due to neurological central or peripheral nerve diseases. Continence and micturition/defecation involve a balance between urethral/anal closure and detrusor/rectal muscle activity. Disorders or troubles of coordination of both functions are responsible for bladder and intestinal dysfunctions.

The most common types of urinary disorders especially in women is stress urinary incontinence that is caused by loss of support of the urethra, which is usually a consequence of damage to pelvic support structures as a result of childbirth. Behind behavior changes and pelvic floor training, treatment focuses on the surgical reconstruction of the normal pelvic anatomy using techniques of vaginal repair or sling procedures. In all other conditions, treatments target on efferent effects by using neuroregulator pharmacotherapies with two aims: the first to reduce high vesical pressures (to avoid retrograde reflux) and the second to restore normal micturition. So alpha blockers target on reduction urethral pressure, whereas antimuscarinics and parasympathomimetic drug respectively reduce or active detrusor contractility. Despite the fact that pharmacological treatments are currently first therapeutic options, adherence on long term is low because of side effects and patient tolerability often challenging (Abrams et al. 2000). Also, intradetrusor injections of botulinum toxin A constitute a powerful treatment of overactive bladder in patients being able and willing to return for frequent postvoid residual evaluation (risk for infections) and to perform self-catheterization if necessary (elevated postvoid residuals). Elevated postvoid residuals responsible for urinary tract infections and repetition of injections for life lead to discontinuation of treatment (Kantartzis and Shepherd 2012). Electrical stimulation of the pelvic nerves has emerged as an alternative and attractive treatment for refractory cases of urinary disorders, as well those due to a hypo- or a hypercontractility of the detrusor and/or of the sphincter, as those due to trouble of urethra-vesical coordination (Tanagho and Schmidt 1988; van Kerrebroeck 1998). Pelvic nerve neuromodulation has been proven effective and is today an established treatment option for patients refractory to or intolerant of conservative treatments for urinary disorders. The method, known as the LION procedure (*Laparoscopic Implantation Of Neuroprothesis*), allows the surgeon to place an electrode directly on the pelvic nerves of interest. Neuromodulation is absolutely minimal invasive and preserves the anatomical integrity of the pelvic nerves, the lower urinary, and intestinal tracts and can be readily reversed. In the technique of Sacral Nerve Neuromodulation, implantation of the stimulation's electrode can be obtained by percutaneous puncture technique. However, behind the fact that most gynecologists are not familiar with such techniques, SNM present several important inconvenience and disadvantages (Possover 2014a). Behind technical aspects, SNM present two major problems:

- Not all pelvic nerves and plexuses are suitable for puncture techniques, only the superficial nerves outside the pelvis or below the pelvic floor.

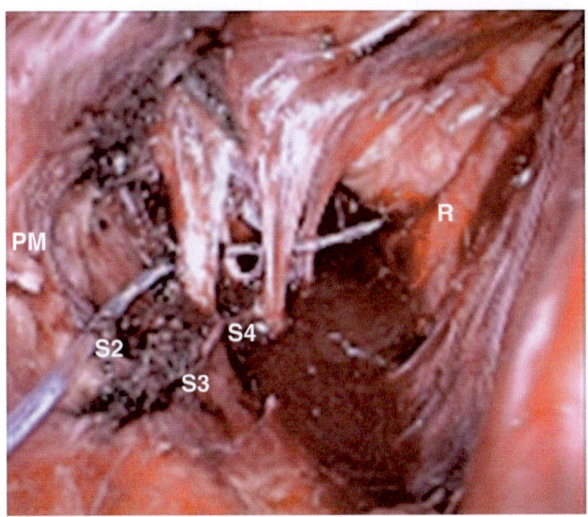

Fig. 21.3 LION procedure to the left sacral plexus. *R* rectum, *PM* pyriform muscle, *S* sacral nerve root

- SNM do not offer etiologic treatment; once neuromodulation is indicated, possible etiologies are omitted. Conservative treatment options and SNM should be classically considered before surgical options are considered. However, when any etiological treatment may exist, even a surgical one, medical and neuromodulative treatment options should be only considered after such an etiologic treatment option has failed. When no etiology can be found, patient's disorders are classified as "idiopathic" or "nonneurogenic." However, some etiologies can only be diagnosed by laparoscopy: so deeply infiltrating endometriosis of the bladder, vesicointestinal adhesions, endometriosis/fibrosis/vascular entrapment of the sacral nerve roots or of the pudendal nerve are all conditions that can induce such urinary disorders, but can only be diagnosed and treated by laparoscopy (Possover and Forman 2012). Etiologic treatment is then not only the treatment of choice but also avoids unnecessary costs for symptomatic treatment options on long term. When by laparoscopy no any etiology can be found, the procedure can be directly used for placement of an electrode to the nerve(s) of interest.

The LION procedure to the sacral plexus (Fig. 21.3) has the advantage to enable neuromodulation of all sacral nerve roots involved in bladder and rectal functions with only one multipolar lead and one pacemaker (Possover 2010c).

Because of failure of SNM in some patients suffering from incontinence and/or overactive bladder, trying to optimize the results of pelvic nerve neuromodulation, pudendal nerve stimulation (PNS) has been proposed as a logical alternative in those patients who fail to respond to SNM and successfully tested. Indeed, because the pudendal nerve rises from S2, S3, and S4, PNS activates afferent innervation over these three sacral segments, thereby providing increased afferent input for best inhibition of bladder and rectum (treatment of OAB). Pudendal efferent stimulation also activates the external urethral and external anal sphincters as well as the levator ani muscles, providing improvement of urinary and anal–fecal incontinence without activation of other fibers present in the sacral nerve roots. PNS also provides a potential modulative effect on bladder voiding function and improvement of sexual functions. Since the pudendal nerve (PN) directly innervates much of the pelvic floor, it is believed to be more optimal stimulation site for treatment of both urinary and anal–fecal incontinence as well as bladder overactivity (Spinelli et al. 2005), with few undesired side effects comparing to SNM and in some nonneurogenic disorders (Peters et al. 2005) may be explained by the more selective stimulation of nerve fibers innervating the external urethral and external anal sphincter muscles. There is no doubt that PNS is the better option for treatments of most frequent bladder disorders: PNS is no longer an alternative after failure of SNM, but has to be proposed in first line instead SNM. Main reasons why PNS has not replaced SNM until now are not problems with indication or efficacy, but technical difficulties. The anatomical location of the nerve, deep inside the pelvis and in proximity to major pelvic vessels, makes implantation by percutaneous puncture techniques extremely difficult and very dangerous. The PNS can be obtained by transgluteal puncture technique assisted by electrophysiological guidance. Location of leads below the pelvic floor by lacking anchoring to fix anatomical structures and permanent exposition to external traumas while sitting, intercourse, or walking exposes for lead migration and cable rupture. The LION procedure is the only technique that enables placement of a lead to the endopelvic portion of the PN by minimal invasive approach (Possover 2014b). Gynecologists are trained in laparoscopic surgery and for most of them, the LION procedure to the pelvic nerves especially to the PN may not present major surgical difficulties; only the anatomical way for exposure the PN must be learned. LION procedures are suitable for day-surgery, take less than 30 min for the entire procedure, while no special instrumentations or equipments (X-rays, electrophysiological guidance, etc.) or training in percutaneous puncture techniques are required, just classical OR instrument setup for laparoscopy.

21.6 Recovery of Pelvic Motor Functions in Spinal Cord Disorders

Spinal cord injury (SCI) dramatically changes the life of the affected person. The loss of control of skeletal muscles and sensations below the injury, together with serious disturbances in autonomic nervous system functions, produce a profound deterioration in the quality of life and loss of autonomy. In view of trends in the epidemiology of SCI, it is becoming increasingly important to develop treatment strategies that can enhance recovery motor function, walking in particular, following SCI. Because a complete biological cure for spinal cord injuries is not foreseeable in the near future, electronic devices that help the victim's recover some functions are urgently needed. None of the previously available devices was able to control both pelvic organ function and leg movements. The LION procedure is actually the only minimal invasive technique of electrode implantation that enables selective placement of electrodes under control of the view and in direct contact to the endopelvic portion of the lumbosacral nerves (Possover et al. 2010; Possover 2004b). Because separate electrodes are placed to the sciatic and femoral nerves, re-education with electrical controlled muscles

eccentric actions and FES-assisted locomotor training can be started few weeks after implantation. Nerve stimulation has major advantages compared to electrical muscles stimulation to induce a more harmonious movement with less fatigue effect. Because electrodes are connected to a rechargeable pacemaker, FES-training and continuous pelvic nerve neuromodulation are both feasible on long term. Both kind of stimulation may induce a building of muscle mass that constitute a major prevention effect to formation of decubitus lesions (Mawson et al. 1993). More than that, previous researches have also suggested that exogenously applied weak electric fields around damaged axons have a role to play in facilitating axonal regeneration, possibly by providing neurotropic guidance to the growing axons (Lu et al. 2008). Other experimental studies also indicated that electrical stimulation can lead to significant functional recovery more due to alternate synaptic pathways (McCaig et al. 2000). In a recent study, we reported on recovery of sensory and supraspinal control of leg movements in four peoples with chronic paraplegia treated by FES-assisted locomotor training and continuous low-frequency pelvic nerves neuromodulation (Possover 2013b). This finding suggests that such a form of rehabilitation may induce changes that affect the central pattern generator and allows supra- and infraspinal inputs to engage residual spinal pathways. Low-frequency neuromodulation of the pelvic nerves has the advantage to provide continuously such afferent inputs without need of active participation of the patient. All these information create a "need for reconnection/regeneration" resulting in a potential neural plasticity and secondary improved functional abilities. Therefore, motivation, re-education of SCI peoples and probably peripheral nerves stimulation will be essential in rehabilitation of peoples with SCI.

Conclusion

All of these new diagnostic and treatment options are the result of our pioneering work in the multidisciplinary field of neuropelveology. At the beginning, we started with laparoscopic nerve sparing techniques in gynecology.

After a short time, it became obvious that laparoscopy is not only an optimal tool for learning and teaching pelvic neuroanatomy but also offers a unique approach to the pelvic nerves. From that point, neuropelveology has overstepped the limits of the gynecology and has opened new ways not only in clinical medicine but also in neuroscience researches. The main dilemma is that knowledge required in neuropelveology is dispersed into completely different specialty areas, which usually have nothing in common. The way is not easy because laparoscopic surgeries to the pelvic nerves require in-depth knowledge of the neuroanatomy of the pelvis and a great deal of expertise in advanced laparoscopic and neurosurgical procedures. Nevertheless, considering the large number of patients who can benefit from this new field of medicine, teaching in the field of neuropelveology should be mandatory for doctors in training.

References

Abrams P, Kelleher CJ, Kerr LA, Rogers RG (2000) Overactive bladder significantly affects quality of life. Am J Manag Care 6:S580–S590

Kantartzis K, Shepherd J (2012) Sacral neuromodulation and intravesical botulinum toxin for refractory overactive bladder. Curr Opin Obstet Gynecol 24(5): 331–336

Lu MC, Ho CY, Hsu SF et al (2008) Effects of electrical stimulation at different frequencies on regeneration of transacted peripheral nerve. Neurorehabil Neural Repair 22:367–373

Mawson A, Siddiqui F, Connolly B, Sharp C, Summer W, Binndo J Jr (1993) Effect of high voltage pulsed galvanic stimulation on sacral transcutaneous oxygen tension levels in the spinal cord injured. Paraplegia 31:311–319

McCaig CD, Sangster L, Stewart R (2000) Neurotrophins enhance electric field-directed growth cone guidance and directed nerve branching. Dev Dyn 217:299–308

Peters KM, Feber KM, Bennett RC (2005) Sacral versus pudendal nerve stimulation for voiding dysfunction: a prospective, single-blinded, randomized, crossover trial. Neurourol Urodyn 24(7):643–647

Possover M (2004) Laparoscopic exposure and electrostimulation of the somatic and autonomous pelvic nerves: a new method for implantation of neuroprothesis in paralysed patients? J Gynecol Surg Endosc Imag Allied Tech 1:87–90

Possover M (2009) Laparoscopic management of neural pelvic pain in women secondary to pelvic surgery. Fertil Steril 91:2720–2725

Possover M (2010a) The neuropelveology: a new specialty in medicine. Pelviperineology 29:123–124

Possover M (2010b) New surgical evolutions in management of sacral radiculopathies. Surg Technol Int 19:123–128

Possover M (2010c) The laparoscopic implantation of neuroprothesis to the sacral plexus for therapy of neurogenic bladder dysfunctions after failure of percutaneous sacral nerve stimulation. Neuromodulation 13:141–144

Possover M (2011) The neuropelveology: from the exposure of the pelvic nerves to a new discipline in medicine. Gynecol Surg 8:117–119

Possover M (2013a) Laparoscopic management of sacral nerve root schwannoma with intractable vulvococcygodynia: report of three cases and review of literature. J Minim Invasive Gynecol 20(3):394–397

Possover M (2013b) Recovery of sensory and supraspinal control of leg movement in peoples with chronic paraplegia: a case series. Arch Phys Med Rehabil 13:1016

Possover M (2014a) The LION procedure to the pelvic nerves for treatment of urinary and faecal disorders. Surg Technol Int 24:225–230

Possover M (2014b) A novel technique of implantation for pudendal nerve stimulation for treatment of overactive bladder (OAB) with urgency incontinence (UUI). J Minim Invasiv Gynecol (in press)

Possover M, Forman A (2012) Voiding dysfunction associated with pudendal nerve entrapment. Curr Bladder Dysfunct Rep 7(4):281–285

Possover M, Forman A (in press) Neuropelveological assessment of neuropathic pelvic pain. Gynecol Surg

Possover M, Lemos N (2011) Risks, symptoms, and management of pelvic nerve damage secondary to surgery for pelvic organ prolapse: a report of 95 cases. Int Urogynecol J 22(12):1485–1490

Possover M, Rhiem K, Chiantera V (2004) The "Laparoscopic Neuro-Navigation"- LANN: from a functional cartography of the pelvic autonomous neurosystem to a new field of laparoscopic surgery. Min Invas Ther Allied Technol 13:362–367

Possover M, Baekelandt J, Chiantera V (2007a) Anatomy of the sacral roots and the pelvic splanchnic nerves in women using the LANN technique. Surg Laparosc Endosc Percutan Tech 17(6):508–510

Possover M, Baekelandt J, Chianteras V (2007b) The Laparoscopic Implantation of Neuroprothesis – LION technique – to control intractable abdomino-pelvic neuralgia. Neuromodulation 10:18–23

Possover M, Baekelandt J, Chiantera V (2007c) The laparoscopic approach to control intractable pelvic neuralgia: from laparoscopic pelvic neurosurgery to the LION technique. Clin J Pain 23(9):821–825

Possover M, Schurch B, Henle KP (2010) New pelvic nerves stimulation strategy for recovery bladder functions and locomotion in complete paraplegics. Neurourol Urodyn 29:1433–1438

Possover M, Schneider T, Henle KP (2011) Laparoscopic therapy of endometriosis and vascular entrapment of sacral plexus. Fertil Steril 95(2):756–758

Spinelli M, Malaguti S, Giardiello G, Lazzeri M, Tarantola J, Hombergh U (2005) A new minimally invasive procedure for pudendal nerve stimulation to treat neurogenic bladder: description of the method and preliminary data. Neurourol Urodyn 24:305–309

Tanagho EA, Schmidt RA (1988) Electrical stimulation in the clinical management of the neurogenic bladder. J Urol 140:1331–1339

van Kerrebroeck PE (1998) The role of electrical stimulation in voiding dysfunction. Eur Urol 34(suppl 1):27–30

Index

O. Istre (ed.), *Minimally Invasive Gynecological Surgery,*
DOI 10.1007/978-3-662-44059-9, © Springer-Verlag Berlin Heidelberg 2015

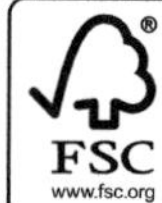